An
Appetite
for Life

An Appetite *for* Life

How to Feed Your Child from the Start

WITHDRAWN

Clare Llewellyn, PhD
Hayley Syrad, PhD

THE EXPERIMENT

NEW YORK

The Experiment, LLC
220 East 23rd Street, Suite 600, New York, NY 10010-4658 | theexperimentpublishing.com

This book contains the opinions and ideas of its authors. It is intended to provide helpful and informative material on the subjects addressed in the book. It is sold with the understanding that the authors and publisher are not engaged in rendering medical, health, or any other kind of personal professional services in the book. The authors and publisher specifically disclaim all responsibility for any liability, loss, or risk—personal or otherwise—that is incurred as a consequence, directly or indirectly, of the use and application of any of the contents of this book.

Many of the designations used by manufacturers and sellers to distinguish their products are claimed as trademarks. Where those designations appear in this book and The Experiment was aware of a trademark claim, the designations have been capitalized.

The Experiment's books are available at special discounts when purchased in bulk for premiums and sales promotions as well as for fund-raising or educational use. For details, contact us at info@theexperimentpublishing.com.

Library of Congress Cataloging-in-Publication Data

Names: Llewellyn, Claire, author. | Syrad, Hayley, author.
Title: An appetite for life : how to feed your child from the start
  / Clare Llewellyn, PhD, Hayley Syrad, PhD.
Description: New York : The Experiment, [2019] | Includes bibliographical
  references and index.
Identifiers: LCCN 2018059799 (print) | LCCN 2019003898 (ebook) | ISBN
  9781615195404 (ebook) | ISBN 9781615195398 (pbk.)
Subjects: LCSH: Children--Nutrition. | Infants--Care. | Diet therapy for
  children.
Classification: LCC RJ206 (ebook) | LCC RJ206 .L52 2019 (print) | DDC
  613.2/68083--dc23
LC record available at https://lccn.loc.gov/2018059799

ISBN 978-1-61519-539-8
Ebook ISBN 978-1-61519-540-4

Cover design by Beth Bugler | Text design by Sarah Schneider
Cover photograph by Jack.Q / Shutterstock
Photograph of Clare Llewellyn by Sian Herbert
Photograph of Hayley Syrad used by permission of the author

Manufactured in the United States of America

First printing May 2019
10 9 8 7 6 5 4 3 2 1

CONTENTS

Introduction

You may be expecting a baby, or you may already have a baby or toddler, and are keen to find out how to give him the best possible start in life. But with all the conflicting advice out there about *what* and *how* to feed your child, you may be struggling to make sense of it all. This book is here to separate the facts from the fads about food, feeding and nutrition during the first 1,000 days of your child's life. From pregnancy and milk-feeding to starting solid foods and dealing with the "terrible twos," *An Appetite for Life* provides you with evidence-based information and practical guidance, from a *scientific* perspective, to help your child establish healthy eating habits right from the start.

As leading scientists in this field, one of our greatest concerns is that much of the advice offered to parents about feeding is based on received wisdom, old wives' tales or simply people's opinion. There is no end of books about parenting and feeding, but most are written by authors with no scientific credentials in this area. In fact, when flipping through the many available books and websites, we were surprised to discover that there is virtually no *scientifically based* information for parents on this topic.

In addition to this, the US currently doesn't have any comprehensive federal guidance on nutrition for women during pregnancy or for infants and toddlers under two years of age. The aim of the "Pregnancy and Birth to 24 Months project" is to develop detailed guidelines for the first 1,000 days, but these are not due to be released until 2020. In the meantime, where should parents go for evidence-based information? This was the impetus behind writing this book; there is a huge unmet need for expectant parents and those with infants and toddlers.

Parents often receive advice that is misguided or, worse, patently wrong. At best, some writers have years of experience, but this is very different from having studied the subject scientifically and having a firm understanding of what is and isn't important and what does and doesn't work when it comes to optimal nutrition and the best feeding strategies. As scientists, not moms, we are going to replace myth with fact, giving you the knowledge and breaking down the science so that you can make your own well-informed decisions about how to feed your child.

Scientists aren't always great at getting research out there into the public domain. Findings tend to be published in scientific journals that either aren't accessible to those who don't pay the hefty subscription fees or are written in such dense scientific language that even we find some of them challenging to read and understand!

Throughout this book we have used the highest-quality evidence currently available to give you the most up-to-date scientific perspective on every topic we cover. There are some issues on which there isn't yet a scientific consensus, because evidence is lacking, and others that we are more certain about. We are frank about this and give you the lowdown on each topic, taking into account everything we know. We have outlined all of the most important scientific findings on eating and feeding your child and have developed guidance and tips based on those findings to help you navigate this important period of your baby's life.

As a side note, throughout the book we refer to the baby as *he*. This is not because we are assuming all babies are male, nor is it an attempt to gender-stereotype, but it helps with flow and ensures there is no confusion when we are referring to the mother as *she*. We also use "person first" language when we refer to overweight and obesity, to avoid labeling children by their weight status, which is considered stigmatizing by many obesity organizations. This means we describe children as *having* overweight or obesity, rather than as *being* overweight or obese; for example, "children with overweight." It may seem a bit odd to read at first, but you soon get used to it.

Who We Are

We are scientists who have been researching the eating and feeding habits of babies and toddlers for over a decade, and we both have a PhD on this topic. Between us, we have read thousands of scientific papers on the subject. But, importantly, we don't just *read* about the science; we actually *do* the science—we have published over a hundred scientific papers and articles on this topic and are leaders in the field. Our research team at University College London (UCL) in the UK, led by Clare, is world-renowned for its knowledge in this area. One of our most significant endeavors has been to help set up the largest ever study into the origins of infant and toddler feeding—the Gemini twin study in the UK. Gemini has greatly advanced our understanding of early eating and feeding behavior and has allowed us to make major new discoveries about the importance of early nutrition and feeding for healthy growth and development. (We describe Gemini in detail, and why it is so important and unique, in Chapter 1.) We met while working together on Gemini and have remained trusted colleagues and firm friends ever since. Throughout *An Appetite for Life* we will offer practical guidance and advice based on this internationally renowned study, as well as on a breadth of other high-quality studies that have been undertaken over decades, to make sure the whole picture is represented. Many other scientific experts in the field have also contributed to this book to ensure its accuracy (they are listed in the Acknowledgments on page 333).

As well as working on Gemini, we both review and evaluate articles for more than twenty scientific journals and have given numerous international talks about work in this area. Clare is an editorial board member of two key scientific journals in the field and teaches research methods and statistics in a master of science program at UCL. She also supervises several PhD researchers in this field. In short, we know how to sift through evidence, cut out the nonsense and get to the crucial information. In this book, we have done all of that work for you, so you don't have to.

Aside from our scientific background, we have both had very different personal experiences with eating, which were a big impetus behind us writing this book. As a child Clare had "failure to thrive" and struggled with excessive food fussiness, which persisted from toddlerhood into early adulthood. She knows firsthand the stress that this causes parents and families, as well as the individual child. We hope that this book will provide information that minimizes the chance of this happening to your own child and that those of you who are currently dealing with a very fussy eater will get the best possible advice on how to deal with it effectively. Hayley, on the other hand, was a model eater growing up and has never had many hang-ups about food. She was always willing to try new foods and, with the odd exception here and there, she always ate what she was given, without over-indulging. She puts this down largely to the feeding methods used by her parents during her early years. (You can read about our stories on pages 7 and 9.)

When we provide you with guidance about feeding your child throughout this book, we have never lost sight of our own experiences, which we hope has ensured that the advice we give you is grounded, realistic, empathic and helpful.

The First 1,000 Days

The first 1,000 days of your baby's life—from conception to his second birthday—are now considered to be the most important in his life. It is widely agreed among scientists worldwide that your baby's experiences during his first 1,000 days will have an enduring influence on his future health and happiness. It is the period during which the foundations are laid for lifelong health, and this is particularly important when it comes to your baby's nutrition. The types of foods your baby receives and the habits he develops can have lasting effects.[1]

There is mounting evidence that *what* you feed your baby is likely to have an important effect not only on his long-term health but also on his food preferences (the foods he likes and dislikes) for years to come. At the same time, *how* he is fed during this very early period may also play a crucial part in forming his appetite regulation (his ability to control how much he eats) and his relationship with food (for example, his tendency to want to eat in response to stress and sadness, and his fussiness). This is a fantastic opportunity to set your child up for life, and this book will help you to do just that.

The first 1,000 days are a time of extraordinary growth and development, unparalleled by any other period of life. By the time your baby turns one, he will have tripled his birth weight. His brain will also undergo significant development—at birth your baby's brain weighs about 13 ounces (370 g), but by the time he is two years old it will weigh over 2 pounds (1 kg) and will be about 80 percent of its adult size.[2] All of this growth and brain development needs to be fueled, and, for babies, this fuel comes first in the form of milk and then, in time, solid food. Optimal nutrition during the first 1,000 days has lasting effects on brain development.[3]

The Book's Philosophy

Healthy eating habits are about far more than simply *what* a child eats. Gemini and a wealth of other scientific studies have shown that healthy eating is also about *how* your baby feeds and eats—how much, how often and the relationship he develops with food all really matter. Evidence suggests that *how* your child is fed during his first 1,000 days plays a role in shaping his appetite regulation—his ability to eat only as much as he needs, and to view food as nourishment rather than comfort, entertainment, or even something to be feared. Eating too much or too little of anything isn't healthy, nor is turning to food to control emotions instead of learning how to regulate them using positive strategies. And being excessively fussy about food often results in a limited dietary repertoire, which can have detrimental effects on health.

It comes as a surprise to many people to discover that our relationship with food may develop soon after we are conceived, through exposure to our mom's diet in the womb. Important habits then start to develop when we begin milk-feeding on the day we are born, and these become more firmly established during the first 1,000 days of life. But babies also bring their own predispositions to the table (pun intended!). Babies are not all born the same—some babies have hearty appetites from the start, while others have poor appetites. When it comes to feeding, understanding what *type* of eater your baby is and responding appropriately is crucial. But at present there is very little information out there about how to respond to your child's unique eating style.

Understanding the *how* of eating is new, so it is no surprise that there is very little information for parents about the strategies you can use to help your baby or toddler develop good appetite regulation, a healthy relationship with food and healthy food preferences that may persist over many years. This is far more than *what* he eats; it's also *how* he interacts with food. This book will provide you with much-needed evidence-based advice about *what* and *how* to feed your child from Day 1.

How the Book Is Organized

We have divided the book into four parts that relate to the main stages of nutrition and feeding during the first 1,000 days: Pregnancy and the Early Days (Part 1); Milk-Feeding (Part 2); Introducing Solid Foods (Part 3); and Early Childhood (Part 4). We have designed it so that you can dip in and out of the chapters that are of the most relevance to you and your child, for the particular stage of feeding that you are at. In each chapter we provide you with the most up-to-date scientific facts about nutrition and feeding, and lots of practical tips to help make sure it goes smoothly.

It isn't possible in one book to cover, in detail, the evidence behind every aspect of early feeding. We have therefore provided a more in-depth discussion of the evidence about topics that have been shrouded in controversy (for example, drinking alcohol in pregnancy) and those that we know parents want a lot more information about (for example, the evidence for the benefits of breastfeeding, how to choose formula milk, and the when, what and how of introducing solid food).

Over the course of writing this book we have spoken to dozens of parents who have kindly shared their own experiences of feeding during the first 1,000 days. Some parents have talked about things that went well, while others have shared their difficulties. The parents we spoke to ensured that we focused on the topics they felt needed more scientifically sound information.

Clare's Story: The "Fussy Eater"

I hope to be able to provide advice, information and comfort to moms with fussy children because I know firsthand how it feels to be an extremely fussy eater. Although I consider myself to be "normal" now (within most contexts anyhow!), from childhood to early adulthood I was a highly selective eater. It drove my parents mad and even reduced my mom to tears on occasion. Nothing is ingrained more clearly in my mind than the many confrontational mealtimes that seemed to define much of my early childhood.

As a fussy eater, every mealtime filled me with all-consuming panic. I would often wake in the morning with a sense of dread about the impending mealtimes. This would persist throughout the day. The problems began when I started solid food. My mom recalls a particular occasion when I was about sixteen months old. She had been trying for hours to no avail to get me to eat just a few mouthfuls of beans. Eventually she gave up and, in her exasperation, asked my godmother, Susie, to come over and help. After an hour she coaxed me into taking a spoonful of three baked beans, whereupon I swiftly fell asleep in my high chair, and that was that. On waking a little while later, I spat out the beans that I had been concealing in the side of my mouth. All hope was lost.

My loathing of food was all the more baffling for my parents whose firstborn (my older brother, Chris) was a breeze to feed. Chris, unlike me, enjoyed mealtimes, didn't make much of a fuss and had a hearty appetite. How could things have gone so wrong with me? Differences between siblings are, in fact, pretty common and point very much toward the problem originating in the child rather than the parents.

By the time I was five years old I was a highly adept fussy eater who had learned all the tricks in the book for concealing how little I had eaten. I would go to great lengths to get rid of food, or hide it, if Mom left me to it, which she had resorted to in an attempt to minimize meal-time stress. The cliché of pushing food around the plate was my go-to strategy. The goal was to create an optical illusion of less food on the plate than there actually was. If I found my efforts unconvincing, I would resort to simply throwing it away by flushing it down the toilet to make the evidence disappear entirely from view. But I didn't always cover my tracks well and would often find myself on the receiving end of a furious and upset parent who had discovered the remnants of my meal floating in the toilet. Often the safer option was simply to give it to my brother, who was on the other end of the appetite spectrum and happy to eat for two.

When I entered middle school at the age of eleven, I was given a medical examination, which was standard for all new students. The school nurse who measured my height and weight was concerned because I had dropped off the bottom of the growth chart. I was taken to the physician and diagnosed with "failure to thrive," as it was called back then—a history of insufficient weight gain over a number of months—and referred to a pediatric growth specialist. After some discussion of the options, the consultant suggested that I should start receiving human growth hormone in two months' time, should the weight faltering continue. This would be delivered via daily injections. The only thing I feared more in life than food was injections. Oh, the horror! The threat of injections was all the impetus I needed to get my act together and eat enough calories to satisfy the consultant's growth target. I ate a small amount of "proper food" in the evenings and on the weekends when I was under supervision, but I controlled my intake at all other times. I succeeded in averting the unthinkable—daily injections. It is interesting to me now looking back that at no point did anyone even so much as broach the question of *why* I didn't want to eat.

By my teenage years I had pretty much reached a place in my life where food anxiety didn't dominate every aspect. And I had my repertoire of foods I would eat quite happily—whether at home or out. But with one caveat: nothing that wasn't simple; an Indian or Chinese restaurant were out of the question. And so things continued. Eventually I left home at eighteen and went to college. I had breakfast and evening meals provided in my halls of residence, but I had about five of these meals in total during my whole first year, preferring instead to hide in my room and eat bowls of cereal or baguettes with butter and mild cheddar slices. And I survived on this for a year. I didn't even get ill. But as I entered the second year everything changed. I moved into a house with four of my really good friends. With this move came some anxiety—how would I hide my weird eating behavior from my housemates? I worried I would be fully exposed. To top it all off, two of my friends were real "foodies" and they often cooked extravagant meals for the household—me included. This led to a total overhaul in my behavior. Over the course of a year, I made the transition from a fairly selective eater to a relatively normal one. This was driven entirely by social pressure. I was so mortified by my eating habits that I complied with expectations and slowly, meal by meal, made extraordinary progress. By the end of the second year I had had my first curry (admittedly, an unadventurous chicken korma, but nonetheless) and eaten a wider variety of foods than I had eaten in my entire life up to that point.

By the time I reached my midtwenties I considered my eating behavior to be normal. And now I will eat pretty much anything. By no means would I consider myself adventurous or a foodie, but I enjoy meals out with friends and look forward to being cooked for, whether or not I know in advance what might be put in front of me. So, do not lose hope! Children can and do learn to manage their fussy tendencies, and it is possible to get to a place where they are eating a good and varied diet, even if it doesn't include every possible food on the planet. Life with an excessively fussy child can be stressful—it can ruin holidays, meals out and family time. But people are also quick to blame the parents for their child's difficulties. I only wish my parents had known then what I know now about problem eating behavior—where it really comes from and the strategies we can use to manage it. This was an important impetus behind this book for me—to help other parents who are already struggling with a fussy child and to minimize the likelihood that it will happen in the first place.

Hayley's Story: The "Model Eater"

My childhood eating habits were very different from Clare's. My parents were the envy of friends who had fussy eaters because all of their children (my younger brother, Jonathan; my older sister, Amy; and I) were model eaters. At seven years old I ate (and enjoyed) snails in France.

Sometimes I can't quite believe I did that, and I am not so sure I would eat them now. Was it that my parents were just lucky to have three children who loved food or was it because of *how* and *what* they fed us when we were younger? I would argue it was a bit of both, because we know that some children have a genetic tendency to be fussy (more on this on pages 24–25), but we also know that fussiness can be a result of early experience with food (the ethos of this book). Interestingly, some of the tips we provide in this book on how to prevent fussy eating were in fact used by my mom and dad when we were babies—for example, offering vegetables as a first food rather than fruit, and not adding salt or sugar to foods. If I was given fruit it was fruit that did not contain much sugar, such as puréed cooking apples or plums.

Once I was ready to move on to typical family food, my parents never gave me kids' meals at home or if we ate out. I was given what my parents were eating, but they did not add salt to the meals during cooking—they added it to their plate once it was served. My mom felt that a baby would find plenty of flavor in the food without the need for extra saltiness.

As a young child I was very occasionally given dessert, but my parents wanted to avoid giving me sugary foods until I was a bit older. I was rarely given snacks, and I didn't make a habit of asking for food between meals. I don't snack much even now and am pretty good at only eating when I am hungry; I look forward to meals, and food tastes so much better to me if I am hungry. But of course, I am human and at times I will eat chocolate if it's offered to me, regardless of whether I am hungry!

My eating habits were not totally perfect as a child, though; I did go through a stage during early childhood of not eating meat and being picky about gelatinous substances, such as the jelly on corned beef or the rind of fat on bacon (I still cut this off). And at the age of eight I remember being adamant that I was not eating my grandmother's cauliflower cheese. Cauliflower cheese was, and still is, one of my favorite dishes, but the sauce really did taste terrible; she had made it using the water from the boiled cauliflower! I was told I would have to sit at the table until I ate it, so I sat there for two hours, on my own, until eventually my grandmother realized I was not going to eat it and admitted defeat.

There are a few foods today that I am not keen on, but I would say I am quite an adventurous eater and eager to try new foods. I view food as something to be enjoyed, whether it's a fresh salad or chocolate cake, and the key for me has always been to eat a balanced diet and to keep active. I was brought up in an era where you cleared your plate, and it is difficult to change the habit of a lifetime, but I have learned how much I can eat without feeling too full and only serve myself that amount.

I have always been fascinated by diet and nutrition. I think that because I have a healthy relationship with food I have been intrigued as to why some people don't. I am passionate about exploring the reasons behind unhealthy eating habits, whether that is excessive fussiness or excessive over- or undereating. Food is such a vital part of our lives, and a person's relationship with food affects both their physical and mental health. Writing this book has provided me with an opportunity to get the science out there to parents and help instill the best practices to set many children on the road to healthy eating. That is my mission.

Babies and toddlers bring their own quirks to the table when it comes to food, so parents' feeding experiences are rarely the same, and the challenges they face depend on their own particular child. Some are a nightmare to feed, like Clare, and others a dream, like Hayley. We have written this book to provide you with helpful and practical advice that is relevant to you and your baby, whatever type of feeder he is and for every stage of feeding.

CHAPTER 1

An Appetite for Life

"There is no love sincerer than the love of food."
GEORGE BERNARD SHAW

You may or may not agree with the above statement, but no doubt you will have heard some friend or family member make a similar declaration, possibly in the midst of a bountiful and glorious feast. But we're not all the same when it comes to food. We all know someone who has very little interest in it, the one who pushes food around the plate and for whom eating is simply a chore. For others, chomping down delicious food is one of the greatest pleasures in life. Just as adults have varying appetites and attitudes toward food, children and babies also differ in their love for (or loathing of) food. Some of you may already have one child who enjoys eating and another for whom mealtimes are a source of enormous stress.

So, why do we have such different relationships with food? This is a question that has intrigued researchers for decades, and it is relevant today, more than ever before, because of the dramatic rise in obesity as well as the growing concern about eating disorders. There is now increasing evidence that your baby's appetite, as well as the foods that he likes and dislikes, are shaped during his first 1,000 days of life—from pregnancy through to around two years of age. And scientists now know quite a lot about how appetite and food preferences develop and the best strategies to use to help babies foster a good relationship with food right from the start. What we know for certain is that *how* a child eats (how he responds to food and interacts with it) is just as important as *what* he eats (the foods he likes and dislikes).

Appetite: How We Eat

Appetite is a catch-all word that researchers use to describe how we respond to food and the opportunity to eat. Appetite—what it is and how it is expressed—has been studied for decades. Differences in people's appetites help to explain why some of us are susceptible to gaining too much weight, while others manage to maintain a healthy and stable weight with virtually no effort. So, why are we so different, and when does this start happening?

Our understanding of children's appetite was revolutionized in 2001, when Professor Jane Wardle, an eminent behavioral scientist, developed the first comprehensive measure of eating styles in children—the Child Eating Behaviour Questionnaire (CEBQ; see Appendix, page 297).[1] This questionnaire enabled researchers to study, for the first time, how much children really differed in their appetite and how appetite related to weight—it allowed us to explore the eating styles of children across the whole spectrum of weight, from underweight to obesity. The CEBQ is a questionnaire that you can use to describe how your child behaves in relation to seven different eating styles, and it can help you to understand your child's appetite:

1. *Food responsiveness* measures a child's tendency to want to eat when he sees, smells or tastes super-delicious foods, even if he isn't hungry—for example, wanting a chocolate bar when he gets to the supermarket checkout and sees a wall of treats.

2. *Enjoyment of food* describes the amount of pleasure a child derives from the experience of eating.

3. *Satiety responsiveness* captures how easily a child fills up once he starts eating, and how long he stays full for before he gets hungry and wants to start eating again.

4. *Slowness in eating* measures how quickly or slowly a child typically finishes a meal or snack.

5. *Emotional overeating* assesses a child's tendency to want to eat more if he has been very upset or cranky.

6. *Emotional undereating* assesses a child's tendency to lose his appetite if he has been very upset or angry.

7. *Food fussiness* measures how fussy or picky a child is when it comes to the types of foods he is willing to eat, and his willingness to try new foods.

The CEBQ led to important discoveries about appetite—children differ enormously in their appetites, and leaner children tend to have smaller appetites while those of a higher weight tend to have heartier appetites. But many crucial questions still remained unanswered. We still didn't know whether appetite really *caused* children to develop underweight or overweight, or whether it was actually their weight that caused their appetite to be big or small. And we knew virtually nothing about babies—whether or not babies also showed differences in these eating styles—and where appetite comes from in the first place. This is the nature-nurture question: Is our appetite caused by our genes, and therefore already there at birth, or is it shaped by our early experience with feeding?

Twins offer a powerful way of answering these questions. This is because identical twins are 100 percent genetically the same, while nonidentical twins are only about 50 percent genetically the same, like regular siblings. But importantly, both types of twins share their environments to a very similar extent; they are gestated in the same mother for the same amount of time, grow up in the same family, are exposed to the same parenting policies and so on. This means that researchers can compare how alike the two types of twins are to find out how much genes are involved in shaping a particular characteristic, such as appetite, or the extent to which appetite is learned. If identical twins are more similar than nonidentical twins for the trait being studied, genes are important in shaping that trait.

Professor Jane Wardle decided that the best possible way to understand appetite properly was to set up a twin study that measured appetite comprehensively in very large numbers of *babies* right from the beginning of life and observe their weight gain over subsequent months and years. This would allow us to answer all of the unanswered questions, and more. It also meant developing a new measure of appetite, like the CEBQ, but specifically for very young babies.

In 2007, Jane Wardle, Clare Llewellyn and a team of other research-ers at University College London established Gemini—the largest study ever undertaken into infant appetite. Since Gemini was set up, we have measured

- the appetites of more than 4,800 British twin babies during the first few weeks of life when they were still fed only milk, and again when they were toddlers
- their weights and heights every three months since the study began
- everything the children ate and drank for three days when they were toddlers.

This comprehensive study has made Gemini one of the richest growth-data resources in the world and has created the largest con-temporary dietary data set for toddlers in the whole of the UK. We have used this information to find out

- if appetite is something that is learned or inherited
- how much babies really differ in their appetites for milk
- how a baby's appetite relates to weight gain
- how a baby's appetite relates to actual food intake
- how a toddler's food intake and eating patterns relate to weight gain.

We developed a new measure of appetite for milk-feeding babies (the Baby Eating Behaviour Questionnaire [BEBQ]; see Appendix, page 295) that allowed us to measure infant appetite in large numbers, in the same way as the CEBQ had allowed us to measure the appetites of large numbers of children.[2] The BEBQ is the first and only comprehen-sive measure of infant appetite and is used widely in research. It cap-tures four different aspects of a baby's appetite:

1. *Milk responsiveness* indicates a baby's urge to feed when milk is offered, even if they are not hungry, and how demanding they are with regard to being fed.

2. *Enjoyment of feeding* assesses how much pleasure the baby experiences during feeding.

3. *Satiety responsiveness* measures a baby's fullness sensitivity; for example, how easily or quickly he fills up once he starts feeding.

4. *Slowness in feeding* measures a baby's typical feeding speed—whether they guzzle their milk in record time or seem to take forever.

The wealth of research that has come from Gemini and other studies has transformed our understanding of babies' and children's appetite and what it means for parents when it comes to feeding them. Alongside other high-quality studies, these findings have formed the basis of much of the advice in this book.

BABIES DIFFER IN THEIR APPETITES FOR MILK

As a result of the BEBQ, we discovered that babies differ enormously when it comes to their appetite for milk. And this is true of both breast- *and* formula-fed babies. Some babies have ravenous appetites, feeding whenever milk is offered (even if they have just been fed) and emptying a bottle of milk in record time. A few will even guzzle milk so quickly that it comes straight back up. At the other end of the spectrum are the picky feeders—the babies who can only manage a little bit of milk at a time and seem to take hours over a single feed or even fall asleep on the job. For moms of these babies, feeding can feel like a constant struggle. Yet other babies seem to have their milk intake perfectly in check. In short, babies really vary in their ability to regulate their milk intake according to their needs.

CHILDREN DIFFER IN HOW THEY RESPOND TO FOOD

Like babies, children also differ a lot in how they respond to food: Some love it, others loathe it, and some are in between. You may have already noticed this if you have two children of your own with quite different dispositions toward food. There are distinct eating styles that characterize a poorer or more avid appetite. If your child has a poor appetite, he is likely to show some of the following characteristics, some of which may drive you crazy:

- He may be very "satiety sensitive," meaning he will fill up very easily once he starts eating and will not be able to eat much in one go. This means that if he has a snack (or even a glass of milk) too close to a meal he might not be able to manage all the food he's offered. He may rarely seem hungry—especially if the available food isn't all that enticing—and is probably far more interested in doing other activities, such as playing on an iPad, than eating his meal.

- He may eat slowly, and it can feel like mealtimes take ages, but he likes to take his time and won't be rushed.

- He may be a fusspot—fussier than other children when it comes to food, especially when trying *new* foods. He may not eat certain foods because of their texture—for example, foods with lumps in them, foods that develop a skin on the top after a while or foods that are slimy—the list is actually endless and may change from day to day! He may also object to foods touching on the plate and may refuse to eat something if it has been contaminated by something else, even if he likes the "something else" on its own (for example, potatoes that have been contaminated with tomato sauce from a side of baked beans, which he apparently likes). He may also declare that he doesn't like a particular food without even having tried it, which of course means he will refuse to taste it.

- After he has been very upset or angry he may completely lose his appetite for a while, so he will eat even less than usual.

If your child has a large and enthusiastic appetite, he will tend to show some of the following behaviors toward food, some of which may prove challenging to manage at times:

- He may be very "food responsive" and constantly ask for food if treats are visible and he thinks he stands a chance of persuading you!

- He will really enjoy snacks and meals and probably makes this shamelessly obvious. For him eating is pure pleasure. In general, this makes mealtimes easy insofar as he is an adventurous little eater who is interested in new types of foods and willing to give anything a go.

- He eats very quickly. Sometimes it seems as though he has inhaled the meal that you just spent hours preparing.

- Not even emotional upset is enough to put him off his food. In fact, sometimes he even eats more than usual when he's upset. Because he loves food and it brings him a lot of pleasure, it's something that makes him feel better when he's upset.

Of course, children don't necessarily fit neatly into one category. In fact, it isn't uncommon for some children to have a hearty appetite when it comes to foods high in sugar and/or fat, but to be incredibly fussy when it comes to other foods (usually the ones you would most like him to eat, such as vegetables). You may be thinking this about your own child. Unfortunately, most children prefer foods high in sugar and/or fat to nutrient-dense foods such as vegetables and fruit—this is a parent's perpetual challenge, especially given the access to these foods that children have today. But in general, children with a big or poor appetite tend to demonstrate distinct eating behaviors such as the ones we have just described. What type of eater do you think your baby or child is? Try completing the BEBQ (for babies up to six months) or the CEBQ (for children over twelve months) in Appendix (pages 295 and 297) to find out.

The fact that children vary so much in their appetites means that each child brings unique challenges to you as a parent when it comes to feeding them. There can be no one-size-fits-all advice about feeding your child—it depends entirely on the type of eater your child is, and your feeding strategy needs to be tailored to suit him and his particular quirks.

APPETITE PERSISTS THROUGHOUT CHILDHOOD

Research that measured the appetites of 428 British children when they were four and again when they were eleven years old showed that appetite is a fairly stable trait that persists throughout your child's development.[3] A toddler with a poor appetite tends also to grow into a child who is less interested in food and who finds activities other than eating more enticing. If you have an eager eater, on the other hand, he will probably grow into a child with a hearty appetite who loves food and derives a great deal of pleasure from eating.

But this doesn't mean that your child's appetite can't be changed. A landmark study called NOURISH has shown that parents who feed their babies and toddlers using certain strategies (called responsive feeding—see Chapter 6 for more on this) can have a lasting impact on their child's developing appetite. So, although a toddler who has a tiny appetite is unlikely to grow into a child with a large and voracious one, the way that you feed him can make an important difference to his relationship with food, the foods he will eat and his ability to eat enough. The same is true for a toddler with a large and voracious appetite, which can be tempered with the right feeding strategies.

A word about food fussiness: We know from research that fussiness seems to follow a pattern in your child's development—it tends to emerge during toddlerhood, increase during the preschool years and gradually diminish during later childhood (although in rare instances it can persist into adulthood).[4] So, don't worry if your child has suddenly become fussy when yesterday he seemed fine. This is very common and is a normal part of development for many children, but that doesn't mean that it isn't stressful! In fact, dealing with fussiness can be one of the most challenging aspects of feeding. The good news is that it's usually just a phase that your child will eventually grow out of and throughout this book we have some great strategies for you to use to help him overcome this.

APPETITE HAS AN IMPACT ON WEIGHT

Research has shown that your child's appetite is one of the most important influences on his early growth. Gemini allowed us to examine in detail for the first time the relationship between a baby's appetite during the first few months of life and his subsequent weight gain. Babies who are more responsive to milk derive greater pleasure from feeding, feed quickly, are less sensitive to their fullness signals and tend to be more prone to overfeeding. These babies gain weight more rapidly and are at greater risk of excessive weight gain. Babies with poorer appetites are more likely to underfeed, gain weight more slowly and are at greater risk of weight faltering (meaning insufficient weight gain over a period of a few weeks or months—see page 78 for detailed information about weight faltering).

When we compared the weight gain of pairs of British twins with very different appetites (one third of all the same-sex non-identical twin pairs), we found that the twins with the heartier appetites grew much faster than their co-twins with poorer appetites from birth to toddlerhood.[5] By the time they were toddlers there was a 2.2-pound

(1 kg) difference in weight between twin pairs who had very different appetites, defined by their food responsiveness and satiety sensitivity. This might not sound like a lot, but the average weight at fifteen months was about 22 pounds (10 kg), so a 2.2-pound (1 kg) difference is a 10 percent difference in body weight. In adult terms, this is the equivalent to being 140 versus 154 pounds, or 60 versus 66 kg. This is a big weight difference. You would certainly notice if you gained or lost 10 percent of your body weight—and the chances are, so would your friends and family.

This study was important because it showed for the first time that early appetite plays a crucial role in how much weight babies gain—it helps to explain why some babies have rapid weight gain, while others have weight faltering. Another study in Singapore replicated our finding in a sample of unrelated babies;[6] and a wealth of studies have shown, pretty much without exception, that toddlers and older children with a more avid appetite carry more body fat, while those with a poorer appetite carry less body fat.[7] We now know that optimal early weight gain is very important for your baby's later health (see Chapter 3), so finding that appetite plays such an important part in this process highlights the importance of helping your baby develop good appetite regulation right from the beginning of life.

You can imagine how being a food-responsive child who really enjoys food can easily lead to overeating in the context of the modern food environment. Children are bombarded with food cues throughout the day via the relentless onslaught of food advertising—for foods high in sugar and fat, not for the more nutritious foods such as vegetables or fruit. In 2017 the University of Connecticut's Rudd Center for Food Policy and Obesity published a report summarizing the extent of food, beverage and restaurant advertising and children's exposure to this advertising on TV and the internet.[8] In 2016, over 20,000 food, drink and restaurant companies spent more than $13.5 billion on food advertising across all media. Preschoolers aged two to five watched an average of ten food ads per day on TV, totaling 3,746 food ads that year. Of all the food and drink advertisements on TV, those for non-core foods (unnecessary foods or drinks high in fat, sugar and salt, including fast food and other candy, sweet and salty snacks, and sugary drinks) vastly outnumbered those for core nutritious foods (foods required daily to ensure optimal nutrition, including dairy, fruit and vegetables), which comprised less than 10 percent.

This may not seem like a big deal for a young child who doesn't yet have the independence to go out and buy the foods that he sees and then eat them, but a review of eighteen experimental studies examining how much people eat after watching ads (either on television or on the internet) found that children eat more at a meal following exposure to food ads.[9] This is because watching food ads is thought to make food-responsive children want to eat, simply by looking at the food. Preschoolers' high exposure to food ads partly reflects the fact that they are watching far more TV (3.4 hours per day[10]) than is recommended by the American Academy of Pediatrics (no more than one hour of high-quality programming for children older than two years of age, and none for children younger than eighteen months).[11] So, cutting down the time children spend watching TV would greatly reduce their exposure to these food ads. But the modern "obesogenic" environment isn't just restricted to the television or internet; it is virtually impossible to walk down a main street without seeing or smelling food as you go about your business. If your child is food responsive, these food cues will make him want to eat. In fact, in Gemini we found that toddlers who were more food responsive ate more often throughout the day.[12] To put some numbers around this, the most food-responsive toddlers consumed about three extra meals per week compared to the least food responsive, equating to a difference of around 540 calories per week and 2,340 calories per month—which is about two and a half extra days of food intake every month (the average daily energy requirement at two years of age in the US is approximately 1,000 calories).

Children with weaker fullness sensitivity (satiety) are also vulnerable to the modern food environment because they have a tendency to carry on eating, as long as there is still food to eat. In Gemini we also found that toddlers who were less sensitive to their satiety consumed a larger amount of food every time they ate.[13] Toddlers who were the least sensitive to their fullness (lowest satiety) consumed about 40 extra calories every time they ate, compared to toddlers who were the most satiety sensitive. Because the children were eating about five times a day (about three meals and two snacks), the net difference between the two types of children added up to almost 200 calories a day, 1,300 calories a week, and 5,600 calories a month (which is about five and a half extra days of food intake every month). Larger portions of food than are needed can prove particularly problematic for these children, in terms of encouraging overeating. Children who are less sensitive to feelings of fullness have a tendency to eat too much if portions are bigger or if they are distracted during eating, such as eating in front of the television or playing with an iPad at the table. This is the sort of information we feel is very important for parents to know. We know that your child's unique appetite needs to be taken into account when feeding him. There are ways to deal with all types of babies and children, to help make sure they neither under- or over-eat. The key to making sure you get it right is *responsive feeding*, and we will explain exactly how to do this for each stage of feeding.

WHERE DOES APPETITE COME FROM?

The age-old question of whether appetite is caused by our genes (nature) or our early feeding experiences (nurture) is a pretty important one for you as a parent. If your baby's appetite is largely shaped by his early feeding experiences, the onus is on you to make sure you get it right. If your baby's genes are important in shaping his appetite, it's more about understanding what type of appetite your baby is born with and making sure you respond to him appropriately.

There is pretty widespread (and largely unsupported) belief among researchers, as well as health professionals, that all babies are born with a natural ability to regulate their milk intake perfectly (they will take only as much milk as they need). In theory this means they are able to feed whenever they are hungry and stop as soon as they are full. The prevailing view is that your baby's appetite regulation is developed through a process of learning, and that you are the main shaper. The theory is that if your baby's signals of hunger and fullness are consistently met by you with a prompt, developmentally appropriate feeding response, he will quickly learn how to regulate his milk intake according to his needs. This is thought to be the pathway through which appetite regulation is developed and optimized. But is it really the case that all babies are born with the potential for perfect appetite control and it is only compromised if interfered with by you? This implies that all babies are born on a level playing field and that appetite regulation is largely learned. It is true that *on the whole* babies seem to be better at regulating their intake according to their needs than older children or adults, but it is certainly not true that *all babies* can do this well. There are still big differences between babies.

In fact, a handful of early studies with newborns showed that there were big differences between how avidly they sucked for milk and how much they drank, suggesting that babies differ quite a lot in their appetite right from birth, which doesn't concur very well with the idea that appetite regulation is learned. In 1968, researchers undertook one of the first ever studies of infant appetite using eight newborn babies, twelve to sixteen hours old.[14] Over eighteen consecutive feeds they observed striking and consistent differences between how quickly and vigorously they sucked for milk; some had avid appetites, and others poorer appetites, right from the beginning of life. Small studies also showed large differences in the amount of milk produced by breast-feeding moms, and this was primarily controlled by the baby, suggesting that the quantity of milk produced reflects to some extent a baby's appetite.[15] One of the most intriguing early studies of newborns' feeding behavior used a really neat design to get a handle on the extent to which infant appetite was genetic. In 1980 Robert Milstein, a psychiatrist at Yale University, selected twenty-four newborn babies (twenty-seven to seventy-four hours old) whose parents either had a healthy weight or had overweight, and he compared how avidly the babies sucked when offered a sweetened solution.[16] Because weight is largely inherited, this design was able to shed light on whether babies at higher risk of developing overweight (according to their parents' weights) show a tendency to want to eat more when the food or drink offered is good-tasting (in this case, sweet). Milstein observed that the babies born at higher risk of overweight sucked more avidly in response to the sweetened solution than did those at low risk, suggesting that wanting to drink more of the good-tasting solution is inherited and may play a role in their susceptibility to overweight. Two other early studies observed large differences in how avidly young babies (two weeks and three months old) would suck for milk, with the more voracious and enthusiastic feeders gaining considerably more weight over the following two years.[17]

These small early studies highlighted that differences in appetite are present right from the beginning of life and seem to vary according to a baby's genetic risk of overweight, suggesting a genetic component to appetite. Differences so early on cannot have been learned, but in 1980, the extent to which infant appetite was truly innate was still unknown. Thirty years on, we were able to answer the nature-nurture question for the first time in Gemini because we studied twins. We found that identical twin pairs were far more alike than nonidentical twin pairs for all aspects of their appetite.[18] This indicated that a lot of the differences between babies' appetites for milk are, in fact, down to their genes. This discovery is new and came as quite a surprise to many researchers and health professionals, although it makes sense given that we know that appetite is actually largely controlled by biology. Two systems in our brain control how hungry or full we feel: the "homeostatic system," controlled mainly by part of the brain called the hypothalamus, and how rewarding and pleasurable we find food— the "hedonic system"—controlled mainly by a pathway in the brain which produces dopamine and other neurotransmitters that control our wanting and liking. Several appetite hormones, such as ghrelin (the "hunger hormone") and leptin (the "satiety hormone"), control our appetites by regulating these systems in the brain.[19] Scientists have also found that the genes that influence our satiety sensitivity and food responsiveness are most highly expressed in areas of the brain that control our appetite.[20] The fact that your baby's genes influence his appetite so strongly has big implications for you as a parent. You need to get to know the appetite he is born with and respond appropriately. In Gemini, we also looked at the nature and nurture of food fussiness, emotional overeating and emotional undereating in *toddlerhood*. It may provide some comfort to you if you have a fussy toddler to discover that fussiness actually has a pretty strong genetic basis—it's not your fault! Some parents with a fussy toddler feel judged or guilty about his eating difficulties. But if you have a fussy toddler, understanding that he has a genetic predisposition toward this might help you to go easier on yourself. Some toddlers are just prone to being a lot more finicky than others.

But when it comes to toddlers eating more or less in response to emotion, genes are *unimportant*.[21] Instead, it is a baby's early experiences that shape this. In fact, after finding almost no influence of genes on emotional eating in Gemini, we were so surprised that we explored this in another sample of British twins, and we found exactly the same thing.[22] We also now know that parents play quite an important role in nurturing this behavior. With researchers from Norway we used a large ongoing study of 1,000 families with very young children to show that a young child who is offered food in order to soothe him when he is upset is more likely to learn to turn to food to control his emotions when he is older.[23] It is important to find alternative strategies to comfort a baby or toddler who is upset, rather than use milk or food. We will explain how you do this in the chapters that follow.

So, if genes are at the root of most aspects of a baby's appetite, does this mean it can't be changed? No. It is a common misconception that if something has a strong genetic basis, it can't be modified. This absolutely isn't the case. Your baby's genes are *not* his destiny when it comes to his appetite. A strong genetic influence on your baby's appetite means that he is born with a *disposition* to have a more avid appetite or to be a more difficult feeder. But the extent to which his genes will have an impact is also dependent on his early nutritional and feeding experiences as well. For example, people with a strong genetic predisposition to lung cancer are very unlikely to develop it if they don't smoke. Your baby's genes set his appetite *potential*, but his early environmental experiences can act as a volume control. The appetite-control systems in the brain start to develop in utero and continue to do so during the first few weeks and months after he is born. Research suggests that during this time, his nutritional and feeding experiences can influence his appetite importantly, and possibly for the rest of his life. This means that Mom's nutrition during pregnancy and your baby's early nutrition and feeding experiences matter. *What* your baby is fed (the foods he is offered) and *how* he is fed (your feeding strategies) can *both* influence his early appetite regulation and relationship with food. What all this really means for you, as a parent, is that it is crucial for you to understand your baby's appetite and to develop strategies that are tailored to his unique eating styles. Understanding your baby's appetite, and responding to him appropriately, is a fundamental part of supporting him in developing long-term healthy eating habits.

Food Preferences: What We Eat

"What is food to one man is bitter poison to others."
LUCRETIUS CIRCA 99–55 BCE

How your baby responds to food—how much and how often he wants to eat—influences his weight gain, but *what* he eats is important, too. Nobody needs to be convinced that diet matters—"we are what we eat," after all. A bad diet is probably responsible for about 10 percent of the entire world's ill health,[24] and research indicates that your baby's nutrition during his first 1,000 days may matter more than at any other time in his life.[25] Your baby's early diet will determine not only his health and development now but also how he fares well into his adult life. In particular, the first two years are unprecedented in terms of brain development, and optimal nutrition is vital for this.[26] But your baby's early nutrition and growth can also "program" his later health, affecting his risk of developing obesity and metabolic diseases, such as heart disease and type 2 diabetes.[27] So, making sure his nutrition is optimal during this developmental window of opportunity will give him the best possible start in life.

It's all very well knowing this, but getting your child to *actually eat* a healthy diet is quite a different matter, as any parent will know. Our food preferences determine *what* we actually eat or avoid. And this is probably even truer for young children than it is for adults. If a baby or toddler doesn't like something, he's simply not going to eat it. And it's unlikely that you're going to be able to negotiate with him, given that babies and toddlers lack the cognitive ability to understand the health benefits of eating something they don't like. So, the real question is, How can you get your baby or toddler to like nutritious foods? If you crack this, he will eat them.

The main hurdle that you will come up against is that the foods that babies and toddlers naturally tend to dislike the most are the nutrient-dense ones that you will want him to eat—the prime example being vegetables and, in particular, the green, bitter-tasting ones, such as spinach. Things also get a bit trickier with little ones because studies have shown that babies and children have a much greater liking for sweetness than adults do—the sweeter the better.[28] Very few babies or toddlers would turn their nose up at a piece of chocolate or a spoonful of ice cream, no matter how picky they might be. In fact, you may have looked on in wonder at the sheer amount of sugary food a young child will put away at a birthday party, given the chance! These taste dispositions make sense in terms of evolution—liking sweet foods and disliking bitter foods are traits that help vulnerable babies and toddlers survive. Sweet foods contain sugar, and therefore calories, which they need to fuel their growth, so it's good for them to gravitate toward these foods. On the other hand, foods containing harmful toxins taste bitter, which signals that something is unsafe to eat, so disliking these tastes helps to protect them from harm. These traits can prove challenging when it comes to encouraging your baby and toddler to like and eat bitter-tasting foods such as green vegetables. But, fear not, there are lots of things that you can do to help your child develop healthy food preferences. For example, when you move your baby from milk to solid food, start off giving him the bitter-tasting vegetables—it is his first experience of food and he doesn't yet know that chocolate exists!

There are also developmental changes in babies' and toddlers' willingness to *try* certain foods. In general, babies are much more willing to try new foods—flavors and textures—and accept them, than toddlers are. At around twenty months of age they become much more wary about eating foods they don't recognize—in fact, they can be put off by even small changes in appearance, from packaging to differences in preparation (for example, cooked rather than raw carrots). This developmental phase is called neophobia—refusing any new or unfamiliar food, usually based on sight—and is pretty common in most toddlers and young children between about twenty months and six years of age.[29] This explains why some toddlers reject a food that they apparently liked only the day before. What this means for a parent is that it will usually take much more effort to get a toddler or young child to try a new food and to like it, than it will for a young baby. Babies are most open to new flavors around the time they are introduced to solid foods, known as complementary feeding.

But age may be an even bigger deal when it comes to *texture*. Babies who have not experienced different textures during their first year of life find new foods difficult to accept after this point. This can persist into later childhood (and, in rare cases, into adulthood). These babies are less likely to accept foods that aren't smooth in texture—those that contain lumps or that require lots of chewing and are harder to swallow, such as fruit, vegetables and protein foods. It can also affect their speech development.

This means that the greater the variety of foods your baby tries early on during complementary feeding the better. But even so, you can expect things to become a little more challenging during the second year. It may help to know that this is a natural part of your baby's development and there are still tricks that you can use to encourage him to try new things. One of the main ways he learns which foods are safe to eat is by looking to you—he wants you to test-drive them first and check they're OK. You may already be aware that your child copies you, and other adults, a lot of the time. The same applies with eating; if he sees you eating something, he is more likely to eat it as well. This is called vicarious learning (see page 233). So, if you want your baby to try a new food, the best way you can encourage this is to eat it yourself, in front of him, without making a fuss. Better still, give the impression that you are thoroughly enjoying it. Being a role model yourself, and using others as role models, works well.

Given that there are general tendencies that we observe across all babies and toddlers, we may assume that what we like to eat is written into our genes and that all babies and toddlers like and dislike the same foods, but actually there are big differences between the food preferences of any two babies or toddlers of the same age. They may all have a *general tendency* to like sweet foods and dislike bitter ones, but this is true for some children more than others. You may even have noticed differences between your own children—one might have no issue at all with eating spinach, while the other one will refuse to eat anything that has even been touched by it on the plate. And the extraordinary thing is that the types of food we eat show a fair amount of stability all the way from childhood to adulthood.[30] This raises the question of where our food likes and dislikes come from in the first place—nature or nurture? We have been able to answer this question using Gemini.

WHERE DO FOOD PREFERENCES COME FROM?

When the Gemini twins were three years old we asked their parents to tell us how much they liked 114 foods, so that we could carry out the largest study to date on the nature and nurture of toddlers' preferences for key food groups: vegetables, fruit, protein (such as meat and fish), dairy (such as cheese and yogurt), starch (such as bread and pasta) and foods high in sugar and/or fat (such as chocolate and ice cream).[31]

We found that genes play a part in shaping toddlers' food preferences, but genes are more important for toddlers' liking of vegetables, fruit and protein than they are for liking of foods high in sugar and/or fat, and dairy and starchy foods. This was an important finding that helped us to understand a bit more about fussy eating, because for fussy children, the biggest problem foods are vegetables, then fruit, then animal-based protein foods (meat and fish)—in that order. They rarely take issue with eating fatty, sugary foods, carbohydrates (such as bread and pasta) and dairy foods (unless we're talking about yogurt with bits of slimy fruit in it). You may have noticed this with your own child if he is fussy—no encouragement is needed at all to get him to eat a cookie, but persuading him to try some green beans is a whole different kettle of fish. This is because many of the genes that cause a child to be fussy are *the same* as the genes that cause him to dislike vegetables and fruit (but they don't cause him to dislike tasty snack foods, dairy or starches).[32] It seems that all of this is part and parcel of an underlying food-avoidance trait—you might think of them as the "yucky genes." This clustering of fussiness and dislike for these types of foods may reflect some kind of hypervigilance among these children, given that protein foods are the main source of bacteria that cause serious illness, and vegetables and fruit sometimes contain toxins that can be poisonous. A hypervigilant child is fearful of anything that might cause him harm, including food. Some children are also fussy because they are particularly sensitive to textures; they're often reluctant to try foods that are anything other than soft and smooth (like ice cream).

For parents, this means that it can be a bit trickier to get your child to eat these foods, because, to some extent, you are battling their biology. But genes are not the full story, and you *can* usually get your child to eat these types of foods; it just takes a bit more effort. Importantly, Gemini also showed us that nurture (early experiences with food, such as the first solid foods, the foods that they see you and others eat, your attitudes toward food, and so on) is at least as important as genes for children's liking or disliking of *every* type of food—including vegetables, fruit and protein. In fact, early experiences are actually by far the most important reason why some toddlers have a penchant for foods high in sugar and/or fat—a taste for these foods is largely learned, not inherited. This means there is a lot of opportunity for you as a parent to shape your child's food preferences and make sure he is as healthy as possible.

CAN I TEACH MY BABY TO LIKE NUTRITIOUS FOOD?

Yes. Two key processes are involved in children learning to like certain foods: familiarity and feeling sure that a food is safe. One of the most powerful ways to get babies and children to like a food is through repeated exposure to it—they need to actually try it and become familiar with its taste and texture.[33] Repeated exposure to different flavors and textures is the journey to familiarity, and therefore to acceptance and liking. A recent discovery that shocked many people was that this process may even begin in the womb: a mother's amniotic fluid is flavored with her own diet, the baby swallows it, and in this process he is exposed to whatever tastes are in there.[34] So, in fact, your baby is swimming in a sea of flavors right from the beginning of his life. His taste buds start to develop at only thirteen to fifteen weeks, and by the third trimester he breathes and swallows about a liter of amniotic fluid every day. Experimental studies have shown that flavors such as garlic, aniseed and carrot can make their way into the amniotic fluid and flavor it for the baby (see page 37).[35] The changing flavor of amniotic fluid might also explain the rather intriguing finding that babies whose moms experienced severe vomiting during pregnancy (hyperemesis gravidarum) seem to prefer saltier foods—the theory being that Mom's amniotic fluid was probably a bit saltier because she was dehydrated.[36]

Exposure to flavors continues on the day your baby is born, when he starts milk-feeding. If he is breastfed he continues to have some exposure to Mom's diet, which also flavors her breast milk. If he is formula-fed he will learn to like the flavor of his main type of formula milk and will be predisposed to like the distinct flavors in that particular formula as an older child, as well.[37] Through the process of complementary feeding, your baby's food preferences will be shaped further by the foods that he gets exposed to. His first foods may be particularly important in terms of his willingness to eat certain foods later on. Giving him plenty of vegetables during this early process is likely to encourage him to eat them later. However, fussy eating and refusal of certain foods is pretty commonplace among toddlers. For many parents, mealtimes mean tantrums, and knowing how to deal with a child who flatly refuses to eat anything other than their favorite foods can be challenging. In Part 3 we will provide you with detailed guidance about *what* solid food to introduce during complementary feeding and *how* to introduce it, because we know from research that these strategies may help to prevent fussiness and encourage children to eat a varied diet.

THE BOTTOM LINE

- Babies and toddlers are not all the same when it comes to milk and food.
- Some babies and toddlers are less sensitive to their fullness; they eat a little bit more, each time they eat. These babies and toddlers are more susceptible to overeating if portion sizes are too large—be it milk in a bottle or food on a plate.

- Some babies and toddlers react more strongly to milk and food; wanting to eat (or eat more) when they see, smell or taste delicious food; they are susceptible to overeating because they are always hungry and will eat at any opportunity.

- Toddlers with poor appetites and little interest in food tend to be pickier eaters who are more prone to being fussy and often dislike vegetables, fruit and protein foods.

- Differences in appetite are probably one of the most important reasons why some babies gain weight more rapidly and others more slowly.

- When it comes to feeding your baby, it's all about understanding what type of eater he is and making sure you respond to his unique appetite.

- Your baby's food preferences can be influenced by his early experiences—and when we say early, we mean this may even start when he is still in the womb!

- Exposure is crucial. Your baby will eat what he knows. He will gain some exposure to Mom's diet during pregnancy and breastfeeding, because it will flavor her amniotic fluid and breast milk. Complementary feeding then shapes his food preferences, and the first foods you offer are key.

The chapters that follow will equip you with evidence-based tips about how to manage every type of eater and how to help your baby develop healthy food preferences that will endure for many years.

PART 1

Pregnancy and the Early Days

F YOU ARE EXPECTING A BABY, you may have discovered that there is a lot of conflicting advice out there about what to eat and drink during pregnancy. With newborns in particular, the guidance on how often babies should be weighed and what healthy weight gain looks like can be confusing—not to mention growth charts!

We now know that Mom's nutrition and weight gain during pregnancy can have an impact not only on her own health but also on her baby's long-term health.[1] With that in mind, we provide you with facts and practical advice about how to eat healthily during pregnancy, and the benefits of this for you and your baby (Chapter 2). We also know that babies' early growth has an important influence on their future health—well into adult life. So, it's important to keep an eye on this. But some moms are unsure about how to monitor their baby's weight gain and what to look out for. In Chapter 3 we explain exactly what healthy weight gain looks like during the first two years of life, how to spot weight gain that is too fast or too slow and why early weight gain is important for a baby's health now and in the future.

CHAPTER 2

Pregnancy:
The First 270 Days

Pregnancy marks the first 270 days of your child's life. It can be exciting but also quite daunting, and you may have some apprehension and many questions. . . .

Will I have cravings?
Will I feel sick?
What should I be eating?
How much weight am I going to put on?

In this chapter we equip you with advice on nutrition during pregnancy and offer information on healthy weight gain. There are a lot of different guidelines on nutrition in pregnancy—we have looked at all of these and summarized the most important evidence-based advice that is relevant for pregnant moms in high-income countries such as the US. We also give you ideas for how to eat healthily even if you feel sick and have cravings. We don't intend for this chapter to be preachy or judgmental; we simply want to give you the guidelines and the evidence behind them so that you can make up your own mind about what is right for you. We hope that you will come away from this chapter feeling a little less daunted and more confident that you have all the information you need for a healthy pregnancy.

Why Your Eating Matters

You will probably already know that healthy eating during pregnancy is vital for the growth and development of your baby. Energy (calories) and nutrients are needed to meet your needs as well as the needs of your growing baby. A good diet in pregnancy is linked to better outcomes for Mom, such as lower risk of iron-deficiency anemia and gestational diabetes, which can cause complications for Mom and baby that include premature labor and birth, and preeclampsia (when blood flow to the placenta is low so the baby doesn't get enough oxygen and nutrients). Benefits for your baby include lower risk of being born with a low or high birth weight, neural-tube defects (such as spina bifida), being stunted, or having accelerated growth.[1] Many people are also surprised to discover that a mother's diet during pregnancy may also influence her unborn baby's appetite regulation and food preferences, which, in turn, can affect the baby's risk of obesity and future health; so it's worth paying attention to your diet during pregnancy, as much as you can.

PROGRAMMING OF APPETITE

Your baby's appetite regulation starts to develop during gestation and continues to mature during the first few weeks and months after birth. Appetite regulation (hunger and satiety, as well as food responsiveness) is largely controlled by the brain and, in particular, a structure called the hypothalamus. A baby's early nutritional experience in the womb may affect the development of his appetite regulation. Moms who are under- or overnourished during pregnancy are more likely to have babies who are small or large, respectively, for their gestational age. Being born too small or too big puts a baby at greater risk of a number of diseases later in life (see Chapter 3 for more on this), and there is some evidence that the appetite pathways in the brains of babies who are born both small and big have been disrupted during their early fetal growth, such that they are predisposed to overeat and to prefer foods that are high in sugar and fat.[2]

Both over- and undernutrition appear to result in permanent alteration to the same neural circuits controlling appetite, and a key appetite hormone—leptin—seems to be involved. Leptin is made by fat cells (the more fat we carry, the more leptin we have) and plays a fundamental role in regulating hunger and satiety in the brain. It is often called the satiety hormone, because the more of it we have, the less hungry we feel, and vice versa. Research—largely with animals (because it's unethical to starve or overfeed pregnant moms!)—has suggested that babies who are born small to mothers who had poor nutrition during pregnancy are born with lower levels of leptin and so are very hungry. They also have a permanent increase in their appetite via changes to their hypothalamus, making them susceptible to overeating.[3] These developmental changes are thought to occur because the body is predicting a famine when the baby is born, so an avid appetite would provide a survival advantage in an environment where food is scarce. It is increased appetite that is thought to drive rapid early growth for babies who are born small for their gestational age (called "catch-up" growth). The problem is that if a baby who is born small enters an environment that is, in fact, rich in food (and not a famine), the result is an increased risk of obesity. For babies born very large, the reason for their increased appetite seems to be that their hypothalamus is somehow resistant to the effects of leptin—they have high amounts of it (as would be expected, given the increased amount of fat), but it doesn't have the appetite-dampening effect on the hypothalamus that it should have. It isn't clear at the moment why this occurs, or even if it has any particular survival advantage, but it appears to increase the risk of obesity. However, this research is based almost entirely on animal, not human, studies.

PROGRAMMING OF FOOD PREFERENCES

There is research to show that the flavor and smell of foods and drinks from Mom's diet during pregnancy make their way into her amniotic fluid. In one study involving pregnant women, half were given a capsule to swallow that contained garlic, and the other half were given a placebo capsule. The odor of the amniotic fluid in women who had the garlic capsules was judged by a sensory panel of adults to be stronger than that of the women consuming the placebo capsules.[4] A small experimental study showed that babies whose moms consumed 10 ounces (300 ml) of carrot juice for four days per week for three consecutive weeks in the last trimester were more accepting of carrot-flavored baby cereal compared to plain cereal and enjoyed it more compared to babies whose moms had only drunk water.[5] This study was small and needs replicating, but it suggests that some programming of babies' food preferences may occur during pregnancy. With this in mind, if you have a healthy diet containing lots of fruit and vegetables during pregnancy, your baby may be more likely to accept and like these healthy foods.

WEIGHT GAIN DURING PREGNANCY

> "You're going to put on weight and that's a fact, so there's no point in getting anxious about it."—**Carla (thirty weeks pregnant)**

During pregnancy consuming a healthy diet is important to ensure that your baby is well nourished, so that he develops normally and has a healthy birth weight. It's also a good idea to keep an eye on your weight gain, as much as you can, because gaining too little or too much weight is linked to an increased risk of certain complications for you and your baby. The US National Academy of Medicine (NAM; formerly the Institute of Medicine) suggests that the optimal amount of weight gain during pregnancy depends on your weight at the start of your pregnancy. Their recommendations are based on your pre-pregnancy body mass index (BMI), which is an estimation of your weight after taking into account how tall you are and is calculated using the following equation: weight (kg) / height (m)^2. As a rule of thumb, if your pre-pregnancy BMI was lower you should gain more weight, and if it was higher you should gain less:[6]

- BMI of less than 18.5: gain between 28 and 40 pounds (12.5 and 18 kg) of weight during pregnancy
- BMI of between 18.5 and 24.9: gain between 25 and 35 pounds (11.5 and 16 kg) of weight during pregnancy
- BMI of between 25 and 29.9: gain between 15 and 25 pounds (7 and 11.5 kg) of weight during pregnancy
- BMI greater than 30: gain between 11 and 20 pounds (5 and 9 kg) of weight during pregnancy.

The baby, placenta and amniotic fluid account for about 35 percent of weight gain.[7] Other increases in weight come from increased maternal blood volume (which increases by nearly 50 percent during pregnancy), breast-tissue development and increased fat—on average women accrue an additional 7.5 pounds (3.5 kg) of fat in order to prepare for breastfeeding (extra energy reserves are required in order to produce milk). A large review of almost 1.5 million women estimated that 47 percent of women gain more weight and 23 percent gain less weight during pregnancy than is recommended by the NAM.[8] The complications arising from gaining *too little* weight during pregnancy (compared to recommended) include

- increased risk of baby being born small for their gestational age (below the 10th percentile); about 5 percent more babies are born small to moms who gain less weight than recommended
- increased risk of baby being born preterm; about 5 percent more babies are born preterm to moms who gain less weight than recommended.

The complications arising from gaining *too much* weight (compared to recommended) include

- increased risk of cesarean delivery; about 4 percent more babies are born by C-section to moms who gain more weight than recommended
- increased risk of baby being born large for their gestational age (above the 90th percentile); about 4 percent more babies are born large for their gestational age when moms gain more weight than recommended
- increased risk of baby being born macrosomic (birth weight greater than 8.5 pounds [4 kg]); about 6 percent more babies are born macrosomic to moms who gain more weight than recommended.

While going a couple of pounds outside the guidelines is probably not a big deal, gaining much more or much less than recommended is not a good idea, so it's sensible to keep an eye on your weight gain. Although, it's fair to say that from this research we don't know if it is weight gain per se that is actually the real cause of the complications or if in fact it is other medical issues that go hand in hand with gaining too little or too much weight. Something to be aware of, too, is that weight gain is unlikely to be steady; most women tend not to gain that much in the first trimester, a lot in the second (due mainly to water so that your blood volume can increase), and then a bit more in the third (which is mainly increased fat on mom and baby), and some women don't gain any weight in the last month.[9]

Another reason to be aware of your weight gain during pregnancy is that fat that is gained can prove tricky to shift after your baby has been born. But weight gain can also be incredibly variable from one woman to the next, and it isn't always a reflection of differences in fat—for example, some women retain an additional 11 pounds (5 kg) of water.[10] It doesn't take a rocket scientist to work out that the amount of weight you gain is partly determined by the amount and types of food you eat during your pregnancy. In particular, excessive gestational weight gain is usually due to eating too much overall and, in particular, eating too many foods high in fat and sugar. So, making sure you eat well is the important thing to focus on during your pregnancy, rather than fixating on your weight. This is important whatever your weight when you start your pregnancy.

Nutrition During Pregnancy

Healthy eating during pregnancy is about eating a balanced diet with a wide variety of foods to ensure you have a good store of nutrients to meet the demands of your baby and keep you healthy. It's also about eating the right amount.

ENERGY (CALORIES)

There is a widely held belief that pregnant women should, or need to, "eat for two," and some women nearly double their calorie intake.[11] However, contrary to this popular belief, women don't need any additional calories at the beginning of pregnancy. The NAM provides daily energy intake (calories) guidelines for women during pregnancy, and you may be surprised to discover that you don't actually need to eat any more than a nonpregnant women until the second and third trimesters.[12] The suggested increases are 340 calories per day during the second trimester and 450 kcal per day during the third trimester, but these are rough estimates and they will be different for each woman—the amount will depend on your pre-pregnancy weight. The increase is needed to make up for the energy used to grow and maintain the baby, the placenta and the mom's tissues, and to ensure sufficient energy stores to make plenty of milk once the baby is born.

FATS

Fats have structural and metabolic functions in the body and are a source of essential fatty acids, which the body cannot make. Fat also helps the body absorb nutrients such as vitamins A, D and E. Fat that you consume that is not used by your body will be stored as body fat. During pregnancy, total fat intake should represent 20 to 35 percent of your overall calorie intake to prevent excessive weight gain.[13] This is actually no different from standard advice for all adults.[14] There are also "good" and "bad" fats. Trans fats (technically called trans fatty acids) are considered unhealthy, and there is consensus about this in the scientific community. They increase cholesterol levels in the blood—in particular, they increase bad cholesterol (LDL) and decrease good cholesterol (HDL)—as well as another form of fat in the blood called triglycerides. This means that they increase the risk of developing heart disease. Trans fats have no health benefits at all and will only cause harm. The NAM therefore recommends that you consume as little as possible. So, limiting the foods that contain trans fats is an important part of keeping yourself healthy, especially during pregnancy. Trans fat occurs naturally in very small amounts in meat and dairy fat, but most dietary trans fat is artificial; it is created industrially by adding hydrogen to liquid vegetable oils to make them solid at room temperature. Trans fats tend to be found in fried and baked processed food such as doughnuts, cakes and frozen pizzas. The reason they are used commercially is because they're cheap, have a long shelf life and give foods a particular desirable taste. The amount of trans fat can vary a lot within different food categories, so the only way to know if there is any in a product is to check both the Nutrition Facts label and the ingredients list. They are called partially hydrogenated oil (PHO) or partially hydrogenated fat in the ingredients lists (a fully hydrogenated fat contains no trans fats, so you only need to avoid *partially* hydrogenated fats)—the higher up these are in the ingredients list, the more trans fat there is in that particular food. Products containing less than 0.5 g of trans fat per serving can be labeled as containing 0 g, so be sure to look at the ingredients list as well as the Nutrition Facts label.

In 2015, the US Food and Drug Administration (FDA) determined that PHOs are not generally recognized as safe, based on extensive research into their health effects. So, since June 2018 manufacturers have not been allowed to add them to foods. However, to allow time for products produced prior to June 2018 to work their way through distribution, these foods have until January 1, 2020 before they are completely phased out.

You may have seen conflicting advice in the media about whether or not saturated fat is unhealthy. Evidence generally points toward high intakes of saturated fat leading to higher total cholesterol and, in particular, higher levels of bad cholesterol (LDL), which blocks arteries and leads to heart disease. A large review of good-quality randomized controlled trials (the highest-quality evidence) carried out by the World Health Organization (WHO) in 2016 concluded that replacing saturated fat with unsaturated fat (such as cooking with vegetable oil instead of butter) leads to health benefits, such as lowering bad cholesterol (LDL).[15] The consensus is that saturated fat should be limited, including in pregnancy. It is mainly found in animal-derived fats, such as butter and cream, but also in some vegetable sources, including palm and coconut oil. Processed foods, such as chocolate, chips, cookies, pastries, ice cream and cakes, are often high in saturated fat.

Unsaturated fats are the good fats, and there are two main types: monounsaturated fats, which are found in olive oil, peanut oil, avocados and most nuts; and polyunsaturated fats (PUFAs), which are found in corn oil and safflower oil. PUFAs are *essential* fats, which means that they are necessary for various functions in the body (for example, making new cells, blood clotting and muscle movement), and you cannot make them. You must therefore have these as part of your diet. They are particularly important in pregnancy for the development of your baby's brain and eyes. There are two types of PUFAs: omega-3 fatty acids and omega-6 fatty acids. Omega-3 fatty acids may help to prevent heart disease by lowering blood pressure, raising good cholesterol (HDL) and lowering triglycerides. Foods high in PUFAs include avocados, oily fish (such as mackerel, sardines and salmon), some vegetable oils (such as flaxseed oil) and some nuts and seeds (such as walnuts and flaxseeds).

CARBOHYDRATES

Carbohydrates provide fuel for the body and help organs and muscles to function properly. They should be the largest source of energy during pregnancy because they are broken down into simple sugars, which pass easily across the placenta and provide energy to you and your growing baby. Try to choose carbohydrates that have a low glycemic index (GI), which means that your blood-sugar levels will rise slowly after eating them. Low-GI foods typically have a GI of 55 or less and include foods such as soy products, beans, whole fruit (not fruit juice or dried fruit), milk, pasta, 100 percent whole wheat bread, oatmeal and lentils. A few whole fruits, such as pineapple and watermelon, have a higher GI; in general, the riper the fruit, the higher the GI. If possible, opt for *whole grain* varieties of foods rather than refined ones—these are foods that include all three parts of the grain (the bran, the germ, the endosperm); refined grains have had the bran and the germ removed, giving them a whiter appearance. Whole grain foods are more slowly digested, absorbed and metabolized and cause a lower and slower rise in blood glucose. This means you are less likely to experience sudden rises or dips in your blood-sugar level (called glycemic control), which is important for the healthy growth and development of your baby. A diet containing low-GI foods during pregnancy halves your risk of having a big baby (large for gestational age) and improves your glucose levels slightly during pregnancy.[16] Low-GI foods can also help you feel fuller for longer (see pages 273–74 for more information on this). It is recommended that pregnant women consume 135 g per day from carbohydrates, which is 35 g per day more than recommended for all adults. Carbohydrates should make up between 45 and 65 percent of your daily calorie intake (i.e., at least half).[17]

PROTEIN

Proteins are one of the building blocks of body tissue, so more are needed in pregnancy. Most adults get plenty of protein so you shouldn't worry, but it's important to ensure you include protein foods in your diet during pregnancy. Good sources include lean meat, fish, chicken, eggs and dairy. If you are vegetarian, include some legumes (for example, lentils and beans), soy foods (for example, tofu and edamame beans), nuts, seeds and nut butters.

FIBER

There are two types of fiber—soluble and insoluble. Soluble fiber dissolves in water and makes bowel movements easier, helping to prevent constipation. Many types of dietary fiber also have prebiotic properties, which means these foods increase the microbiota ("friendly bacteria") in the gut and improve our gut health. It's found in grains (such as oats and barley), fruit (such as bananas and apples), beans and pulses (such as baked beans and chickpeas) and root vegetables (such as carrots and potatoes). Insoluble fiber doesn't dissolve in water; it passes through your intestines without being broken down and helps other foods move through your digestive system more easily. This keeps your bowels healthy. It is found in high-fiber breakfast cereals, whole wheat bread, pasta and brown rice, nuts and seeds.

Constipation is, unfortunately, pretty common during pregnancy because of an increase in the hormone progesterone, which relaxes smooth muscle in your body and makes food pass through your intestines more slowly. Increasing your fiber intake, drinking plenty of fluids and doing some gentle exercise can help with this. There is also some evidence to suggest that fiber might reduce the risk of gestational diabetes and preeclampsia,[18] but very little research has been carried out on the impact of fiber specifically on pregnancy outcomes. The beneficial effects in this study may come from the fact that foods high in fiber tend to also be low GI and rich in lots of other nutrients. Pregnant women in the US are recommended to consume around 28 g of fiber per day.[19]

FOLIC ACID (FOLATE)

Folic acid (folate in its natural form) is a B vitamin that is vital for the formation of red blood cells. It is particularly important before and during the first few weeks of pregnancy. Babies rapidly develop spine and nerve cells in the early stages of pregnancy, and inadequate folic acid during this important period increases the baby's risk of developing a neural-tube defect, such as spina bifida. A review of studies of folic acid supplementation found that it prevents neural tube defects but does not have a clear effect on other birth defects such as cleft lip and palate.[20] In line with the *2015–2020 Dietary Guidelines for Americans*, the American College of Obstetricians and Gynocologists (ACOG) therefore recommends that pregnant women consume 600 mcg of folic acid daily from fortified foods or supplements.[21] It's also a good idea to make sure you eat foods naturally rich in this vitamin and foods that have been fortified with folic acid, such as some breads and breakfast cereals. Folic acid is destroyed by heat, so if you cook foods high in folic acid it is best to steam them (which has a minimal impact on the folate content) rather than boil them (which destroys most of the folate). The following are good food sources of folic acid.

- Spinach
- Kale
- Cabbage
- Broccoli
- Beans and legumes
- Oranges and orange juice
- Wheat bran and other whole grain foods

VITAMIN B12

Vitamin B12 helps to keep the body's nerve and blood cells healthy and helps make DNA; deficiency during pregnancy can cause severe and permanent neurological damage. It is found in animal products such as fish, meat, poultry, eggs, milk and milk products. Pregnant women need 2.6 mcg per day,[22] but women can become deficient in vitamin B12 if they don't consume any animal-based foods. The American Dietetic

Association therefore recommends that vegans and lacto-ovo vegetarians take a vitamin B12 supplement during pregnancy to ensure that enough is transferred to the fetus and infant.[23]

VITAMIN D

Vitamin D is essential for healthy bones, teeth and muscles. During pregnancy vitamin D is important for the development of a baby's bones and immune and nervous systems and growth. Lack of vitamin D during pregnancy can affect how much vitamin D your baby stores for the first few months of his life.[24] Most of our vitamin D actually comes from the sun; our skin makes it when exposed to sunlight. But most people don't get enough sunlight during the winter months to make adequate amounts, and many adults tend to be deficient in vitamin D given the public health advice to wear sunscreen and stay out of the sun during the summer. Vitamin D is found naturally in very few foods (mainly oily fish, such as salmon and mackerel, and fish oil, and in smaller amounts in beef liver, cheese and egg yolks), but it is in such small amounts that it is virtually impossible to get enough of it through these foods alone. In the US, most dietary vitamin D comes from foods that have been fortified with it, which includes most milk brands (usually fortified with 100 IU per cup), although most other dairy products (for example, cheese and ice cream) tend not to be. Other fortified foods include most ready-to-eat breakfast cereals and some brands of orange juice, yogurt, and margarine. A large national survey in the US that estimated how much vitamin D people were consuming from food and from supplements found that most people were not consuming enough vitamin D from food only, but those taking supplements (37 percent of adults) were getting the recommended amount.[25] Reviews have found that taking vitamin D supplements during pregnancy might reduce the risk of preeclampsia and of having a baby with a low birth weight, and it improves infant growth during the first year of postnatal life without causing any harm.[26] Guidelines vary in the US, but the NAM recommends that all pregnant women should have 15 mcg (600 IU) of vitamin D per day.[27]

Vegetarians/Vegans

If you are a vegan or vegetarian you may already be aware that many essential nutrients—such as iron, calcium, vitamin B12 and vitamin D—are found in animal-based products (such as red meat, fish, milk and eggs). It's possible to get the nutrients you and your baby need without eating animal-based foods, but you will need to eat fortified foods and take supplements just to be safe. It's a good idea to speak to your physician so that they can help establish what you need. Below are some good sources of nutrients if you follow a vegetarian or vegan diet:

- Protein: legumes, soy foods, nuts, seeds and nut butters
- Iron: fortified breakfast cereal with added iron, whole grain bread and other grains (for example, brown rice, oats and wheat), legumes (such as lentils and chickpeas), tofu and other soy foods, green vegetables, dried fruit (such as apricots) and eggs (for vegetarians)
- Calcium: calcium-fortified almond or soy milk, breakfast cereals, white beans, tahini and calcium-set tofu, almonds or sesame seeds, kale, broccoli and bok choy
- Vitamin D: fortified plant milks and grains, and eggs (for vegetarians)
- Vitamin B12: unsweetened soy milk and fortified breakfast cereal.

VITAMIN C

Vitamin C, another important nutrient during pregnancy, is needed to make collagen, a protein that builds up cartilage, tendons, bones and skin. During pregnancy vitamin C requirements are increased slightly, to about 85 mg per day,[28] so it's a good idea to make sure you eat some foods rich in vitamin C—including citrus fruits, green vegetables (such as broccoli and kale)—and grains fortified with it.

VITAMIN A

Vitamin A plays a crucial role in maintaining healthy vision and the immune system. It comes in two forms:

1. Retinol, found in meat, fish, dairy foods and eggs

2. Beta-carotene, found in fruit (for example, apricots) and vegetables (for example, carrots, green vegetables such as broccoli and kale, and sweet potato), which the body then converts into vitamin A.

There is a risk of abnormal development of a baby's eyes, skull, lungs and heart if Mom has too much or not enough vitamin A. The recommended daily intake of vitamin A during pregnancy is 770 mcg (2,565 IU) per day.[29] But vitamin A is something that can also be harmful if you have too much of it—in particular, be careful about eating liver, because it contains high amounts (about 6,500 mcg per serving; 28,000 IU), and the maximum total intake (from both food and supplements) that is considered safe in pregnancy is 3,000 mcg (10,000 IU) per day.[30]

IRON

Your body uses iron to make hemoglobin, a substance in red blood cells that transports oxygen throughout your body. During pregnancy, your body produces more blood to support the placenta and to supply oxygen to your baby, so the demand for iron goes up to keep up with the increase in blood supply. This increase in blood means that without enough iron your organs and tissues won't get enough oxygen. This can increase the risk of your baby being born with a low birth weight and preterm delivery, both of which are linked to stunted growth in later life.[31]

A large survey of American women carried out between 1999 and 2006 found that 30 percent of pregnant women were iron deficient in the third trimester,[32] so it's important to make sure you include some iron-rich foods in your diet, such as lean red meat, poultry, seeds, dark green vegetables, and fortified foods (such as grains and breads). Certain substances make it harder for your body to absorb iron from non-meat sources, including tannins (found in tea), calcium (found in milk), polyphenols (found in coffee) and phytates and oxalates (found in wheat bran and pulses). Try to avoid drinking tea and coffee at the same time as eating iron-rich foods. At the same time, eating foods that are high in vitamin C with your main meal—such as peppers, or simply adding lemon juice to salads—can aid iron absorption. The NAM-recommended daily intake of iron during pregnancy is 27 mg per day,[33] but organizations take different views as to whether or not you should routinely take a supplement. The ACOG suggests that pregnant moms should be screened for iron deficiency and only anemic moms should take a supplement,[34] but the CDC (Centers for Disease Control and Prevention) recommends that all pregnant women take a low-dose supplement (30 mg per day) and be screened for anemia. They recommend that those with anemia take a higher dose (60 to 120 mg per day).[35] The NAM also recommends routine supplementation for all pregnant women.[36] A review of studies of iron supplementation indicated that when women were given iron supplements versus not, there were slightly fewer babies born with a low birth weight (8.4 percent versus 10.2 percent), and the average birth weight was slightly higher (but only by 31 g).[37] Given the fairly small impact of supplementation on babies' outcomes, and that high levels of iron can also be harmful, we would recommend that you get screened for iron deficiency and take a supplement only if you need to, or if your physician advises you to.

CALCIUM

Calcium is needed to keep bones healthy, and there is some evidence that supplementation reduces the risk of preeclampsia by 55 percent, and is of most benefit to women at high risk of the condition and those with inadequate calcium intakes in their daily diet (less than 900 mg per day).[38] Although calcium needs are increased during pregnancy, the body adapts to ensure more calcium is absorbed. Calcium can be found in dairy products such as milk, cheese and yogurt, and eating these foods regularly during pregnancy will ensure you get enough. Nondairy sources of calcium include spinach, tofu, peas, beans and lentils, oranges and egg yolk. If you only eat plant foods, choose soy products and other nondairy drinks that are calcium enriched. The recommended daily intake is 1,000 mg per day, but the ACOG, along with most organizations worldwide, only recommends supplementation for pregnant moms who consume less than 600 mg per day through their normal diet. For these women, a daily supplementation of 1,500 to 2,000 mg per day is recommended to prevent preeclampsia.[39] The upper safe level for pregnant women is 2,500 mg per day.

IODINE

Iodine helps make thyroid hormones and plays a role in regulating metabolism. It is also important for healthy brain development, and insufficient iodine in pregnancy is the main cause of mental retardation worldwide. Both a national survey of pregnant women in the US and a small study of healthy pregnant women in Boston suggested that a substantial proportion (about half) of pregnant women had insufficient levels of iodine.[40] The true impact of slightly lower iodine intakes than recommended isn't known, but a large British study of pregnant women found that mild deficiency was linked with children having a slightly lower verbal IQ and reading ability, although the design of the study means that it isn't possible to know if this link was due to low iodine levels or some other factor that wasn't accounted for in the analysis.[41] In North America, dairy products constitute the major source of iodine, and women who don't consume any dairy products are at greatest risk of deficiency, but seafood, meat, and iodized salt also provide iodine. However, it is also harmful to consume too much iodine, and some types of seaweed have very high concentrations of it, so it is best not to eat this during pregnancy. The NAM has recommended a total intake of 220 mcg of iodine per day for pregnant women (from food and/or a supplement), with an upper safe level of 1,100 mcg per day.[42] The American Thyroid Association recommends taking a supplement of 150 mcg of iodine in daily prenatal vitamin/mineral supplements during pregnancy, [43] but be aware that in the most recent survey only about half of all prenatal multivitamins on the US market contained iodine. Don't assume you are getting iodine from your multivitamin if you take one; you need to check the label.[44]

ZINC

Zinc plays a role in enzyme and insulin production, and it helps to form a baby's organs, skeleton, nerves and circulatory system. It is found in meat, fish, eggs, milk, pulses, nuts and most grains. There is no need to take a supplement.

Supplements

The ACOG suggests taking a prenatal vitamin supplement to ensure that you are getting all of the vitamins and minerals that you need, but this isn't strictly necessary over and above folic acid, iodine and vitamin D. Iron supplementation during pregnancy is not routinely recommended for all pregnant women by all organizations, so we recommend that you speak to your physician about whether or not you need to do this. A well-rounded diet should supply all of the other vitamins and minerals you need during pregnancy, but if you follow a restricted diet (e.g., vegetarian or vegan) you should seek advice from your obstetrician or a dietitian because you may need additional supplements. The Special Supplemental Nutrition Program for Women, Infants, and Children (WIC) provides food and nutrition support to low-income women (see page 256 for more on this).

Healthy Eating During Pregnancy

You don't need to go on a special or unusual diet to get all the nutrients you and your baby need during pregnancy; it's about making sure you eat a *balanced* diet, although this can be tough if you are feeling sick or exhausted, fighting cravings and trying to juggle lots of things in your life to prepare for your new arrival. To get all of the nutrients you need during your pregnancy, the American Dietetic Association recommends that each day you ensure you eat something from each of the five food groups: grains, fruit, vegetables, dairy (and dairy alternatives) and proteins.

The amount you need to eat in a given day from each food group will be different for every person because it depends on your current stage of pregnancy, your age, your height and weight and how physically active you are. In order to make this easier the US Department of Agriculture (USDA) has created an online tool called the MyPlate Plan that will tell you the types of foods and the amount that are exactly right for you, once you enter your basic information: choosemyplate .gov/myplateplan. The ACOG recommends using this to help you plan your meals while you're pregnant. As a very rough guide, everyone is encouraged to fill half the plate with fruit and vegetables (slightly more vegetables than fruit) and the rest of the plate with starchy and protein foods (slightly more starchy than protein foods), with a bit of dairy on the side.

Aside from the crucial nutrients that you will get from the five food groups, it is a good idea to limit the amount of food you eat that's high in fat and/or sugar. Foods high in fat and/or sugar will displace those that are nutrient dense and make it difficult for you to get all the nutrients you need for your pregnancy without eating too many calories. Ideally, only 20 to 35 percent of your total calories each day should come from fat, but less than 10 percent should come from saturated fat.[45] Try to opt for foods low in saturated fat and, where possible, opt for polyunsaturated fats instead.

You should also aim to limit added sugars in your diet to less than 10 percent of your total calorie intake. Added sugars are those that are added to foods to sweeten them (e.g., adding sugar to tea, or manufacturers adding sugar during processing), as well as the sugars found naturally in honey and syrups. Sugars found naturally in *whole* fruits, vegetables and grains are not added sugars, so these are fine. Unsweetened fruit juices and dried fruit are actually fairly high in sugar so it's a good idea to limit these; in fact, in the UK the sugar in fruit and vegetable juices is not distinguished from other added sugars. The main sources of added sugars in the diets of Americans are soda, energy drinks and sports drinks (which account for 36 percent of all added sugar intake); grain-based desserts (13 percent); sugar-sweetened fruit drinks (10 percent); dairy-based desserts (6 percent); and candy (6 percent).[46] Since 2016, nutrition labels have gradually started to include both the amount of total sugars and added sugars in a food; the sugar contained in whole fruits and fruit juices are captured under "total sugars" (see page 251 for more on this). As a guide, most desserts (cakes, cookies, chocolate) contain added sugars. If you have sugar in your tea or coffee, pregnancy is a great time to give it up by gradually reducing the amount you add each day.

Try to eat less fat overall, and less saturated fat. You can reduce your saturated-fat intake by cutting the fat off meat and buying lean cuts of meat; grilling, baking or poaching foods rather than frying them; taking the skin off poultry meat; opting for lower-fat dairy products, such as reduced-fat milk and low-fat yogurt; using less spread on bread; having fewer processed foods such as cakes, cookies, fried snacks and takeout.

FOOD SAFETY

During pregnancy it is very important to be aware of food hygiene to avoid the risk of food poisoning, which you are more susceptible to and which can sometimes be harmful to you and your baby. It will also be particularly unpleasant while you are pregnant, especially if you are already suffering from sickness or nausea—oh the horror! Some cases of food poisoning can be very serious if you are pregnant, such as listeria, which can be found in some uncooked meats.

- Wash all fruit, vegetables and salad (even prepackaged salad), as soil can contain toxoplasma (see the following, "Foods to Avoid"), which can lead to miscarriage, stillbirth or damage to the baby's brain or other organs such as the eyes.

- Wash all surfaces, utensils and your hands after preparing raw foods such as meat, poultry and fish and keep raw foods separate from ready-to-eat food to avoid contamination and food-poisoning germs, such as salmonella, campylobacter and E. coli.

- Use a separate knife and chopping board for raw meats.

- Cook all meat thoroughly so that there is no trace of blood or pink meat, especially poultry, pork, sausages and chopped meat.

The FDA suggests four steps to food safety during pregnancy:[47]

1. **Clean:** Before, during, and after food preparation, wash hands and kitchen surfaces often with hot water and soap.

2. **Separate:** Keep raw meats separate from other foods, such as fruit and vegetables.

3. **Cook:** Thoroughly cook meat, poultry and seafood. Thoroughly cook and reheat food to a safe internal temperature before eating.

4. **Chill:** Your refrigerator should register at 40° F (4° C) or below. Place a refrigerator thermometer in the refrigerator and check the temperature periodically. Store perishable foods that are precooked or ready-to-eat in your refrigerator and eat them as soon as possible.

If you would like more information about food safety in pregnancy, see the FDA's *Food Safety for Pregnant Women* (fda.gov).

FOODS TO AVOID

There are certain foods you should limit or not eat while pregnant because they can cause harm to your baby. The two biggest concerns for pregnant women are listeriosis and toxoplasmosis. Pregnant women are ten times more likely to get listeriosis than a nonpregnant adult,[48] and the CDC estimates that there are around 1,600 cases of it in the US every year with up to a quarter of these occurring during pregnancy (mainly during the third trimester when immunity is most suppressed)—between 1 in 6,000 and 1 in 12,000 pregnancies are affected each year.[49] Listeriosis is very serious, especially during pregnancy— 260 people die from it every year (including perfectly healthy adults),[50] and it can have scary consequences for your baby if you are pregnant— with miscarriage, preterm labor, stillbirth or neonatal death occurring in 10 to 50 percent of infected moms.[51] The risk of listeriosis to Hispanic women is much higher than it is for the general population; pregnant Hispanic women are twenty-four times more likely to get it.[52] Apparently, this is because of the cultural tradition of eating Mexican-style soft cheeses like *queso fresco*, which, in many Latin American countries, are often made from unpasteurized milk.[53]

Toxoplasmosis is caused by a parasite (*Toxoplasma gondii*) that is found in undercooked or contaminated meat (especially pork, lamb and venison). Cats are a nuisance for spreading it—they eat infected rodents, birds and other small animals and contaminate soil when they poop! Unwashed fruits and vegetables that have been in contact with contaminated soil or water can also infect you with toxoplasmosis. If you get infected when you're pregnant it can pass to your baby and cause serious problems later in life such as eye and brain damage leading to blindness, severe mental disability and epilepsy.

But the good news is that very few babies are born with it in the US; a recent study of 521,655 births in California between 1998 and 2012 confirmed only two cases of it.[54] And it's also pretty easy to avoid—just make sure you cook meat thoroughly, wash your fruit and vegetables, and wash knives, chopping boards, utensils and surfaces after contact with raw meat and unwashed fruit and vegetables. Oh—and avoid cat poop and litter!

The other main causes of food poisoning—salmonella, campylobacter and *E. coli*—are potentially very unpleasant in pregnancy but are far less likely to harm your baby. To avoid any of these causes of food poisoning, avoid the following foods:

- Soft cheeses with mold-ripened white rinds—such as queso fresco, *panela*, asadero, *queso blanco*, Camembert, Brie—or goats' cheeses and soft blue cheeses such as Gorgonzola and Roquefort. Thorough cooking should kill any bacteria, though, so these are fine to eat if they are cooked. Hard cheeses such as Parmesan and cheddar are fine, as are other soft cheeses that have been pasteurized—such as cottage cheese, feta, mozzarella, ricotta, cream cheese and *halloumi*—and processed cheeses such as cheese spreads. Bear in mind, however, that soft cheeses are less acidic than hard cheeses and contain more moisture, so they can be an ideal environment for harmful bacteria, such as listeria, to grow in. Make sure you store them carefully in the fridge once they have been opened and don't eat them past the use-by date. The FDA also recommends not buying homemade cheese.[55]

- Unpasteurized milk or foods made from them (they can contain listeria).

- Pâté (any type, including vegetable), as it can contain listeria. Liver pâté also contains high levels of vitamin A, which can harm your baby (see pages 47–48).

- Raw eggs and food containing raw or partially cooked eggs—such as homemade mayonnaise, hollandaise or Béarnaise sauce, Caesar salad dressing, homemade ice cream or tiramisu—should be avoided due to the risk of salmonella, which causes a type of food poisoning leading to diarrhea and vomiting. Only eat eggs that have been cooked until both the white and yolk are solid. The FDA also considers pasteurized eggs safe to eat, even if raw or only partially cooked.[56]

- Raw and undercooked meats, as they can cause toxoplasmosis (see page 54). This even includes the meats that would normally be fine to eat slightly pink, such as steak. Some cold meats—such as salami, chorizo, Parma ham and pepperoni—are cured rather than cooked and may contain toxoplasma. Freezing cured meats for at least four days or cooking them will kill most parasites, and the meats will be safer to eat. Prepackaged cooked meats such as ham and corned beef are safe to eat.
- Raw shellfish, such as oysters, as they can be contaminated with harmful bacteria and viruses that could cause food poisoning. Cooked shellfish—such as mussels, lobster, prawns and crab— and white fish, such as cod, and smoked fish, such as smoked salmon, are safe to eat during pregnancy.[57]

Another thing to be cautious about is eating fish that contain high levels of mercury. Mercury can harm a baby's developing nervous system, and maternal exposure has been linked to lower intelligence and impaired language, attention and memory in children. High levels can cause mental retardation.[58] Big fish at the top of the food chain contain the highest amounts, so avoid shark, swordfish, king mackerel and tilefish from the Gulf of Mexico (if you are partial to eating these!), and limit the amount of white (albacore) tuna to 6 ounces (170 g) per week.[59] Try to eat plenty of oily fish, however, which are extremely nutritious and excellent for your baby's development in pregnancy; just avoid the types of oily fish that are too high in mercury (a good option is salmon).

Caffeine

Some organizations advise women to limit caffeine in pregnancy because several studies have linked high intakes with detrimental outcomes.[60] A large review of fifty-three studies found that an increase of 100 mg of caffeine per day (about one cup of coffee) was linked with a 14 percent increased risk of miscarriage, 19 percent increased risk of stillbirth, 7 percent increased risk of low birth weight (being born less than 5.5 pounds/2.5 kg) and a 10 percent increased risk of babies being small for gestational age (less than 10th percentile). However, they also found that these effects were pretty small within the lower intake range (up to 200 mg per day). A big problem with these studies is that they are observational and not experimental—this means that they simply look at how much caffeine women drink in pregnancy and link it to outcomes, but it could in fact be other factors that actually cause the poor outcomes among women who consume higher levels of caffeine. In particular, studies do not and cannot fully account for the level of nausea women experienced (this is subjective), which affects *both* their consumption of caffeine (the sicker women feel, the less coffee they drink) *and* their likelihood of having a healthy pregnancy (the worse the nausea, the lower the risk of miscarriage). In fact, one study found that higher consumption of *decaffeinated* coffee was linked to higher risk of miscarriage, suggesting that the coffee-miscarriage link has little to do with the caffeine in coffee and much more to do with nausea being a good predictor both of who will stop drinking coffee and the likelihood of miscarriage.[61]

Miscarriage is the main concern about high caffeine during the first trimester, but in the second and third trimesters the focus is on fetal growth and risk of stillbirth. However, there is a robust study of caffeine intake during the second trimester and pregnancy outcomes that gets around the problems inherent in the observational studies of caffeine and miscarriage. Rather than simply linking women's caffeine intake with pregnancy outcomes, the researchers randomly allocated more than 1,200 pregnant regular coffee drinkers (three or more cups per day) from Denmark to either reduce their caffeine consumption by about 180 mg per day (the equivalent of nearly two cups of coffee) during the second and third trimesters, or continue drinking it as before.[62] They did this by supplying all the women with either caffeinated or decaffeinated coffee and asked them to drink this in place of their usual coffee, but the women didn't know which type of coffee they were given. This study found no difference in the birth weights, length, head circumference or number of preterm births across the two groups, indicating that reducing caffeine did not affect these outcomes. However, the researchers didn't look at stillbirth and focused solely on caffeine from coffee but not from other sources (such as tea, some sodas or chocolate).

So, at the moment the link between caffeine and birth outcomes is not clear, especially for the risk of miscarriage during the first trimester.

For this reason organizations such as the ACOG tend to err on the side of caution and recommend that you should have no more than 200 mg of caffeine per day,[63] which is approximately three cups of instant coffee or tea, or one cup of filter coffee. Also be aware that some sodas contain caffeine, as does chocolate.

Alcohol

Drinking alcohol in pregnancy is a controversial topic that has received no end of media attention over the years. You may be wondering what the evidence really says, and whether or not you should have anything alcoholic to drink at all. Or you may feel worried if you didn't know you were pregnant in the first few weeks during which you were still drinking, and you are wondering if this is likely to have caused your baby any harm.

There is clear evidence that chronic (very regular) heavy drinking in pregnancy increases the risk of miscarriage, stillbirth and fetal alcohol spectrum disorders (FASD). FASD affects between 1 and 2 percent of babies born to heavy drinkers (defined by the ACOG as three or more drinks per occasion or more than seven drinks per week) and can include a range of developmental problems, such as learning difficulties; physical disabilities (movement and coordination problems called cerebral palsy); mood, attention and behavioral problems (such as autism and attention deficit hyperactivity disorder); problems with the liver, kidney, heart or other organs; hearing and vision problems; poor growth (small birth weight, slow growth and shorter height in adulthood); small head size; and distinctive facial features. What is less clear is whether there is any harm from low or moderate amounts of drinking. In other words, is there any level of alcohol that is safe to drink in pregnancy? A comprehensive high-quality review of the evidence of the impact of alcohol consumption on birth weight and preterm birth concluded that there is no effect on low birth weight or being born small for gestational age with intakes up to 10 g of pure alcohol per day (which equates to a bit less than one small drink per day according to standard drink sizes—see below), and no effect on preterm birth with intakes up to 18 g of pure alcohol per day (which equates to just over one small drink per day).[64] Another thorough review focused on alcohol consumption and neuropsychological outcomes, including academic performance, cognition, information processing ability, attention, behavior, memory, language, motor skills, vision, hearing, emotion regulation and social skills.[65] The three highest-quality studies (those that accounted for other important factors such as whether or not Mom smoked; her age, intelligence, wealth and education; and so on) showed a small detrimental effect on child behavior at nine months to five years among women who drank up to six drinks per week versus up to three drinks per week (with each drink including 13.7 g of pure alcohol, which equates to roughly one standard drink); problem behaviors included increased demand for attention, poorer interactive play skills, more difficulty regulating behavior and increased demand for attention. When they looked across all of the studies—regardless of quality—they found a small detrimental effect of binge-drinking (four or more drinks on at least one occasion) on child cognition between six months and fourteen years of age, but when considering only the studies of high quality this finding was found to be unreliable (statistically, it could be a chance finding). They found no other links between binge-drinking and any other outcomes. So, the evidence suggests that light drinking (up to three drinks per week) is unlikely to be harmful to your growing baby, but moderate or heavy drinking is a bad idea.

However, none of the studies have been designed in such a way that it is possible to know for certain if drinking any alcohol during pregnancy is safe. Many studies have relied on women reporting their alcohol consumption retrospectively after pregnancy, which makes the information unreliable because of the difficulty of remembering accurately. But even when considering studies that asked women during pregnancy, it is also possible that women who drink during pregnancy and those who abstain completely are different in important ways that also affect their health—for example, the extent to which they follow all sorts of health advice; education; and other pressures on their lives. In particular, studies largely show that women who drink lightly in pregnancy are more highly educated and wealthier than those who don't, but these women are also more likely to have children who fare better in life on a whole range of outcomes; this is a big problem that can mask the damaging effects of alcohol on their children's outcomes. The only way to study this fairly would be to randomly allocate women to drink or not to drink in pregnancy and compare the outcomes (a randomized controlled trial), but this type of study would be unethical.

A recent high-quality review attempted to use only the studies with the strongest designs to establish whether even light drinking in pregnancy is safe. Researchers concluded that moms who drank up to 32 g of alcohol per week (just over two standard drinks according to US guidelines) had a slightly increased risk (8 percent) of having a baby born small for their gestational age but found no other detrimental effects at this low level of drinking. However, their main conclusion was that there are insufficient studies that have been designed well enough to make any robust conclusions.[66] This means we can't be sure if there is any level of alcohol that is really safe to drink, particularly during the first trimester when fetal development is probably most adversely affected. Alcohol passes through your blood into the placenta, so if you drink, your baby does, too. But it is certainly not going to harm your baby if you *don't* drink. This is the reason why the *2015–2020 Dietary Guidelines for Americans* and the ACOG both recommend that pregnant women should not drink alcohol during pregnancy.[67] If you do drink, limit yourself to no more than one or two units of alcohol, once or twice a week, but it's probably best to abstain during the first trimester when your baby's development is most likely to be adversely affected by drinking.

What if you were drinking before you found out you were pregnant? Try not to feel overly worried if you didn't know that you were pregnant and were still drinking regularly; the likelihood is that everything will be fine. But aim to stop as soon as you find out you are pregnant.

One standard drink is 0.6 fluid ounces—or 14 g—of pure alcohol and is the equivalent of

- a 1.5-ounce (45 ml) shot of 80-proof spirit, such as vodka at 40 percent
- a 12-ounce (355 ml) can of regular beer at 5 percent
- a 5-ounce (150 ml) glass of table wine at 12 percent.[68]

It can be very difficult to give up habits that have taken years to acquire—for example, if it has become routine to share a bottle of wine over dinner on a Friday night. If you are finding it hard to cut down, there's a lot of support out there to help you. Rethinking Drinking is a National Institute on Alcohol Abuse and Alcoholism website that provides information about self-help groups you can join (rethinkingdrinking.niaaa.nih.gov), and Alcoholics Anonymous also provides information and advice by phone (212–870–3400) or online (aa.org). It may prove very difficult to do, but both you and your baby will benefit enormously if you manage it, so do seek help and support if you feel you need it to stop drinking.

Achieving a Healthy Diet

It's one thing knowing what a healthy, balanced diet is during pregnancy, but it's quite another to actually make sure you achieve it. It can be challenging, especially when there are lots of other things to think about during this time, or if you are experiencing cravings and sickness. There are a few strategies that research has shown to be helpful in achieving a healthy diet, including during pregnancy: setting healthy food goals, having structured meal plans and monitoring your dietary intake.[69]

SETTING FOOD GOALS

Goal setting is an important part of making sure you actually do something, so this is a fantastic way to try to make small, healthy changes to your eating habits when you're pregnant. It involves a four-step process:

1. Recognize a need for change. For example, increase the amount of fruit and vegetables you eat during pregnancy.

2. Establish a goal. For example, eat three servings of vegetables per day.

3. Adopt a goal-directed activity and monitor it. For example, instead of eating a bag of chips as a midmorning snack, have carrot sticks with hummus and monitor your food intake using an app.

4. Reward your goal if you achieve it. For example, put one dollar into a jar each day if you eat five fruits and vegetables. (A few examples of other nonfood-related rewards include an evening out, a new piece

of clothing, a new baby gift, a spa treatment or a trip to the hairdresser.) Try not to use food as a reward—for example, a bar of chocolate as a treat.

The key to goal setting is to make them SMART (Specific, Measurable, Achievable, Realistic and Timely):

- **Specific:** For example, specify that you want to eat three servings of vegetables and two servings of fruit each day.

- **Measurable:** You must be able to measure your goals—for example, by tracking your fruit and vegetable intake in a lifestyle app.

- **Achievable:** The goal you set for yourself must be achievable or you are setting yourself up for failure. If you currently only eat one serving of fruit or vegetables per day, aim to start increasing this to two or three and gradually increase your intake.

- **Realistic:** If your goal is not realistic—for example, going to the gym every day before work if you are so tired you are already struggling to get out of bed when your alarm usually goes off— then it will not be achievable.

- **Timely:** You need to set a time frame for your goal so that you have a fixed time limit in which to reach your goal. With pregnancy this is perfect because you have nine months set out for you. But you can also set shorter time periods than this. For example, over the next week aim to eat one extra piece of fruit each day as your midmorning snack.

STRUCTURED MEAL PLANS AND BREAKFAST EVERY DAY

Planning and structuring meals will not only help to ensure that you obtain essential nutrients and food groups for you and your baby, but it can also make life easier because your meals are planned from day to day or week to week. Try to plan lunch and dinner for four to five days of the week and, when you do the weekly shopping, stick as close to the ingredients you need as you can. Planning meals in advance reduces the number of decisions required when it comes to food choices, and this may help you make sure you don't eat unnecessary unhealthy snacks or foods. Shopping online can also save you time and means you don't have to lug bags all the way home.

Try to establish a routine of eating breakfast every day. If you miss breakfast you may be tempted to snack midmorning on high-fat and high-sugar foods, which means missing out on the nutrients that most healthy breakfast foods provide, such as fiber, iron and zinc. Try to eat three meals per day with healthy snacks in between (see page 65 for ideas for healthy snacks). This will help to keep your hunger at bay. Choosemyplate.gov helps make it easier to plan meals and make healthy food choices at each mealtime.

DAILY MONITORING OF DIETARY INTAKE

Monitoring the food you eat helps you keep track of the food groups and nutrients you are consuming. There is now a huge range of apps available for smartphone devices that will track your daily intake over the course of a day, and some are specifically designed for use during pregnancy. Research suggests that monitoring your dietary intake can help prevent excessive weight gain, and it is thought that this is because it increases people's awareness of their behavior and the circumstances that surround their eating behaviors.[70] However, bear in mind that many of these apps focus on calorie counting, which we do not advocate during pregnancy, as dieting is not recommended. In addition, some apps are badly regulated and are of poor quality, so make sure you go for one from a reputable organization.

SICKNESS AND CRAVINGS

Nausea and/or vomiting, especially during the first trimester, occur in about 70 percent of pregnant women, according to a large review of studies from all over the world—33 percent have nausea with no vomiting, but unfortunately 24 percent are still vomiting in the third trimester.[71] The severest form of nausea and vomiting (hyperemesis gravidarum) affects about 1 percent of pregnant women. Nausea and/or vomiting can occur at any time of the day—not just in the morning. It can be triggered by food smells, perfume and cigarette smoke. The cause of nausea and/or vomiting in pregnancy is not well understood, although the consensus is that it is caused by biological changes relating to pregnancy (such as hormones). Some researchers have suggested that it has a protective function in making sure harmful foods or substances are avoided or expelled from the body. There is some evidence to support this theory; for example, symptoms are strongest during the first trimester, when your baby's development is most susceptible to harm, and worse nausea is associated with a lower risk of miscarriage.[72] Nevertheless, the symptoms can be very difficult to cope with, especially if they are severe. So, what can you do to alleviate them? A high-quality review of forty-one studies of different treatments for mild to moderate symptoms up to twenty weeks' gestation concluded that there is little consistent evidence favoring any treatment, although there was some evidence for P6 acupressure (on the wrist), auricular acupressure (on the ear) and ginger being helpful. The researchers also didn't find any consistent evidence of the effectiveness of any one particular prescription medication for mild to moderate symptoms, nor did they find evidence of acupuncture being helpful. What they revealed more than anything was a lack of well-designed studies into strategies to help with sickness, and they found no studies at all of dietary or lifestyle interventions, which seems like an oversight.[73]

So, if you are struggling with nausea and/or vomiting, then it might be worth trying some ginger tea, which may provide some relief. However, this review was of studies for treating mild to moderate symptoms only; if your symptoms are very bad you should definitely speak to your physician, who may be able to prescribe medication that will help. A British charity (First Steps Nutrition) that provides independent advice about nutrition and eating for pregnant moms suggests three other tips that are worth trying:

1. Have small bland or dry snacks regularly (for example, dry toast or rice cakes).
2. Have a dry snack upon waking (keep some crackers next to your bed).
3. Avoid fatty or spicy foods, or foods with strong smells.

As well as sickness, some women experience strong aversions to foods, such as tea, coffee and fried foods. Intense cravings, or strong urges for foods, also often occur during pregnancy. It is thought that between 50 and 90 percent of women experience cravings at some point during pregnancy. Cravings for high-fat, high-sugar foods (for example, sweets, desserts and chocolates) during pregnancy may result in increased overall calorie intake and, in turn, can lead to excessive gestational weight gain (see pages 38–39). One study found that the only thing that predicted excess gestational weight gain among African American women was food cravings.[74] This is a relatively understudied area, so it is not entirely clear what causes strong urges (or aversions) for specific foods during pregnancy, but it has been suggested that hormonal fluctuations or the nutritional needs of mother and baby may play a role. It may also be an adaptive mechanism to protect the baby from toxins, hence the commonly reported aversions to meat, fish, caffeinated drinks and alcohol. Regardless of the cause of cravings, you will know if you have had them that they are very difficult to resist! Try your best to opt for healthy snacks (see below for some healthy snack ideas) if you can.

Healthy Snack Ideas

Try to combine two food groups in snacks to maximize nutritional value.

- Fresh fruit and low-fat plain yogurt
- Carrot, celery and cucumber sticks with hummus
- A small low-fat cream cheese and tomato sandwich
- Hard-boiled egg with one slice of whole wheat toast
- Crackers with cottage cheese
- A piece of whole fruit and a handful of unsalted mixed nuts
- Rice cakes with hummus
- Pita bread with guacamole
- A small bowl of whole grain cereal with reduced-fat milk
- A slice of whole wheat toast with a thin layer of nut butter

THE BOTTOM LINE

- Excessive weight gain during pregnancy is linked to poorer outcomes for both Mom and baby, and it can be difficult to shift afterward. A balanced diet is key to achieving healthy weight gain.

- Do not eat for two: Only 340 calories extra per day are needed during the second trimester, and only 450 kcal during the last trimester.

- Eat a healthy, balanced diet rich in fruit, vegetables, whole grains, lean protein foods, and low-fat dairy (or other calcium-rich dairy alternatives). There is no substitute for a healthy, nutritious diet in pregnancy.

- All women should take supplements of 600 mcg of folic acid, 150 mcg of iodine and 15 mcg of vitamin D daily during pregnancy.

- Ask your physician if you should take an iron supplement, but you may not need to.

- Those who follow a vegetarian or vegan diet should take a vitamin B12 supplement during pregnancy, and seek advice from their physician to ensure adequate nutritional support.

- Do not take vitamin A supplements.

- Limit alcohol and caffeine.

- A good way to make sure you eat well during pregnancy is to set goals.

- Be aware of food hygiene and avoid high-risk foods during pregnancy to minimize the risk of food poisoning.

CHAPTER 3

Your Baby's Early Growth

Concern about your baby's growth is a natural part of being a parent. Many parents are uncertain about how much weight gain is too much or too little (especially if your baby is breastfed and you can't "see" how much milk he is taking), when it really becomes a problem, and how to read and interpret growth charts. We have known for decades that poor fetal growth in pregnancy and insufficient weight gain in the first few months after birth can cause health problems for children later on. And, in recent years, the spotlight has also turned on excessive weight gain. It is now well established that *both* a healthy birth weight *and* optimal early weight gain in the first two years after birth set the stage for lifelong health. Growth is also a good barometer for your baby's general health—lack of, or excessive weight gain, can sometimes indicate that your baby has an underlying health problem that is causing the slow/rapid weight gain. It's therefore useful to keep an eye on your baby's weight gain during the early weeks and months after birth. In the US, there are regular routine postnatal care appointments so that your health care professionals can check that your baby is developing well—it won't just be left to you.

Your baby will grow extraordinarily quickly during his first year of life, which means he needs to eat an awful lot of calories (mainly in the form of milk) to fuel his growth. This is why feeding can feel like an endless activity during the early weeks and months. By one year of age, your baby's growth will have slowed down considerably.

Your baby's weight gain will be far from constant, as he will grow at very different rates during certain developmental phases. The usual growth pattern is for your baby to lose weight initially after birth but to regain his birth weight by two to three weeks of age. After this he will gain weight very quickly, with the fastest weight gain of all at about six weeks of age (called peak weight velocity), after which his rate of weight gain will slow to a plateau at around six months. Weight gain from six months will be much steadier. You will also notice that your baby's weight will increase a lot more than his length during the first year. On average, at one year of age he will have increased his weight by a whopping 300 percent but will have grown in length by only 50 percent. This is why one-year-old babies look squat, chubby and adorable! This complex early growth pattern means that the only way to check if your baby's weight is healthy at any one time is to compare it *over time* to that of other babies of exactly the same age and sex, and to look at his weight in the context of his previous weight gain. This is what the WHO growth chart is for—to see your baby's weight (and length) *in context*.

How to Interpret a Growth Chart

The WHO growth chart can be used to monitor your baby's weight and length gain over his first few months and years. Interpreting your baby's weight and length gain using the chart can be tricky, so it's good to be armed with information about what it is and how and why it was developed. Growth charts are developed by measuring the weights (and other things, such as length and head circumference) of a very large number of male and female babies and children at all different ages. This provides a reference against which the weights of other babies can be compared. The measured weights of all the babies of the same age and sex are organized into ten bands called percentiles. These percentiles tell you the proportion of babies' weights that fell at or below the weight of a particular percentile in the sample that was measured. There are equivalent percentile charts for length as well as head circumference.

So, when you plot your baby's weight and find his percentile, this tells you where his weight sits *relative to all of the babies in the sample* that were measured. The 50th percentile weight is the average—half of babies in the sample had a higher weight and half a lower weight. The 50th percentile is not "normal" weight, just average. This means that around half of the babies in the sample had a healthy weight that was above or below average. The 95th percentile indicates that 5 percent of babies in the sample had a higher weight than this, but 95 percent had the same or a lower weight. The 5th percentile is at the other end of the spectrum—five babies in every hundred, based on the sample, would have a *healthy weight* the same or lower than this weight, but most babies (95 percent) had a higher weight. This means that for some babies having a weight at the 5th or 95th percentile is likely to be *perfectly healthy*, especially if they are also around the same percentile for length, have always been around these percentiles and have shorter or taller than average parents respectively.

THE WHO GROWTH CHART

In the US the WHO growth charts are used to monitor growth in infants and children up to two years (from two to nineteen years of age, growth is then measured using the CDC growth charts). The sample of babies used to develop the WHO growth chart were from six countries (Brazil, Ghana, India, Norway, Oman and the US), and they were healthy, full-term and predominantly breastfed for at least four months (and still breastfeeding at twelve months), so supposedly they represent the *optimal growth pattern* for all babies—how babies *ought* to grow under the best possible conditions. These growth charts have therefore become the standard against which all babies should be compared, whatever their ethnicity and whether or not they are breast- or formula-fed. You will see nine percentile lines on the chart. The lowest percentile line (2nd) represents the lowest threshold, below which only one out of fifty healthy children will fall, followed by the 5th, 10th, 25th, 50th, 75th, 90th, 95th and 98th.

While the WHO growth standard is considered by most countries to be the best way to monitor the growth of healthy term babies, there is no international consensus regarding how best to monitor the growth of preterm babies, or even what "healthy" growth looks like for a preterm baby. This is surprising given that 8 to 9 percent of all babies are born between thirty-three and (just less than) thirty-seven weeks' gestation (babies born very preterm at less than thirty-two weeks' gestation represent only 10 percent of all preterm births).[1] There are several growth charts specifically for preterm infants, but some are better than others. The INTERGROWTH-21st Preterm Postnatal Growth Standards is the only chart that is equivalent to the WHO growth chart insofar as it is based on a large sample of international preterm babies who had healthy growth during pregnancy and no complications, and it has linked postnatal growth to a range of health outcomes at two years of age. A recent review concluded that this is the most robust growth chart for babies born between thirty-two and (just less than) thirty-seven weeks and can be used until your baby is sixty-four weeks' gestational age (which equates to six months' corrected age—i.e., six months of age if he had been born at forty weeks), after which he can be measured using the WHO growth standard without needing to make any adjustment for his gestational age.[2] However, given the lack of consensus on this topic, your pediatrician may decide to use a different preterm growth chart for your child, especially if he was born at less than thirty-two weeks' gestation.

WEIGHT, LENGTH, HEIGHT AND BODY MASS INDEX

Growth is about far more than just weight gain—it is length gain and head size, as well, and in the US your pediatrician will regularly measure all of these during the first two years of your baby's life (the health professional responsible for monitoring your baby's growth and the measurements that are taken vary by country). Length and height are not quite the same—because length is measured lying down and height standing up, height will always be slightly less than length, as gravity compresses the spine slightly. But in reality, they don't differ that much. Your baby's height will not be routinely measured before he's two years old because it's too difficult to measure it reliably in children younger than this (most toddlers less than two years old—and even those over the age of two—are too wriggly!). So, prior to the age of two, your baby's length will be measured instead, though measuring his length accurately is sometimes still a challenge. The WHO growth chart shows length percentiles up to two years of age rather than height percentiles for this reason. From two years of age, your baby's growth will be measured using the CDC growth chart instead. From this point onward his height will be measured instead of his length, and his height and weight will be used to calculate his body mass index (BMI). BMI is a ratio of weight to the square of height—your baby's weight taking into account how tall he is—and is a crude measure of his body fat. It is calculated using a simple equation: weight (kg) / height (m)^2.

The BMI percentiles can be used to classify the weight status of children two years of age and older: underweight (less than the 5th percentile), healthy weight (5th percentile to less than the 85th), overweight (85th to less than the 95th) and obesity (equal to or above the 95th percentile). The CDC has an online calculator at cdc.gov that will estimate your child's BMI from his weight, height, sex, date of measurement and date of birth. The CDC website also contains useful instructions on how to measure his weight and height accurately, if you want to do this yourself.

Monitoring Your Baby's Growth

Growth rates (especially weight gain per week) are incredibly variable from week to week for an individual baby. They also vary enormously between babies, even siblings. It is very important not to compare and make judgments about your baby's growth based on the weight gain of babies of other family members or friends, even if they are the same age. Your baby's growth will depend on a lot of things, including the height and weight of parents and other family members. Weight gain is not a competition, and greater weekly weight gain is not a valid sign of a healthy baby "doing well" or one baby doing better than another.

Babies' weights are like adults' weights in that they can fluctuate during the day depending on whether or not they have just been fed or if they have just peed or pooped. If you want to weigh your baby yourself, it's therefore a good idea to try to weigh him under the same conditions each time—for example, just before a feeding or right after changing his diaper (a full diaper can account for quite a lot of weight!). Always weigh your baby without his diaper and with no clothes on. This isn't always the most pleasant experience for a baby, so be sure to keep him warm before and after. The weighing scales you use can also make a difference to the weight. Home weighing scales designed for adults are not always accurate and don't usually have small enough units for you to be able to see small increments in your baby's weight gain (it can also be tricky keeping your baby on them!), so we wouldn't recommend using them. It is much better to weigh your baby using a baby scale if you have one or wait for your pediatrician to weigh him for you.

WEIGHT DURING THE FIRST FEW DAYS AFTER BIRTH

A baby's weight gain during the first two weeks is hugely variable, and some degree of weight loss is common in the first few days after birth, especially among exclusively breastfed babies and those who are born by cesarean section. Exclusively breastfed babies receive a very small amount of nutrition in the period when they are getting only colostrum, before your milk comes in (which should have happened by about seventy-two hours after he's born). A healthy-term baby can tolerate a very brief period of relatively low nutrition, but some babies develop complications such as low blood sugar level (hypoglycemia), jaundice and dehydration (also known as hypernatremia, where a baby's blood has too high a level of sodium [salt] in it). Unfortunately, there are no hard and fast rules as to exactly how much weight loss is OK, and individual babies vary, but higher amounts of weight loss increase the risk of complications. Because complications can result in serious brain injury during this very early period, health professionals will be checking him very regularly.

How Much Weight Is OK for My Baby to Lose After Birth?

There are conflicting opinions about what should be considered an acceptable amount of weight loss and, for exclusively breastfed babies, when supplementation with formula should be considered. The AAP considers up to 7 percent weight loss to be normal and not a cause for concern in most cases, but more than 10 percent to be excessive.[3] But clinicians and hospitals sometimes differ on what they consider an acceptable amount of weight loss. Most weight loss seems to have occurred by the second and third days after birth and is much higher for exclusively breastfed babies than formula-fed ones, especially those also born by cesarean section. For exclusively breastfed babies born vaginally, weight loss peaks at about forty-eight hours after birth, and these babies lose on average about 7 percent of their birth weight. For exclusively breastfed babies born by cesarean section, weight loss peaks at about seventy-two hours, and these babies lose on average about 8.6 percent of their birth weight.[4] Weight loss is considerably lower for babies who are exclusively formula fed; it peaks at forty-eight hours both for those born vaginally (2.9 percent) and by cesarean section (3.7 percent), and weight loss greater than 7 percent is uncommon for formula-fed babies, regardless of delivery mode.[5]

The AAP's policy is that breastfeeding will be evaluated for exclusively breastfed babies who have lost more than 7 percent of their birth weight in the first seventy-two hours, and your baby will be monitored very closely to ensure he is getting sufficient milk (this will involve careful observation of your baby's position at the breast, his latch and his sucking, among other things). Your baby's weight will also be monitored very closely while you're in the hospital, whether he is breastfed or formula-fed. On average babies are weighed five times during the first thirty days (six times for those born by cesarean section).[6] The Newborn Weight Tool (newbornweight.org) is a fantastic free resource that allows parents to monitor their baby's weight loss during the first month of life, to check that things are going OK.

How Many Babies Lose More than 10 Percent of Their Birth Weight?

A US study of 108,907 exclusively breastfed term newborns found that about 5 percent of those born vaginally had lost at least 10 percent of their birth weight forty-eight hours after birth. However, a substantial number of babies who were born by C-section had lost more than 10 percent of their birth weight (25 percent of babies by seventy-two hours).[7] So it's actually fairly common among exclusively breastfed babies who are also born by C-section.

How Quickly Should My Baby Regain His Birth Weight?

Health professionals focus on making sure that your baby regains his birth weight by ten to fourteen days, and the AAP and the American College of Obstetricians and Gynecologists advise that feeding needs to be carefully evaluated for babies who have not regained their birth weight by two weeks of age. But the largest American study to date on timing of weight regain in almost 150,000 newborns indicates that it could take a bit longer than this for some babies, especially those born by C-section.[8] There isn't much information available about the health outcomes of babies who take longer than ten to fourteen days to regain their weight, so we don't know for certain if this is a problem or not.

What Causes Excessive Weight Loss During the First Few Days?

The usual cause of excessive weight loss (more than 10 percent of birth weight) during the first few days is that your baby isn't feeding properly. A study of neonatal weight loss found no underlying medical problems among infants who lost more than 10 percent of their birth weight, suggesting that it was feeding problems that were the most likely cause.[9] Some moms experience a delay in their milk coming in or have a low milk supply (see page 110).

How Do I Know If My Baby Is Getting Enough Milk?

Key signs that your baby is feeding properly during the first few days (and weeks) are his weight gain, diapers and feeding patterns. In the first four weeks (from Day 5 onward, after your milk has come in) he should be producing six or more wet diapers per twenty-four-hour period. If he is producing fewer than this he may be dehydrated (in the first forty-eight hours, he is likely to have only two or three wet diapers). A wet diaper should contain the equivalent of 2 to 4 tablespoons of water. Most breastfed babies are also producing three bright yellow poops every twenty-four hours by Day 4 or 5 (formula-fed babies can produce fewer than this). If you are worried about your baby's milk intake in the first few days, speak to your pediatrician and get him checked out.

ROUTINE WEIGHING DURING THE FIRST TWO YEARS

The US health prevention program Bright Futures is led by the AAP. It entitles all babies, children and adolescents in the US to have regular, free well-child care visits, which are health assessments carried out by a pediatrician and include growth monitoring, among many other things. This ensures that if there are any problems with your baby's growth they can be picked up early, and you can be supported to get him back on track. Lots of parents only see the pediatrician when their baby is sick, but these health checks are just as important for healthy babies. They're a valuable way to make sure your baby is thriving. If something isn't quite right, it can be picked up early and dealt with before it becomes a more serious problem. You can also use the opportunity to ask your pediatrician about anything to do with your baby's development. Your baby's growth is probably the most important piece of information about his health during the early years, so we strongly urge you to take advantage of these free checks. The AAP recommends that you take your baby for a well-child care visit at the following ages, during the first two years* (the checks extend up until twenty-one years of age).[10]

- Two to five days old
- One month old
- Two months old
- Four months old
- Six months old
- Nine months old
- Twelve months old
- Fifteen months old
- Eighteen months old
- Two years (twenty-four months) old

It is common for healthy babies to move up and down the growth chart quite a bit in their first few weeks, so don't feel alarmed if your baby isn't tracking steadily during this early period. In particular, if your baby was born big he may fall slightly (called "catch-down" growth), and if he was born small he may move upward (called "catch-up" growth), before settling. After six weeks there is less movement and your baby's position on the chart will usually become a bit more stable, although a big drop in his weight after minor illnesses is common and

---

* Many babies are also seen for a weight check between ten days and two weeks of age, and some babies with excessive weight loss have many visits in the first two weeks.

nothing to worry about, as long as when he regains the weight he goes back to his "usual" percentile, which normally happens within two to three weeks. It is only *persistent* and *substantial* changes in weight that should concern you (after *repeated measurements* consistently show downward or upward crossing of percentiles); so don't panic if on one occasion your baby's weight has moved up or down.

RAPID WEIGHT GAIN

Rapid weight gain is gaining too much weight too quickly. It can compromise your baby's health so is worth looking out for. A baby is considered to have rapid weight gain if he crosses *more than one major percentile space upward* on the growth chart, regardless of what percentile he started on. In most countries there are no guidelines on how best to manage rapid weight gain, and, as such, many health professionals don't flag it with parents.

How Common Is Rapid Weight Gain?

We don't actually know how many babies in the US have rapid weight gain according to the WHO growth chart because there are no population-based estimates. But a study of 1,971 babies found that 24 percent of term babies (born at thirty-nine weeks or later) had rapid weight gain from birth to four months, 39 percent from birth to one year, and 42 percent from birth to two years.[11] Rapid weight gain in infancy in the US seems reasonably common.

Why Is Rapid Weight Gain a Problem?

Rapid weight gain in infancy has been linked to metabolic diseases in adulthood including obesity, cardiovascular disease and type 2 diabetes. One study found that babies with rapid growth were nearly four times more likely to have obesity as children than babies staying on the same percentile. Rapid early growth even predicted adult obesity as late as sixty-six years of age. Importantly, the effect of rapid growth on obesity was the same for breastfed and formula-fed babies, boys and girls, and for those born with a large, small or healthy birth weight.[12] As well as having increased risk for obesity, babies who grow very quickly tend to gain fat around their middle and are less sensitive to the effects of insulin during the first three years of life, which is an important marker of metabolic health and is involved in the development of type 2 diabetes and cardiovascular disease.[13] Rapid growth in the first few months after birth also promotes earlier puberty, which may seem unimportant in itself, but it is related to reproductive cancers, metabolic diseases and all-cause mortality (dying from any cause).[14] Optimal growth during the first two years is therefore an important part of your baby's later health and is something to keep an eye on.

What Causes Rapid Weight Gain, and What Can You Do If It Happens to Your Baby?

Babies with rapid growth tend to have larger appetites and high demands around feeding. Part of your baby's appetite is due to his genes (genes influence his appetite and therefore his weight gain),[15] but *how* your baby is fed can also influence his appetite and his response to milk and food. Babies' appetites and relationships with food develop through a complex interplay between their own genetic predispositions and their early experiences with milk, food, feeding and eating—*what* and *how* he is fed can also affect his milk and food intake. If your baby is experiencing rapid growth, it's worth making sure you are not encouraging him to overfeed (see pages 175–78).

What About Catch-Up Growth?

Many babies who are born small for gestational age or preterm experience catch-up growth in the first six to twelve months of life. It is a form of rapid growth but is important for survival and the prevention of infection, stunting and other developmental problems, such as lower IQ. If catch-up growth doesn't occur during this early window, about half of the babies will be shorter as adults than expected if they had not been born small for their gestational age.[16] So, if your baby was born small or preterm, it is likely that he will have faster growth so that he can catch up and reach a healthy weight. However, growth can sometimes be excessive, and if this happens your health professional may flag it. The strategies that we suggest in the subsequent chapters of this book for *how* and *what* to feed your baby will help you support him in developing good appetite regulation and a healthy relationship with food, whether he was born with a low, normal or high birth weight.

WEIGHT FALTERING

Weight faltering (which used to be called "failure to thrive") is when your baby is gaining weight more slowly than he should, which can compromise his health and development. It is not uncommon for parents (and health professionals) to worry about this during their baby's first two years. There isn't an overall accepted definition and it is complex to diagnose, but most health professionals become concerned if your baby's age- and sex-adjusted weight crosses a certain number of major percentile spaces downward. Some health professionals suggest that crossing downward through *two major percentile spaces* (based on at least two weights measured at least four weeks apart) should be a red flag. Others have the view that it depends on which percentile the baby was on before the weight problems started, and that there should be less allowance for babies already on a low percentile (downward crossing of only one percentile space should be a red flag for a baby who is already small—e.g., on the 5th percentile) and more leeway for babies already on a high percentile (e.g., a big baby on the 95th percentile can cross several percentile spaces downward before anyone needs to worry too much).

However, if there is any concern about your baby's weight, then his head circumference, as well as his length (or height if he is two years old or older) will also be taken into account (along with other measures of his body fat). Healthy growth is about far more than just his weight gain. In particular, head circumference is critically important in assessing a child's growth. A head that is growing too big or one that isn't growing fast enough can suggest an underlying serious condition that requires evaluation. If your baby's head is growing normally, but he has *both* a low weight percentile *and* a low length percentile, this can indicate *growth faltering*, which usually means that he is not consuming enough calories. However, a low length or height percentile can also reflect your baby's genetic predisposition to be of a shorter stature. If you and your partner are short, then it is likely that your baby will be short, too (his adult height will typically be an average of both parents). If you are both pretty tall and your baby's length is low, this is more concerning. If your pediatrician is worried, then your baby's weight and length may be monitored more regularly. Bear in mind that, in general, it is babies and children who are already of a *very low* weight or BMI (e.g., below the 5th percentile) who need to be monitored very carefully. Those with low weight/length/BMI *as well as* weight faltering need to be assessed. Your pediatrician will take many different things into account if there is any concern about your baby's growth.

If your baby's weight is faltering, your pediatrician may suggest some feeding strategies to help get him back on track. In the chapters that follow we provide tips on how to feed your baby if he has a poor appetite for milk or difficulty eating solid food, to make sure that he is getting enough (see pages 207 and 286). Your baby is considered to have recovered when he goes back to within one to two percentile spaces of his previous position, which can take several months.

How Common Is Weight Faltering?

Weight faltering in infancy tends to be mild when it occurs in affluent countries such as the US, so try not to feel overly anxious about this happening to your baby. Weight faltering tends to be most common during the first two years of life when growth is fastest, and in high-income countries it affects between 1 and 10 percent of infants under two years of age.[17] The US does not have up-to-date robust statistics on the number of babies and toddlers who have weight faltering in the population, but studies have estimated that about 5 to 10 percent of outpatient doctor visits in primary care are due to weight faltering.[18]

Why Is Weight Faltering a Problem?

Health professionals take weight faltering seriously because if it is *prolonged* and *severe* it can cause developmental problems. Many studies of babies and children have reported that *severe* weight faltering is linked to[19]

- IQ deficits of 3 to 5 points (this is a very small impact)
- reduced academic performance
- stunting
- smaller head size
- lower immunity and increased infection
- gastrointestinal problems
- heart problems.

However, as we have said, in the US weight faltering is usually mild in comparison to the more severe cases that are seen in developing countries in which many of these studies are undertaken. Early treatment and recovery can reverse the problems with immunity and gastrointestinal and heart problems, although children are often still shorter and have a slightly lower IQ and academic performance.[20]

What Causes Weight Faltering, and What Can You Do If It Happens to Your Baby?

Many years ago weight faltering was called the "maternal deprivation syndrome" and was believed to be caused by emotional and physical neglect of the child. In fact, it is only in rare cases that weight faltering is caused by parental neglect, mental-health problems or addiction (about 5 percent of cases).[21] Most children with weight faltering are not neglected. As you might expect, poverty is the single most important risk factor for weight faltering.[22] It is rare for it to be caused by an underlying disease—up to 86 percent of children who are hospitalized for weight faltering have no underlying disease that is causing it, and this percentage is probably much higher for children who are diagnosed by their pediatrician at a standard appointment.[23] It is especially unlikely that there is an underlying disease if your baby or child seems otherwise well in every other respect. So, what does cause poor weight gain?

What we have learned over the last thirty years is that weight faltering has a *predominantly nutritional cause*—it most often happens because your baby or toddler isn't consuming as many calories as he needs. This accounts for the vast majority of cases. There is increasing evidence that poor weight gain is related to your baby's appetite and feeding and eating behavior.[24] In many cases children with weight faltering have a poor appetite, and this can lead to difficult mealtimes, increasingly stressful interactions, and spiraling difficulties with feeding and eating. If your baby is a difficult feeder, there are lots of strategies that you can use to make sure you support him in getting the nutrition that he needs (see pages 207–08).

Birth Weight

Your baby's early growth is important during his first few months of life, but his weight at birth matters, too. Birth weight is thought to indicate the quality of his nutrition during pregnancy. If your baby has a low birth weight (less than 2.5 kg/5.5 pounds) he may have had undernutrition in pregnancy, but there are ethnic differences in birth weight, too, and many South Asian babies are born small, which is probably genetic. If your baby has a high birth weight (more than 4 kg/ 8.8 pounds), called macrosomia ("large body" in Greek), he may have had overnutrition. But because boys are born slightly heavier than girls, and gestational age influences birth weight enormously—a baby born at forty weeks will have a higher birth weight than a baby born at thirty-seven weeks—both of these are taken into account when classifying your baby as having a low or high birth weight. Being born "small for gestational age" (SGA) is usually considered to be a birth weight in the lowest 9 percent of babies of the same gestational age and sex (*below* the 10th percentile) and "large for gestational age" (LGA) is a birth weight in the highest 9 percent (*above* the 90th percentile).

In spite of many alarming headlines about birth weight increasing,[25] this simply isn't supported by research. In fact, in the US, the average birth weight has been *decreasing* since 1990[26] (as it has in many other countries as well, including the UK, Canada, France, Denmark, Korea, Japan and China[27]). This is partly because length of gestation has decreased due to more medical interventions such as inducement, and very premature babies are more likely to survive. These factors bring the average birth weight down. In addition, in the US since 1997 the number of babies who are born SGA has increased, and the number born LGA has decreased, suggesting that fetal growth has actually slowed down over recent years.[28] And when you dig down, the weight decreases seem to be highest among African American women and, in particular, among those with risk factors such as high blood pressure and obesity.[29] It looks as though decreases in birth weight partly reflect growing disparities in health.

WHY IS A LOW OR HIGH BIRTH WEIGHT A PROBLEM?

The largest and most comprehensive review ever undertaken into birth weight and later health found convincing evidence for a link between birth weight and a range of health outcomes:[30]

- low birth weight and increased risk for dying from any cause
- SGA and childhood stunting
- higher birth weight and better bone health in the hip (higher bone mineral concentration), and lower risk for mortality from cardiovascular diseases.

They also found highly suggestive evidence for a link between

- low birth weight and increased infant mortality *in developing countries*; wheezing disorders in childhood (such as asthma); coronary heart disease; lower rates of overweight and obesity in adulthood; and slightly lower IQ in adolescence
- high birth weight and all types of leukemia; overweight or obesity in adulthood; and lower risk of coronary heart disease.

However, the authors concluded that the effects of birth weight on all of these health outcomes were pretty small. So, don't panic if your baby was born small or large—it doesn't mean that he is definitely going to have any of these health problems; it just increases his risk very slightly. We also have no idea if birth weight actually causes these outcomes or if they are simply a marker for other things that are the true cause (such as socio-economic position, maternal health, and genetics—to name just a few).

WHAT CAUSES A BABY'S BIRTH WEIGHT TO BE LOW OR HIGH?

There are some things that we know influence a baby's birth weight that can't be changed (called unmodifiable) and others that can (modifiable). Unmodifiable influences include[31]

- a baby's own genes (although this only has a small influence on his birth weight)
- sex (boys are heavier than girls)
- Mom's racial or ethnic origin (lower birth weights tend to be seen in Africa, India and East Asia, and higher weights among Europeans and white Americans)

- Mom's height and pre-pregnancy weight (taller moms have heavier babies, and those with a lower pre-pregnancy weight tend to have lighter babies), and Dad's height and weight (taller, heavier dads tend to have bigger babies)

- order of birth (first babies tend to be lighter than subsequent babies) and weights of previous babies

- general health and bouts of illness during pregnancy.

Modifiable influences include

- gestational weight gain (moms who gain more weight tend to have heavier babies)

- gestational diabetes (moms who develop this are more likely to have heavier babies)

- alcohol (heavy alcohol consumption is linked with lower birth weight)

- smoking (smoking in pregnancy is one of the most important risk factors for low birth weight in developed countries and doubles the risk).

So, we have seen that early growth is important for your baby's health and development, and it's worth trying to make sure that he grows at a healthy rate. The chapters that follow are packed full of information and advice about how to establish good feeding and eating habits as soon as your baby is born and over the following two years. At each stage of feeding we consider all types of babies and children—from the babies with poor appetites who may be prone to weight faltering, to the eager eaters who may be prone to rapid weight gain.

THE BOTTOM LINE

- Growing (weight and length) at an optimal rate during the early years is important for lifelong health and development.

- It's a good idea to take advantage of the regular checks offered to you to have your baby weighed and measured during the first two years.

- It is common for babies (especially if they are exclusively breastfed) to lose weight in the first two to three days after birth, but if he loses more than 10 percent of his birth weight, he needs to be assessed. It is important that your baby regains his birth weight within two to three weeks.

- Babies tend to move around on their percentile position in the early weeks but usually settle on a more stable percentile position from around six weeks onward.

- Rapid growth in the US is common, especially in babies born small who experience catch-up growth, while weight faltering is less common.

- Growing too slowly or too quickly usually has a nutritional basis, and your baby's appetite plays an important part in his early growth.

PART 2

Milk-Feeding

F EEDING A YOUNG BABY CAN SOMETIMES feel daunting, especially when you are doing it for the first time. A new parent has to
make lots of different decisions, largely relating to

- *what* to feed: whether to breastfeed or use formula, or use a
  mixture of both, and which type of formula to use

- *how* to feed: how often and how much to feed, and how to manage
  the actual feeding interaction (for example, feeding to a schedule
  or "on demand").

There is a lot of strong opinion when it comes to milk-feeding. The
information out there isn't always evidence based, and there is an awful
lot of information for parents to sift through. Scrutinizing every little
detail available on the internet can seem like an insurmountable task,
especially during the first few weeks after birth, when sleep deprivation
is at its most brutal, and you really just want practical, properly
researched advice. As scientists, we have found it time-consuming and
hard-going navigating the swathes of claims and exploring the scientific
evidence for each one. We cannot imagine how we could have done this
without the time or training we have had, and this was one of the main
reasons we decided to write this book.

The topic of breast- versus formula-feeding is one that often arouses
emotive discussion, and many moms will have found themselves on
the receiving end of those voicing strongly held opinions about what
they should or shouldn't be doing. This can be very stressful to say the
least and makes it difficult to know the facts when it comes to
milk-feeding. Some moms who don't manage to breastfeed, or who
choose not to, feel guilty, judged or that they have failed their baby.
Other moms are put under pressure by friends or family members to
stop breastfeeding before they are ready or are made to feel that it's
inappropriate to breastfeed a baby in a public place. This can lead to

moms giving up or not even starting in the first place. It is also surprisingly difficult to find good scientific information about formula, yet this is crucial for parents to make an informed decision about the type and amount of formula to feed, if this is necessary.

The decision to breast- or formula-feed is highly personal and, importantly, in some situations it isn't possible, suitable or adequate to breastfeed. We are not judging your decision; as we see it, only one thing matters when it comes to feeding your child, and that is doing the right thing for you and your baby. We hope that by providing you with the most up-to-date evidence-based information, we can support you in making the decision that is right for you. The tips and advice that we provide in Chapter 6 on *how* to feed to support your baby's development of good appetite regulation will apply whether you decide to breast- or formula-feed, or use a mixture of both.

CHAPTER 4

Breastfeeding

The American Academy of Pediatrics (AAP), in line with the World Health Organization (WHO), recommends that babies are breast-fed *exclusively* for the first six months (twenty-six weeks) after birth[1]—this means that babies should receive no other food or drink (not even water), except for vitamin D supplementation (and any necessary medication). The AAP also recommends that breastfeeding (and/or formula, if used) should continue from six months until one year of age (and that moms should breastfeed for longer if they and their baby wish to continue), alongside the introduction of solid food. The WHO advises that from six months babies should be given nutritious complementary food and continue to be breastfed up to two years or beyond. These are pretty uncompromising guidelines. So, what is the evidence for such a strong stance? In the next few pages we will explore the scientific facts about breastfeeding so you can make an informed decision about what is best for you and your baby.

The Challenges of Breastfeeding Research

Before we summarize the scientific findings of studies that have examined the benefits of breastfeeding, it is worth reflecting briefly on the considerable challenges in this field of research. The first obstacle relates to measurement of milk-feeding. Trying to obtain detailed and meaningful information about the amount of breast milk versus formula babies receive for the duration of infancy is not an easy task. A lot of the time the questions need to be asked retrospectively—weeks, months or even years after breast- and formula-feeding has finished—and it is difficult for parents to remember the details of how they fed their baby when it wasn't simply one method or the other (which is actually the majority of moms). And although many studies consider all formula milks to be pretty much the same as one another, they really are not. Formula differs quite a lot across countries, and sometimes even within a country (for example, standard cow's milk formula versus soy-based—see Chapter 5), and the composition of formula has changed enormously over time. So, grouping all babies drinking "formula" together in research is messy at best.[2]

The second major challenge—and this is a big one—relates to the study designs. The vast majority of research is observational, not experimental. Observational research is when scientists study large numbers of babies from birth over many years and compare the outcomes of those who were breastfed and formula-fed. The main problem with this type of study is that moms who breastfeed their babies often differ from moms who formula-feed in important ways, such as income, education level, health, IQ, age, social support and so on. This means that differences in the health outcomes of breastfed and formula-fed babies could, in fact, have been caused by any of these other factors and not necessarily by how they were fed. Some researchers have tried to get around the social and economic issues by comparing studies in countries where breastfeeding rates are unrelated to social class—such as Brazil. If breastfeeding is related to later health in these countries, it suggests that it is breastfeeding and not social class that is linked to different outcomes. Another neat approach is to compare the health outcomes of siblings who were fed differently, because siblings are completely matched for all stable family factors (such as Mom's IQ); this means that researchers can study the effects of feeding method on health outcomes without any "interference" from potentially important family-level influences. However, sibling studies aren't perfect either. For a start, a family's circumstances can change quite a lot from one baby to the next (for example, parental education and income). There can also be important reasons why Mom feeds two siblings differently that relate to the health of the child; for example, a baby with underlying health problems may be more likely to be formula-fed than his brother, and differences between siblings' early life health can influence how they both fare later in life, regardless of how they were fed.

In an ideal world, in order to be certain that breastfeeding really *causes* certain health benefits, studies would *randomly* allocate some women to breastfeed their babies and others to formula-feed (called a randomized controlled trial, or RCT) and compare the health outcomes of babies. The process of *randomization* is key; it is the best way to ensure that the two groups are more or less the same in every respect, except for breastfeeding or formula-feeding. If the breastfed babies are better off in the long run, researchers could be pretty sure that breast-feeding *caused* better outcomes because the two groups weren't differ-ent in any other respect. This is all very well except it isn't ethical (or feasible) to randomize babies to *not receive* breast milk, given the many proposed health advantages. However, as recently as the early 1980s, far less was known about the benefits of breastfeeding, and some studies were therefore able to randomly allocate premature babies on neonatal units to receive either banked breast milk or formula through a tube. These babies have now been followed for many years and their health outcomes compared. Findings from these studies are important, because they are the only babies who have been truly randomized to receive breast milk versus formula.

An alternative approach has been to randomly assign women to receive breastfeeding promotion, with the assumption that those receiving more promotion are more likely to breastfeed or to do it for longer and more exclusively. In the mid-1990s the Promotion of Breast-feeding Intervention Trial (PROBIT) was established in Belarus and did exactly this, and as such it is one of the most important studies ever undertaken in the history of breastfeeding research. It randomized sixteen maternity hospitals to promote prolonged and exclusive breast-feeding, through intensive retraining of all medical and nursing staff. The control group included fifteen maternity hospitals that continued with their usual practices (i.e., they did not routinely promote breast-feeding). Via these hospitals, a total of 17,046 moms who gave birth in 1996 to 1997 and who had already started to breastfeed were randomly allocated to the intervention group or the control group, and the children have been followed up into late adolescence.[3] Belarus was chosen for two key reasons: (1) the environment was comparable to other developed nations insofar as women had access to clean water, good medical care, high rates of vaccinations, adult literacy, nutritious food and relatively low infant and child mortality; and (2) hospitals did not routinely promote breastfeeding, so an intervention to support breastfeeding would be more likely to increase breastfeeding rates in Belarus than in countries that strongly promoted it already, such as the US. As expected, the proportion of moms who exclusively breastfed was much higher in the intervention group than in the control group at both three months (43 percent versus 6 percent) and six months (8 percent versus 1 percent). This study has provided invaluable insights into the importance of breastfeeding for both the short- and long-term health and development of infants. However, all babies in the control group were breastfed to start with, and a substantial number of babies in both groups were either predominantly breastfed at three months (28 percent of babies in the control group versus 52 percent in the intervention group) or breastfed to some degree (60 percent of babies in the control group versus 73 percent in the intervention group). So, the findings from this study are by no means conclusive—it can tell us a bit about the benefits of *more versus less* breastfeeding in the population, but the benefits of breastfeeding are probably diluted.

As you can see, in reality, measurement of breastfeeding in most studies is pretty crude, by necessity, and it is tricky to design studies that can really tell us if breastfeeding *causes* better outcomes. This means that we can't always be completely sure about the benefits of breastfeeding versus formula-feeding. At the same time, if researchers haven't found a clear link between breastfeeding and a particular outcome, it doesn't mean there definitely isn't one; it may just have been too difficult to find it because of the challenges of research in this area. This must be borne in mind when weighing up the evidence for the various claims that are made. It is also fair to say that it is difficult to find another area of research that has been so intensely scrutinized, because it is a topic that evokes such emotional debate.

The Advantages for Your Baby

On balance, research suggests that infants benefit from being breastfed. And there are also practical advantages for parents that are not to be understated: It's free and readily available and there's no need to sterilize bottles.

Research has suggested that babies who are partially or exclusively breastfed (usually for a minimum of three to four months in studies) are at an advantage in terms of a number of different health benefits, although we don't know exactly why yet for all of the outcomes. These advantages may be both short-term (during the time the baby is being breastfed) and longer-term (after breastfeeding has stopped). It would be fair to say, though, that the evidence for the shorter-term benefits is much clearer. There may also be advantages for moms, as well, although these are less well supported by the evidence.

SHORTER-TERM BENEFITS

- Fewer respiratory, ear and gastrointestinal infections (and fewer hospital visits)
- Reduced risk of sudden infant death syndrome (SIDS)

Protection from Infection

Biologically it makes sense that breast milk protects against infection —it contains a vast array of immunological and antimicrobial factors that support the development of a robust immune system and fight infection (see pages 95–96). And there is pretty convincing evidence that breastfeeding provides protection against infection during infancy. This is certainly true when it comes to gastrointestinal infections (which cause diarrhea and vomiting). This benefit comes into its own particularly in poorer countries where universal access to clean water is not the norm, making formula preparation and sterilization of bottles challenging, and where infections can quickly become serious and life-threatening because of inadequate medical care. In richer countries, while it is far less likely that infections will cause deaths, they are still common in infancy and are a source of distress, anxiety and time off work for parents if they are severe enough to result in the baby needing medical treatment.

In 2016 the *Lancet* commissioned the most comprehensive review to date of the short- and long-term benefits of breastfeeding, using studies from all over the world.[4] Based almost entirely on observational studies, the review concluded that about half of all diarrhea episodes and a third of respiratory infections in babies might be avoided by breastfeeding. When it comes to preventing hospital admissions from these infections, the protective effect seems to be even more pronounced—it estimated that 72 percent of all infant hospital admissions for diarrhea, and 57 percent for respiratory infections, could be prevented by breastfeeding.[5] Ear infections, in particular, are reduced considerably for breastfed babies and toddlers less than two years old, and the amount of breast milk the baby gets, and for how long, both seem to matter. Babies who are exclusively breastfed for six months are 43 percent less likely to have an infection by two years of age than partially breastfed or formula-fed babies; and those who were "ever" versus "never" breastfed are 33 percent less likely, as were those who were "breastfed at all" for *more than* three or four months.[6]

But even in industrialized countries, where water contamination is not an issue, infections are common in early life; and a review of observational studies conducted in developed countries only suggested that breastfeeding was linked with fewer gastrointestinal infections, hospitalization from respiratory infections, and ear infections.[7] The PROBIT trial in Belarus also found that fewer of the infants in the intervention group (with higher breastfeeding rates) had one or more gastrointestinal infections during the first year compared to those in the control group (9 versus 13 percent), so this is a robust benefit that is almost certainly caused by breast milk and is relevant even for infants with access to clean water. But there wasn't any difference in rates of ear infections (6 percent in both groups had at least one infection) or respiratory tract infections (39 percent in both groups had at least two), which included chest infections (such as croup and pneumonia), ear infections or wheezing. Nor were there any differences in rates of hospitalizations from infections between the intervention and control groups. But bear in mind that the findings from the PROBIT trial can't really tell us if breastfeeding versus not breastfeeding offers protection from infection, because a sizeable proportion of babies in *both groups* were breastfed to some extent. It's also difficult to know how much these findings could be generalized to the US, because moms in Belarus got a lot of maternity leave, and they tended to look after their babies at home—i.e., babies didn't go to day care, which is where they often get sick from coughs, colds and ear infections. As a result, there were far fewer of these common infections in Belarus compared to the US. However, more recently a very large study of more than 70,000 Norwegian babies (including 21,000 sibling pairs) looked at breastfeeding and infection during the first eighteen months.[8] Fewer babies were hospitalized if they were breastfed at all for twelve months or more, versus less than six months (8 percent versus 10 percent), and fewer had frequent infections, gastrointestinal infections or pneumonia. But there were no differences in either hospitalization rates or in rates of any type of infection for *siblings* who were breastfed for different durations. This suggests that the lower rates of infection seen among breastfed babies in high-income countries may partly reflect differences *between* families whose babies are breastfed for longer, as well as the breastfeeding itself.

One important area where human breast milk has indisputably proven benefits over formula is the prevention of necrotizing enterocolitis (NEC)—a serious life-threatening gastrointestinal illness that affects about 9 percent of very premature and low-birth-weight babies (those born at twenty-eight weeks or earlier and weighing 1.5 kg/3.3 pounds or less).[9] A recent high-quality review of all randomized trials to date comparing the outcomes of preterm and low-birth-weight infants given formula or human breast milk from a screened donor found that those given breast milk had half the risk of developing NEC (only 3.7 versus 7 percent).[10] This is a big deal; these babies should be given breast milk—whether the mom can provide her own or it comes from a screened donor.

Protection from Sudden Infant Death Syndrome
A review of observational studies estimated that breastfeeding is linked with a 45 percent lower risk of SIDS for babies who receive any breastfeeding at all (versus none),[11] and a 73 percent lower risk of

SIDS for babies who are breastfed exclusively versus partially. But studies also indicate that there is a critical minimum duration of two months' breastfeeding—any less than this confers no protection against SIDS.[12] This suggests that babies receiving *any* breastfeeding for more than two months seem to be protected against SIDS to some extent, and the longer the duration, and the more exclusive the breastfeeding, the greater the protection. However, it isn't possible to know if it is breastfeeding itself that protects against SIDS, or if there are other factors that cause *both* lower breastfeeding *and* an increased risk of SIDS—such as living in poverty. The trial in Belarus (PROBIT) reported fewer deaths by SIDS in the intervention group versus the control group (one versus five), but because of the tiny numbers of deaths in either group this was not a statistically significant difference, meaning we can't be certain if this finding was due to chance.[13] There are fairly plausible biological reasons for breast milk conferring some protection against SIDS. Breastfed infants wake more easily than do formula-fed infants during the period of highest risk (two to three months), and being easily roused seems to be protective.[14] Breast milk protects against infection, and it is possible that SIDS is caused by an underlying infection that results in breathing or heart problems, fever, shock, low blood sugar and deeper sleep.[15]

Thankfully, SIDS is still extremely rare in high income countries. In 2016, in the US, there were approximately 38 deaths per 100,000 live births.[16] So, if breastfeeding prevents SIDS, a 73 percent reduction would mean that exclusive versus partial breastfeeding for six months could reduce the death rate to 10 per 100,000.

LONGER-TERM BENEFITS

Understanding how breastfeeding relates to longer-term health outcomes is more complicated because of the many challenges already described that make it difficult to link early-life feeding with health outcomes many years later. The following long-term health benefits have been studied:

- reduced risk of allergies
- reduced incidence of childhood leukemia

- reduced risk of type 2 diabetes
- reduced risk of obesity
- reduced risk of cardiovascular disease in adulthood
- higher intelligence.

Allergies

The evidence that breastfeeding prevents most allergies or asthma is weak—although health organizations commonly report this as a benefit. This was a conclusion reached from the large *Lancet* review of observational studies, the PROBIT intervention, and sibling studies.[17] Other than reduced risk of rashes (12 versus 18 percent) in the first year of life and of eczema in the first year of life (3 versus 6 percent) and at sixteen years of age (0.3 versus 0.7 percent), PROBIT found no differences in asthma or allergies during infancy, childhood or adolescence for those in the intervention and control groups.[18]

Childhood Leukemia

A review of observational studies concluded that babies who were breastfed at all, for six months or longer, had a lower risk of childhood leukemia than those who were either not breastfed at all or were breastfed for less than six months (breastfeeding is linked only to acute lymphoblastic leukemia [ALL], not to acute myeloid leukemia).[19] It estimated that 14 to 20 percent of leukemia cases could be prevented by breastfeeding for six months or longer, and 9 percent of cases could be prevented by breastfeeding at all versus never. The findings were similar for high- and low-income countries. The authors suggested that the biological properties of breast milk may be what offer protection. Unlike formula, breast milk contains a number of active components that are thought to support the development of a strong immune system, promote a healthy gut microbiome (the bacteria that live in a gut) and reduce inflammation. A relatively recent theory is that infections can trigger ALL if a child's immune system has not been fully "primed" (exposed to microbes) in the first year, because their immune system is not taught to respond to pathogens correctly. And because breastfeeding promotes the rapid reproduction of healthy bacteria in the gut, this has been proposed as the reason why it may help protect the child from an infection going on to cause ALL.[20]

However, the design of these studies makes it difficult to be certain that breastfeeding itself really prevents leukemia. These studies rely on researchers asking moms of children who have been diagnosed with leukemia to remember how they fed them, often years afterward. Not only does this mean that it is difficult to remember what they did with accuracy, but moms may also be influenced in their responses by their own beliefs about the role that breastfeeding may have played in their child's ill health. A major criticism of this particular review was that it didn't adequately take account of other potential causes of leukemia—such as Mom's age at the child's birth. The other point is that the actual reduction in risk for any individual child is very, very small, because ALL is (thankfully) so rare in the first place. In the US, during the years 2001 to 2014, thirty-four cases per 1 million children were diagnosed with ALL.[21] This research suggests that breastfeeding for a minimum of six months could possibly have reduced the rate to twenty-seven cases per 1 million, and breastfeeding at all versus never may have reduced the rate to thirty-one cases per 1 million. The low incidence of ALL also means that PROBIT will never be able to tell us if breastfeeding protects against the condition, because even that large trial is far too small to find differences in such a rare illness. You would need a trial of several hundreds of thousands of children to be able to see any meaningful differences in the rates of ALL in the intervention and control groups, but that would never be feasible.

Overweight and Obesity

A review estimated that any breastfeeding resulted in a 13 percent reduction in later overweight or obesity, according to the highest-quality studies.[22] So, in the US, where about 18 percent of children and adolescents aged two to nineteen years have obesity,[23] this would mean that for every hundred babies who were breastfed, about sixteen would develop obesity, compared to eighteen babies who were breastfed for a shorter duration (or not at all). However, in high-income countries it is not possible to rule out the possibility that this difference results from the fact that babies who are breastfed for longer tend to come from families with higher incomes and education levels and so on. In fact, in countries like Brazil, where income and education levels are unrelated to breastfeeding rates, there is no difference in rates of childhood overweight and obesity for babies who were breast- or formula-fed.[24] Nor do studies tend to find any difference in the BMI or obesity rates of siblings who were fed differently, suggesting that the link between breastfeeding and obesity in some observational studies is actually due to other factors such as social class.[25] The most robust evidence of causality comes from trials, and these indicate no effect of breastfeeding on obesity risk. The PROBIT trial did not reduce BMI or rates of overweight or obesity at 6.5 years, 11 years or 16 years, either.[26] In fact, there were slightly *more* adolescents with overweight and obesity in the group whose moms were given breastfeeding support. The trials of preterm infants randomized to receive donor human breast milk or formula did not show any difference in childhood weight, either, at 18 months or 7.5 years.[27]

So, the evidence that breastfeeding protects against overweight and obesity is not convincing, and when studies have found a relationship it may just reflect other differences between the moms who do it and don't do it. There are probably other more important risk factors for overweight and obesity, such as a baby's early growth (discussed in detail in Chapter 3), which relates to *how* he is fed as well as *what* he is fed (see Chapter 6), and genetic factors.

Type 2 Diabetes

There aren't many high-quality studies that have looked at the link between breastfeeding and children's later risk of type 2 diabetes. A review of observational studies indicated that breastfeeding *may* reduce the risk of type 2 diabetes by about 24 percent, but the small number of high-quality studies (only three) means that this finding isn't reliable (it was not statistically significant, meaning it could have been due to chance).[28] In fact, one study showed a protective effect, one showed that breastfeeding actually increased the risk of type 2 diabetes, and one showed no effect. The PROBIT trial found no effect of breastfeeding on blood sugar, insulin or adiponectin levels (which are all important indicators of risk of type 2 diabetes) at 11.5 years of age.[29] So, at present, we don't know if breastfeeding offers any protection against type 2 diabetes.

Cardiovascular Disease

A review of observational studies did not find any conclusive protective effect of breastfeeding on markers of cardiovascular disease (high cholesterol and high blood pressure) in childhood, adolescence or adulthood.[30] The PROBIT intervention also found no effect of breastfeeding on later blood pressure in childhood (6.5 years) or adolescence (16 years) or on a marker of "good" (HDL) cholesterol (at 11.5 years of age).[31] However, a UK trial of preterm babies who were randomized to receive breast milk versus formula through a tube found a small reduction in blood pressure in adolescence (at 13 to 16 years) and a better cholesterol profile in terms of the ratio of "bad" (LDL) to "good" (HDL) cholesterol (about 14 percent lower) for babies who received breast milk.[32] This suggests that breast milk may be of some benefit for preterm babies, but findings from preterm infants can't necessarily be generalized to healthy term babies. The protective effect of breastfeeding on blood pressure and cholesterol, if there is any at all, is very small. There are much more important risk factors, such as family history, weight and lifestyle, to consider.

Intelligence

This area has long been of interest to researchers. As long ago as 1929, two researchers reported that breastfed babies had higher intelligence scores from seven to thirteen years of age.[33] There have also been various reports of superior development (for example, earlier walking) for babies who are exclusively breastfed for longer.[34] This is an outcome with evidence for breastfeeding playing a causal role, but the effect is probably pretty modest and may not persist into adulthood. A recent review of observational studies estimated that IQ is about three points higher among breastfed than formula-fed babies, after taking into account Mom's intelligence (an important consideration because IQ is fairly heritable and also related to whether or not moms breastfeed).[35] To add further weight to these findings, studies have also found superior school attainment and IQ in breastfed babies from both the UK (where social class is related to breastfeeding rates)[36] and those from Brazil (where social class in *unrelated* to breastfeeding rates).[37] And some[38] (although not all[39]) sibling studies have found that those who were breastfed have higher cognitive ability than their formula-fed siblings. These cross-country and sibling comparisons point toward breastfeeding per se being responsible for higher IQ, not social class or other background influences that tend to go hand in hand with breastfeeding.

In the PROBIT trial in Belarus, verbal IQ was about 7 points higher in the intervention group at 6.5 years of age (performance IQ was about 3 points higher, and overall IQ about 6 points higher, but these differences weren't statistically significant, meaning they could have been due to chance).[40] Interestingly, there was no difference between babies exclusively breastfed for three or six months, suggesting all of the benefit occurs in the first three months. However, the very big difference in verbal IQ scores was criticized because the pediatricians who assessed IQ knew which children were in the intervention and control groups, so it is possible that they were biased toward giving the children in the intervention group a higher score.[41] The kids' teachers, on the other hand, were totally independent—but there were much smaller differences in teacher-assessed IQ scores between the groups, which were not statistically significant. When the children were followed up in adolescence, there was still a difference in verbal ability (1.4 points)— albeit much smaller than at 6.5 years of age—but no differences in any other ability, suggesting the impact of breastfeeding on IQ diminishes with increasing age.[42] Trials of preterm infants randomized to receive donor human breast milk or formula have also reported on several neurodevelopmental outcomes including cognition, language ability and motor development at one to two years of age, but no differences have been found.[43] So, these benefits don't seem to generalize to babies born very preterm, even in early childhood.

It seems that breastfeeding somehow boosts IQ a little bit, but perhaps only for healthy term infants, and the advantage may or may not persist beyond childhood. Of course, the question of interest is *how* breastfeeding could influence intelligence. There are several plausible explanations. Breast milk itself is compositionally different from formula (see page 121). In particular, it contains certain long-chain polyunsaturated fatty acids—docosahexanoic acid (DHA) and arachidonic acid (AA)—that are important for brain development, and breastfed babies have higher concentrations of these than formula-fed babies. Breast milk also contains lactoferrin, which is a protein that binds to iron and may play a role in preventing iron-induced oxidative damage to the brain. But the behaviors involved in breastfeeding versus bottle-feeding may also be important; the very act of breastfeeding is different from feeding from a bottle, and moms may talk to their baby more or interact with them slightly differently or for longer during breast- versus bottle-feeding (simply because it takes longer to breastfeed than to bottle-feed a baby). However, it's a small effect—probably about three IQ points.

The Advantages for Mom

All of the same challenges inherent in research into the long-term benefits for breastfed babies apply to maternal outcomes for breastfeeding moms. It is not possible to know for certain if breastfeeding itself causes beneficial health outcomes for moms who do it, because women who breastfeed tend to differ in important respects from those who don't. On the whole they are wealthier, more educated, tend to follow all sorts of other health advice and have the social and structural support in place to allow them breastfeed at all or to do it for longer. These social differences confer many advantages, including better lifelong health and happiness; breastfeeding may simply be a behavior of someone who is likely to fare pretty well in life for all sorts of other reasons. Unfortunately it isn't possible to take account of all of these factors in observational studies. As yet, the PROBIT trial has only reported on a few health outcomes of the moms, but as time goes on, this trial will provide important insights into the likelihood that breastfeeding per se plays a causal role in several aspects of women's lifelong health. Notwithstanding these limitations, studies suggest that breastfeeding has a number of possible benefits not only for baby but for Mom as well.

NO PERIODS (AMENORRHEA)

Women who exclusively or predominantly breastfeed prolong the delay of their periods because it inhibits ovulation. This finding is pretty well established, is supported by both observational studies as well as the PROBIT intervention and has sound biological plausibility. As you might expect, the effect is stronger for exclusive and predominant breastfeeding than for partial.[44] However, this doesn't mean that you definitely can't get pregnant even if you exclusively breastfeed—you *can* still ovulate, so you do still need to use contraception to prevent pregnancy while breastfeeding.

REDUCED RISK OF BREAST CANCER

As long as 300 years ago, people noticed that more nuns got breast cancer than anyone else—the disease was in fact described as an "accursed pest." In fact, an analysis in the 1960s found that after eighty years of age, a nun's risk of breast cancer is three times higher than other women's, and this is probably because they don't have children (which itself probably increases the risk of breast cancer) and never breastfed.[45] A 2015 review estimated that if you ever (versus never) breastfed, you have a 7 percent reduced risk of breast cancer based on the highest-quality observational studies (only of women who had ever had a pregnancy, which is important because this by itself reduces your risk of breast cancer) conducted in high-income countries.[46] Breast cancer is the most common cancer in the US, affecting about one in eight women in their lifetime (12.4 percent of women).[47] At a population level, the reduction in cases would be considerable, although it's only a very small reduction in risk for any individual. There were around 242,476 new (female) breast cancer cases in 2015 in the US,[48] so breastfeeding may have prevented about 17,000 of them (7 percent of the total number of cases). And for you, if you ever breastfeed, it means your risk goes from 1 in 8 to about 1 in 8.6.

There are a few possible mechanisms through which breastfeeding might protect against breast cancer. Estrogen is involved in the development of some breast cancers, and because breastfeeding reduces the number of menstrual cycles a woman has (because it inhibits ovulation) women are exposed to less estrogen over their lifetime. The process of making milk may make breast cells more resistant to abnormal changes. Women tend to drink less alcohol and smoke less (and may have a healthier diet, too) while breastfeeding, and these lifestyle choices are also linked with lower breast cancer risk. But a complicating factor with this research is that breast cancer is not one single disease—in fact there are several subtypes that are likely to have different causes. Put very simply, there are some that grow in response to certain hormones and others that don't. One particular subtype that accounts for about 13 percent of all female breast cancers in the US is not responsive to these hormones (called "triple negative");[49] it is more common among younger women and has a worse prognosis. A review of breastfeeding and breast cancer risk by subtype found a protective effect for this particular type of breast cancer (a 22 percent reduction in risk), but not for any of the others.[50] This is an important and evolving area of research, but it still has some way to go before we have any real clarity on whether or not breastfeeding truly protects against breast cancer, which types and why.

REDUCED RISK OF OVARIAN CANCER

There appears to be a much larger reduction in risk of ovarian cancer than of breast cancer from breastfeeding. Based on the highest-quality observational studies (only of women who had ever had a pregnancy), a review estimated that any breastfeeding versus none reduced the risk of ovarian cancer by 18 percent.[51] But in comparison to breast cancer, ovarian cancer is rare; it affects only about one in seventy-eight women in the US in their lifetime (1.3 percent).[52] In 2015, in the US, there were 21,429 new cases, so breastfeeding may have prevented about 4,000 of them.[53] And for you, it means your risk goes down from one in seventy-eight to one in ninety-two. It is unlikely that the PROBIT trial will be able to shed light on whether breastfeeding reduces ovarian cancer risk because it is too rare and the sample is too small. It has been suggested that breastfeeding may help to prevent ovarian cancer because it inhibits ovulation. The theory is that the more ovulations occur, the greater the risk of cell mutation in the ovaries, which can trigger the development of cancer.

REDUCED RISK OF TYPE 2 DIABETES AND LOWER WEIGHT

A review of six large observational studies found that women who breastfed the longest (which varied from study to study) had a 32 percent reduction in their risk of type 2 diabetes, and this was over and above other important risk factors such as BMI, physical activity, education, income and even their family history of diabetes.[54] Given the effect of breastfeeding on type 2 diabetes, one would also expect to see an effect on the mother's body fat, but surprisingly few studies have looked at the long-term effect of breastfeeding on later-life weight. A large study of 740,000 British women found that for every six months of breastfeeding, a woman's weight was 1 percent lower,[55] but the PROBIT intervention found no differences in the weights of the moms in the intervention and control groups eleven and a half years after having the child.[56] So, all in all, it's pretty unlikely that breastfeeding has any meaningful effect on later weight.

Other reviews have concluded that some of the benefits of breastfeeding that you may have heard about—reduced risk of depression,[57] protection from osteoporosis[58] and higher postpartum weight loss (weight loss immediately after pregnancy)[59]—are not well supported by the evidence. In particular, a number of studies have reported that women who breastfeed have lower rates of depression, but this does not necessarily mean that breastfeeding per se helps to protect against depression; rather it may indicate that women who develop depression (or those who have an underlying predisposition toward depression) are less likely to breastfeed or more likely to stop. It may also indicate that breastfeeding difficulties can lead women both to stopping breastfeeding and to developing postpartum depression. But again, this is work in progress.

THE BENEFITS OF BREASTFEEDING IN A NUTSHELL

Taking all of this into consideration, there is strong evidence that breastfeeding offers some protection against infection during infancy, and it probably boosts intelligence a little bit, too; it may also protect against SIDS. However, the longer-term benefits for health are less clear. But it is possible that breastfeeding has advantages for your baby's and your longer-term health, which haven't been detected by existing studies because of the considerable challenges in this area of research. So, taking all of this into account, if you want to breastfeed and there are no reasons why you should not, it is a fantastic option. And research suggests that your baby will benefit, even if you only partially breastfeed him.

How Long Should You Breastfeed For?

The AAP recommends breastfeeding exclusively for six months and continuing to breastfeed up to twelve months after solid food has been introduced. The WHO recommends breastfeeding for up to two years and beyond. But what does the evidence say? When it comes to the short-term benefits of breastfeeding—i.e., protection against infection—it is generally agreed that protection is largely conferred only for the period during which your baby is receiving breast milk, and any amount helps. It is harder to know about the longer-term benefits of breastfeeding for longer; aside from the fact that we can't be sure if breastfeeding truly provides longer-term benefits, studies haven't always compared different durations of feeding. The review of SIDS suggested no protection for babies who were breastfed for less than two months, so this appears to be the minimum duration needed, but a baby doesn't need to be *exclusively* breastfed for two months to get some protection. For childhood leukemia, protection appears to be greater for babies breastfed for six months or longer, but there was also a lower risk for those who were "ever" versus "never" breastfed; this suggests that any amount of breast milk will help. The take-home message from all of this is that any amount of breast milk will benefit your baby, and the longer they receive it, the greater the benefit, especially in terms of immunity. But the amount of time you breastfeed for also depends on your own particular circumstances and how long you would like to do this for.

Mixed Feeding

Mixed feeding is using both breast and formula milk. Formula itself won't cause your baby any harm, but it displaces breast milk, which means your baby will get fewer of the potential health benefits from breast milk, such as protection from infection. There are indications of a *dose-response effect* (more breast milk means more protection) for some outcomes when it comes to protection from breastfeeding—exclusively breastfed babies may have greater protection from SIDS and infections than babies who are partially breastfed. So, it looks like during the first six months, the more breast milk, the better.

However, it's fair to say that the topic of mixed feeding is an under-researched one, even though plenty of people do it—in fact, it's so common in some Hispanic communities that it has its own name: *las dos* (meaning "both").[60] Some moms who used this method told us that they opted for mixed feeding because it meant:

- feeling sure that their baby was getting enough milk (some moms were worried they weren't producing enough milk themselves) or getting enough nutrients
- going back to work and being unable to pump enough for all the milk feedings
- getting a break from breastfeeding from time to time
- being able to spend time away from baby, to do something else.

There are no high-quality studies that rigorously evaluate how combination feeding affects breast milk supply, once your milk has come in. But, although there is little evidence to base advice on, most experts in this field tend to suggest that you get your milk supply up during the first month to six weeks (especially the first two weeks) before you introduce formula, if you can. This is because breast milk production is all about supply and demand—if your baby takes less, you produce less. Regular pumping will help you to keep it up if you have to be away from your baby. However, some lactation consultants have concerns that pumps may not be as efficient as a baby at getting the milk out. Few studies have looked at this, but a small study of thirty Australian moms and babies found that the average volume of breast milk consumed by a baby during a breastfeed (assessed by weighing the baby before and after the feed) was similar to the volume expressed in a five-minute period using an electric pump (72 ml versus 60 ml). However, there were big differences between moms; some expressed far more milk than their baby consumed at a breastfeed, indicating that the pump drained the breast more efficiently than their baby did; but some expressed far less milk than their baby took during a breastfeed.[61] Given the dearth of research on this topic, it is conservative to recommend that you try to feed directly from the breast (rather than feeding pumped milk or formula in a bottle) in the early weeks, while you are building up your milk supply. Of course, that is in an ideal world. If you have to be away from your baby for a period of time, then use your breast pump or supplement with formula without guilt.

It is worth mentioning that some babies who lose a lot of weight during the very early days are given formula supplementation, and health care professionals and moms often worry that this will prevent breastfeeding from being effectively established. In fact, the impact of early *limited* formula supplementation on breastfeeding at three and six months has been tested in several trials, with very reassuring results.[62] In a US trial, fifty babies twenty-four to forty-eight hours old who had lost more than 5 percent of their birth weight were randomized to receive either 2 teaspoons (10 ml) of formula after each breastfeed (until milk had come in) or to continue exclusively breastfeeding (the controls). More of the babies who received small amounts of formula were breastfeeding at three months compared to control babies (79 versus 42 percent), and they were also using less formula than controls at one week of age (10 versus 47 percent). A more recent and larger US trial used the same approach to randomize 164 newborns with substantial weight loss to receive either limited formula supplementation or continue to exclusively breastfeed; this study also found no differences in exclusive breastfeeding rates at one month, nor were there any differences in the gut microbiomes (the type and amount of bacteria living in the gut) of babies in the two groups. A third trial undertaken with 104 babies in the Czech Republic used the same approach and found no differences in the rates of exclusive or any breastfeeding at hospital discharge, three months or six months. Much more research is needed to test the impact of early supplementation on breastfeeding, but these studies should reassure you that if your baby has been given formula in the first few days or weeks, it doesn't necessarily mean that you won't be able to breastfeed him afterward or that there will be any long-term changes to his gut microbiome. But bear in mind that these studies provided only a limited amount of formula, not a complete feeding, and only following each breastfeed.

Why Women Stop Breastfeeding

It's clear that most women want to try to breastfeed, but few manage to keep it up for the full six months, at least not exclusively. The US National Immunization Surveys 2016 and 2017 reported that although 83 percent of women start breastfeeding their baby at birth, by three months only 47 percent are still *exclusively* breastfeeding, and only 25 percent *exclusively* breastfeed at six months.[63] However, more than half of US moms are still breastfeeding to some extent at six months (58 percent), even if this is only one feeding per day. These rates might sound low, but compare these to the UK, where only 17 percent are exclusively breastfed at three months, and only 1 percent at six months.[64]

The most perplexing statistic is that 60 percent of women in the US stop breastfeeding before they initially planned to, prior to having the baby.[65] Why? The Infant Feeding Practices Study II (IFPS II) is a large national survey of more than 2,000 new moms that was conducted between 2005 and 2007 to find out all sorts of things about early feeding, including the reasons why moms stop breastfeeding. It turns out that the biggest barriers were concerns that the baby wasn't getting enough milk, and physical difficulties. The following were the top reasons reported by 30 percent of women or more and were especially important during the first month or two.[66]

Nutritional concerns

- Mom didn't have enough milk.
- Breast milk alone didn't satisfy the baby.
- Mom had trouble getting the milk flow to start.

Physical difficulties

- Baby had trouble sucking or latching on.
- Nipples were sore, cracked or bleeding.
- Breastfeeding was too painful.

These can be really challenging problems, and most moms need more support and guidance, especially during the first few days and weeks, when you and your baby are getting the hang of it. This should initially come from the hospital staff and health care providers, but supportive family members and friends can make a big difference, too. It's important to seek help and advice *early* if you are struggling and would like to breastfeed.

NUTRITIONAL CONCERNS

Not having enough milk is one of the most common reasons reported by women who choose to stop breastfeeding and switch to formula or introduce solid food early (and not just in the US—in many other countries, too, such as the UK). In the IFPS II, insufficient milk was one of the main reported reasons for stopping breastfeeding; it reported that 52 percent of moms stopped within the first or second month and 54 percent stopped between three and five months.[67]

There are two potential (but related) issues with milk supply; both are under-researched, and high-quality data on the true prevalence of milk supply problems is lacking. The first issue that some moms experience is a delay in their milk "coming in" after their baby is born—called "delayed onset of lactogenesis 2." For most moms milk should come in by about thirty to forty hours after birth, but it is considered delayed if it takes more than seventy-two hours. A few studies have estimated that between 17 and 41 percent of moms in affluent countries (mainly the US) experience a delay in their milk coming in, although the studies haven't always included large representative samples of women, so it's difficult to know what the stats really are.[68] The following factors are linked to delayed milk production, probably because they affect the hormones that control it: diabetes; hyperthyroidism; high blood pressure; having a BMI higher than 30; caesarean section; preterm birth;

stressful labor or birth; second stage of labor taking longer than an hour; being stressed or in pain after birth; being a first-time mom; taking hormonal contraception during the first week after birth; delay in baby's first breastfeeding after birth; not feeding the baby frequently enough in the first few days; baby being given other liquid foods (such as sugar water) before Mom's milk comes in.[69] The most important of these are being a first-time mom, having a C-section, and frequency of feeding. If you are affected by any of these risk factors, it doesn't necessarily mean that you will experience a delay in your milk coming in; it just increases the risk of this happening.

The second issue can be low milk supply (not enough to meet the nutritional needs of the baby) or not producing any milk all—called "failed lactogenesis 2" (an awful name!). This is even less studied than delay in milk coming in. We have seen various claims made by reputable organizations that this is rare (such as the Mayo Clinic[70]), but they offer no evidence to support this. In truth, we don't actually know how many women produce insufficient milk—or no milk at all—because high-quality data on breast milk production hasn't been collected in large population-based samples that include all types of women. Collecting and checking the milk volume for hundreds or thousands of women is a pretty challenging task, and breast milk production reflects a complex interaction between Mom's natural ability to produce it, the baby's ability to suck and latch, the technique being right and the frequency of feedings. So, what do we really know about this, if anything? A recent review of breastfeeding challenges reported that existing studies of US women suggest between 10 and 15 percent of women don't produce enough milk.[71] Of these, the only reasonably sized and high-quality study tracked the weight gain from birth of healthy term babies born to 319 healthy first-time moms who were intent on breastfeeding for at least a month, who were supported and who were following the recommended best practice protocol ("rooming in," initiating breastfeeding within one to two hours of birth and feeding at least eight times in the first twenty-four hours, feeding on demand every two to three hours thereafter, and not supplementing with formula or water). All women were visited at four to seven days and again at nine to fourteen days to check breastfeeding, provide support to maximize their milk production and weigh the baby. In this ideal scenario, 15 percent of babies hadn't met their twenty-one-day weight gain target of at least 28.5 g per day.[72] Infant growth is not a great measure of maternal milk supply, because other issues such as latch difficulties or tongue tie can cause feeding problems, but it is the best we have so far.

If not dealt with, the causes of delayed onset of milk can also cause low milk or no milk supply going forward. So, what causes low or no milk supply? There are almost certainly genetic differences between people that influence production,[73] and there are also established medical causes (although again, none of these necessarily mean that you won't be able to breastfeed—they are just risk factors):[74]

- Insufficient glandular tissue (also called breast hypoplasia): This is a rare condition where there is not enough glandular tissue in the part of the breast that produces milk, due to insufficient development during adolescence; breasts tend to look narrow, long and tubular (rather than round), are often asymmetrical (one much larger than the other), widely spaced (more 1.5 inches or 4 cm flat space), and don't grow or change during pregnancy or after birth; they may be large or small—the overall size is largely determined by the amount of fat rather than glandular tissue
- Major breast surgery that involves the nipple area, including some breast implants and breast reductions
- Some medications, including hormonal contraceptives and over-the-counter cold and flu meds that include pseudoephedrine
- Smoking
- Polycystic ovary syndrome (PCOS)
- Parts of the placenta being retained after birth
- Excessive blood loss during birth
- Thyroid or pituitary problems
- Type 2 diabetes.

Aside from a few established medical causes, the most common causes of low milk supply for most moms are low feeding frequency and difficulties getting the latch right (usually moms can produce enough milk if the right techniques are used). The frequency (and duration) of feeding is probably the most important influence on milk supply. If you are keen to breastfeed, it is crucial that you offer a feeding whenever your baby is hungry, especially during the first couple of weeks. The more milk is removed from your breasts in the first week, whether by direct nursing or expression, the more milk your breasts will make, and a lot of stimulation of your breasts during the first few days is the key to making sure you have an ample milk supply further down the line. If possible, try to breastfeed within the first hour or two after giving birth, and feed no less than eight times and preferably twelve times or more per day (twenty-four hours). If you start substituting whole breastfeeds with formula too early, your milk supply will diminish. When milk is removed, your body receives hormonal signals to make more. If you are worried about the amount of milk you are producing, you can get a rough estimate by expressing it. A small study showed that expressed milk was a good indicator of the amount the baby took at the breast, but the study also showed that some babies seemed more adept at getting the milk out than the pump,[75] so you may in fact be producing more than you express. Weighing the baby before and after a feed is also generally accepted as a good measure of how much milk per feed your baby is getting.[76] The most important thing during the early days and weeks is to keep an eye on your baby's weight gain, diapers and feeding.[77] In the first few days after birth he should be producing two to three wet diapers each day. After the first four to five days (after your milk has come in), he should be producing at least six wet diapers and three small poops every twenty-four hours. After four weeks, babies poop a bit less often, but they should still pee regularly (a wet diaper should contain the equivalent of about 2 to 4 tablespoons of water). He should also start to gain weight after the first four to five days of life and should regain his birth weight by the end of the second week. After this he should be gaining weight at a steady rate on the growth chart (see Chapter 3 for details about early growth). If you are worried about your baby's milk intake during breastfeeding, take him to your pediatrician or a lactation consultant to get him weighed before and after a breastfeeding. When you see your pediatrician or a lactation consultant, also ask them to check that your baby's latch is right, and take the opportunity to discuss your breastfeeding management techniques such as responsive feeding, understanding your baby's hunger cues and using both breasts (see Chapter 6 for more about responsive feeding).

"I struggled to breastfeed both my children. They're now five and three, but I still find it difficult thinking back to the early days, which were totally overshadowed by feeding dramas. Nothing in the world can prepare you for it, but when breastfeeding doesn't work it can make you feel dreadful and like you've failed from the start. I still wince when I see one of my friends whip their boob out and effortlessly feed their baby. For me breastfeeding was a fiasco full of double pumps, multiple different types of feeding pillows, endless trips to baby cafés and clinics, and well-meaning breast milk advocates breathing down my neck.

"I ended up pumping for a year with my first baby, right up until I went back to work, so I was never able to really relax and enjoy the time that we had. You're on such a strict schedule when you pump that you can't really stray far from home. When I had my second child I was determined the feeding was going to work, and for a while it did, but my milk disappeared at six weeks and my daughter ended up in the hospital, unable to drink anything at all as she'd never learned how to take a bottle. So then the pumping started again, but it was even harder this time as I had a toddler as well. I only did it for about eight months the second time round, but that was long enough.

"I don't know whether the breastfeeding guilt/shame, or whatever it is, is ever really going to leave me, and when I look back a large part of me wishes that I hadn't spent all that time pumping. However, when you're faced with a newborn baby and flooded with crazy hormones it's easy to feel overwhelmed by all of the pro-feeding propaganda there is out there. I found it very, very hard to step away from the pump and accept formula instead."
—**Katherine, mom of Isabelle (five years) and Beatrice (three years)**

Katherine's story highlights the challenges—emotional and physical —that some moms endure when breastfeeding their baby from their own breast hasn't been possible. If you are worried about your milk supply, get some expert advice on how to measure it and how best to manage this. If you have low milk supply and are keen to breastfeed your baby, it may still be possible for you to do this by supplementing with formula. In high income countries like the US, it is generally considered safe to feed your baby formula exclusively. It is incredibly important that your baby receives adequate nutrition to grow and develop well during this crucial period of his life. It is also important that you feel happy and confident, can enjoy caring for your baby, and feel that your attachment is strong and growing.

PHYSICAL DIFFICULTIES

Women are routinely told that breastfeeding shouldn't be painful—at least not after the first few days. But we have struggled to find many women who didn't experience at least some pain during the first few weeks, and most lactation consultants agree that a bit of pain (and certainly sensitivity) is normal during the very early days. A common cause of pain during breastfeeding is that the baby isn't latching on correctly. A state-of-the-art ultrasound study in 2014 revealed that babies "get the milk out" by suction, rather than squeezing and kneading the nipple with their mouth (breastfeeding is not the same as milking a cow!).[78] So, if your nipple is distorted when your baby comes off, then he isn't latching on correctly.

A common cause of cracked, painful nipples is a shallow latch; if your nipple isn't far enough back in your baby's mouth, his tongue will rub or press on your nipple, which can cause the problem. If your baby is latched well, the nipple should go right to the back of his mouth where his tongue action won't hurt it. It is worth seeking help if you have very painful nipples during the early days. Ask your midwife, a lactation consultant or someone at a local breastfeeding support group to help you and your baby get into a position where he is able to draw in a large enough mouthful of your breast to get going. It is worth trying out a few different positions to see if you can find one that causes you less discomfort; it might be that tweaking your position just a tiny bit is all that is needed to make it less painful. If your nipples have become cracked and very painful, you can apply some highly purified lanolin until they have healed again. This will keep them moist, feel soothing and help prevent scabs from forming. There is no need to remove this before you breastfeed again, and you can apply it as often as you need to. Some women also find that applying some expressed breast milk onto their nipples after a feeding helps relieve soreness.

Many professionals in this field don't usually recommend a nipple shield for "protecting" a damaged nipple, although some moms use them this way. Nipple shields tend to be more useful when a baby cannot latch onto the breast—for example, if a mom has a flat or inverted nipple. But nipple shields can sometimes lead to other complications—the shield can open cracks (ouch!), it can be harder for your baby to get the milk out and it can be difficult to move your baby back to your bare breast once he's become used to the shield. But if you have tried everything else and not found a solution, a nipple shield is certainly worth a try.

If a part of your breast is excruciatingly painful, red and inflamed, and you feel very unwell with a fever and/or flu-like symptoms, you could have mastitis. Mastitis develops when part of the breast doesn't drain properly and bacteria begin to grow and cause an infection. The AAP advises using warm compresses, frequent breastfeeding or expressing, which helps to drain the breast and stop the infection from spreading (your baby will not be harmed), lots of fluids, pain meds and taking time to rest (as much as you can with a young baby!). If it doesn't get better quickly, do go see your physician, as you may need antibiotics. The antibiotics prescribed for mastitis don't generally cause any problems for your baby so you can continue to breastfeed as normal, unless your physician tells you not to.

"With Grace I was able to breastfeed her with no obvious problems. With Thomas he was diagnosed with tongue tie, as I was having a lot of problems with him latching on and him appearing hungry after he had fed for a long time.

"However, this diagnosis didn't happen until he was three days old, by which time I was extremely sore and felt unable to breastfeed him. I felt that health care professionals up until this point had not listened or taken my requests for help and support seriously. I was so sore from feeding Thomas when he was three days old that, as soon as the supermarket opened, I went and bought formula.

"This had never been my intention as the way to feed him, but I felt that was the only option at the time. I felt so upset at buying the formula and as though I was a failure. I remember crying as I walked out of the supermarket with it.

"I didn't want to formula-feed Thomas. Because of this I decided to keep trying with the breastfeeding and I struggled on for around two weeks, despite being in absolute agony and Thomas clearly not getting enough milk. I cried every day and found that I was mentally deliberating breastfeeding versus formula-feeding and what was 'right' and 'wrong.' I would make my mind up that breastfeeding just wasn't working and that if Thomas had formula he would still grow up to be a happy, healthy baby. But then I would see someone else (other than me and his dad) giving him a bottle and my heart hurt because I am his mom and I felt that I was the only one that should be feeding him and that I was failing him as a mother. I felt that I was letting him down in a huge way and that because I couldn't and he couldn't breastfeed he was not going to bond with me.

"I spent a huge amount of those first few weeks completely beating myself up about the situation and feeling so low with the guilt of failure when it should have been a time of complete happiness with Thomas. All the leaflets on breastfeeding that I had from the hospital/midwife shouted out about how good breast milk is for the baby and how much better off the baby is. I remember thinking, 'Thomas will end up in hospital unwell if I don't breastfeed him.' Thinking back, that's terrible and no mother should be made to feel that way, especially when ultimately the decision is taken out of their hands for the sake of their baby's health and well-being."—**Amy, mom of Grace (eighteen months) and Thomas (four months)**

The decision to stop breastfeeding can be devastating, as Amy's story demonstrates. If you are struggling with breastfeeding, please don't struggle alone. There is support available, so do seek it out. Our advice to you would be to do this sooner rather than later if you want to breastfeed; many moms find that if they get enough support in the early days and weeks, they are able to get the hang of it in the end. However, some moms still can't manage to breastfeed, after valiant efforts for many weeks and months. If you have made the decision to stop, it is not the end of the world. *How* you feed, as well as *what* you feed, is important. Parenting is not defined solely by the method you used to feed your baby.

Breastfeeding Myths

Most women (although not all) are physically able to breastfeed to some degree, even if not exclusively—and even if formula supplementation is needed in the early days before your milk comes in. All you need is one functioning breast—some women successfully exclusively breastfeed twins, with one on each breast. Your ability to breastfeed has nothing to do with any of the following: the size of your breasts before pregnancy, your age, your ethnicity or your relatives' ability to breastfeed. Most women (again, not all) are still able to breastfeed if they have had breast implants, have a nipple piercing, have flat or inverted nipples, or are diabetic. There are a lot of commonly held myths about breastfeeding that are not supported by evidence. The following four myths have sometimes been powerful enough to put women off breastfeeding altogether.

BREASTFEEDING WILL CHANGE MY BREASTS AND MAKE THEM SAGGY

Until 2007 it was commonly believed—even by medical professionals—that breastfeeding causes breasts to sag (called ptosis).[79] It wasn't until Dr. Brian Rinker, a plastic surgeon at the University of Kentucky, carried out the first research into this question that this myth was debunked. Anecdotally many of the women who were seeking corrective breast surgery at his clinic attributed their ptosis to breastfeeding, so he decided to find out if this was really true. He interviewed 132 women who were seeking surgery to augment or lift their breasts and gathered detailed information about their medical history, as well as the number of pregnancies, breast size before pregnancy, BMI and whether or not they smoked. He found that the number of pregnancies was an important factor, but not breastfeeding itself.[80] During pregnancy, estrogen and progesterone stimulate the milk-secreting glands to develop, and these become engorged with milk and stretch the skin around the breast; they also stretch the ligaments that support your breast. It is these pregnancy processes that lead to breasts sagging, not breastfeeding.

BREASTFED BABIES DON'T SLEEP AS WELL AS FORMULA-FED BABIES

Disrupted sleep and ongoing sleep deprivation are some of the toughest challenges faced by parents with a new baby. There is strong popular opinion that formula-fed babies sleep for longer, and as such women are often advised by well-meaning friends or family either to "top up" with a formula feeding to aid sleep through the night or move to formula altogether. In fact, the jury is out when it comes to the evidence for this, which is very unclear and not of great quality—and, surprisingly, there is no review of this topic. Sleep is also a complex behavior, and research focuses on different aspects such as total duration, quality and number of nighttime wakings. It is true that several studies have found that breastfed babies sleep less during the night, wake more often and wake for longer than formula-fed babies, but researchers have also found no differences between breast- and formula-fed babies. To add to the confusion, over the last decade some studies have reported that breastfeeding babies *and* their moms sleep for longer, that moms manage to get back to sleep more quickly after waking up in the night, and that there are hormonal mechanisms involved in breastfeeding that may, in theory, aid better sleep quality.

But there may also be differences in parenting styles between those who formula feed and those who breastfeed, which account for some of the differences in infant sleep. One of the largest and most detailed studies undertaken in this area examined the sleep patterns of 10,321 babies from across the Asia-Pacific region.[81] Breastfed babies woke up more frequently during the night and for longer than formula-fed babies and had less consolidated sleep, but—and this is a big but—only the ones who were routinely fed to sleep. This large study indicated that feeding your baby to sleep at night is not a good idea if you want him to sleep through, and this is far more common among breastfeeding moms than those who feed formula. A subsequent high-quality randomized controlled trial of 279 parents backed this up (see page 158 for more detail on this study).[82] Parents randomized to the intervention group when their baby was two weeks old were given guidance for establishing good sleep practices, in line with recommendations, including a consistent and short bedtime routine (thirty to forty-five minutes) with early bedtime (7 to 8 PM); avoiding feeding or rocking baby to sleep and instead putting baby down awake but drowsy and allowing him some time to self-soothe; and not routinely waking baby in the night to feed. At two, four and ten months of age these babies slept for about half an hour longer at night than control babies. And, notably, at ten months the babies who had a bedtime of 8 PM or earlier and self-soothed to sleep slept for a whopping one hour and twenty minutes longer than those who went to bed later and didn't self-soothe; importantly, the study included both breastfed and formula-fed babies. So, there are definitely ways to help your baby to sleep better at night that have nothing to do with breastfeeding or formula-feeding.

Sleep research also relies on moms reporting how long their babies slept for, which is difficult if babies are waking several times a night for varying lengths of time, and if moms are exhausted. A rather intriguing recent study compared the nighttime sleep duration of breastfed and formula-fed babies using moms' reports as well as a piece of equipment called an actigraph, which can measure a baby's sleep duration with greater precision.[83] According to the actigraph, there were no differences in the sleep duration of breastfed or formula-fed babies from four to eighteen weeks of age, but the moms of formula-fed babies overestimated their babies' sleep duration from ten weeks of age onward—perhaps because of the commonly held belief that formula-fed babies sleep for longer. Perhaps the biggest myth that needs to be challenged is that babies *should* be sleeping through the night by the time they are six to twelve months old. A British study of 715 babies this age found that 78 percent will wake at least once in the night and 61 percent will have at least one milk feeding,[84] and there was no difference in the number of night wakings or night feedings between moms who were breastfeeding or formula-feeding. What they did find was that babies who were consuming more calories during the day (whether in the form of breast milk, formula or solid food) were less likely to feed at night, but they were no less likely to wake up. So, it seems that regardless of feeding method it is, unfortunately, pretty normal for babies to wake in the night during the first year.

BREASTFEEDING IS EASY

Just because it's natural doesn't mean breastfeeding is easy. Like any new skill, it needs to be learned—by mom and baby—and almost everyone needs help when they are starting out. It is absolutely crucial to ensure you get the positioning right in the early days, so it's a good idea to make sure you seek help and guidance during the first few days or weeks—and there is usually plenty of help around locally. Community drop-ins are available in most areas, where there will be volunteer moms and/or lactation consultants. Private lactation consultants can also come out and see you at home. However, they are not required to be medically trained so cannot assess the health condition of your baby—medical decisions should be made by your physician. The National Office on Women's Health and Breastfeeding Helpline can also provide advice over the phone. So, do seek help if you are struggling; this is especially important during the early weeks when we know moms find it hardest. If you haven't had your baby yet, it is worth knowing where to get support from before he arrives. This could even be friends who are currently breastfeeding or have breastfed before. In fact, get friends and family to help with other things as much as you can, too—doing the dishes, going to the grocery store, cooking meals, doing the laundry, changing diapers, bathing the baby, to name a few! Having someone take care of these tasks can make feeding issues much more manageable because it will allow you to focus on yourself and your baby.

YOU CAN'T BREASTFEED IN SOME PUBLIC PLACES

Anywhere in the US, a woman is permitted to breastfeed her baby in any public or private location in which she and her baby are legally allowed to be.[85] Thirty states, DC, Puerto Rico and the Virgin Islands also have laws exempting breastfeeding from public indecency laws. This doesn't mean that you're going to be arrested for public indecency in the other twenty states;[86] no woman has ever been prosecuted in any state for indecent exposure for breastfeeding in public. You can feed your baby in a restaurant, on an airplane, in the grocery store, in a park, or wherever you happen to be when your baby is hungry; you are not legally required to cover up or go hide in the restroom. In fact, it is unlawful for any member of staff to ask you not to breastfeed on their premises or to refuse to serve you because you are breastfeeding your baby. Although you might feel embarrassed or worried about breast-feeding in public, it is your legal right to do so. Some moms do feel self-conscious, though; feeding scarves are a really good way to feed discreetly in public if you're nervous about it—you can also use a pash-mina or shawl if you have one.

Breast Milk Composition

Breast milk is a dynamic substance, as it adjusts to a baby's changing developmental needs and contains many living cells. It changes over the course of a feeding, from one feeding to the next, in response to environmental changes and with the age of the infant. Important nutritional changes occur over the first few days of milk production. The very first milk to be produced is called colostrum; it is thought that its main purposes are to protect the vulnerable newborn baby from infection and boost development. It is yellow in color and produced in very small amounts but is compositionally rich, providing a large injection of antibodies. Nutritionally, it contains about 54 calories per 100 ml and is relatively high in protein compared to later breast milk. "Transitional milk" is then produced between Days 6 and 14 after birth, which differs from colostrum to support the changing needs of a rapidly growing baby. It contains around 58 calories per 100 ml and has lower protein content than colostrum.

Mature breast milk is established by about two weeks after birth and becomes the milk that supports the baby throughout the following few months. Mature breast milk contains around 65 calories per 100 ml. In general it contains about 3.8 g fat per 100 ml (the fat provides about 50 percent of the baby's calories), but the fat content changes substantially over the course of a single feeding.[87] The initial milk is more watery and contains less fat, but as the feeding progresses the milk becomes richer, containing about double the amount of fat. But change in the amount of fat also varies in relation to the number and size of feedings that babies take. For example, the fat content changes from about 4.3 percent to 10.7 percent for babies taking six to nine large feedings per day; but the initial milk tends to be richer for babies taking more frequent smaller feeds (fourteen to eighteen feedings per day), changing from about 4.8 percent to 8.2 percent fat. This probably ensures that whatever the feeding pattern, breastfeeding babies get roughly the same amount of fat.[88]

But breast milk is not just fuel. It's a complex bioactive fluid that plays a number of roles in supporting the health and development of your baby. Aside from providing optimal nutrition, it contains hundreds of bioactive molecules that contribute to immunity and development. These are not present in formula because they can't be manufactured in a laboratory and/or they don't survive the production process. Although the exact composition of breast milk is still unknown, we do know a fair bit about many of its properties, which include cells and agents that protect the baby against infection and support immune development (for example, immunoglobulins, macrophages, antiviral and antibacterial agents, living white blood cells); lactoferrin, which also has antibacterial properties and helps babies absorb nutrients; fatty acids, which promote development (including the brain); and growth factors. It also contains agents that may play a role in regulating wakefulness and sleepiness (nucleotides), the levels of which change at different times of the day and that may help to establish a baby's body clock.

Vitamin D and Iron

The National Academy of Medicine (NAM) estimates that babies need about 400 IU (15 mcg) of vitamin D per day during the first year of their life for healthy development.[89] Because breast milk typically contains only 25 to 78 IU of vitamin D per quart/liter, babies who are largely receiving breast milk need to take a supplement to ensure they receive sufficient levels.[90] The AAP therefore recommends that exclusively and partially breastfed babies are given are a daily vitamin D supplement of 400 IU per day unless they consume at least 32 ounces (1 L) of vitamin D–fortified formula or whole milk per day (whole cow's milk should not be introduced as the main drink until your baby's first birthday—see page 209). Babies who are exclusively breastfed for several months without vitamin D supplementation are at increased risk of rickets, particularly dark-skinned babies whose moms are deficient in vitamin D (most vitamin D comes from sun exposure, and dark-skinned individuals need more sun exposure to make sufficient amounts).[91] See pages 46 and 224–25 for more information about vitamin D.

Full-term babies (those born at thirty-seven weeks or later) who are born healthy have sufficient iron stores to keep them going for the first four months of life after birth. But at four months of age their iron stores start to deplete, so they need to start sourcing it from their diet. Breast milk is low in iron, so the AAP recommends that babies who are exclusively breastfed or partially breastfed (given breast milk for more than half of their feedings) be given a liquid iron supplement from four months of age to guard against iron deficiency.[92] The recommended dose depends on your baby's weight, and supplementation needs to continue until your baby is eating enough iron-rich food. Making sure the dose is right can be a bit tricky (it depends on your baby's weight), so the AAP suggests you consult your baby's pediatrician. Premature babies often have lower iron stores because iron is largely acquired during the third trimester of pregnancy, which means they often need additional iron beyond that which they get from breast milk or formula. If your baby was premature your pediatrician will be able to advise you on how to supplement your baby's iron.

APPETITE REGULATION

The appetite-control centers in the brain start to develop in utero but continue to develop in the first few weeks and months after birth. The composition of breast milk may also play a role in supporting the development of optimal appetite regulation, by influencing the appetite-regulatory systems in the brain. This is less widely known, but evidence is growing. Breast milk contains many of the hormones that determine hunger and fullness in adults and children.[93] These hormones are not present in formula (or are present in very small amounts) due to the different composition of cows' milk and the processing of formulas to ensure that they are safe and have a long shelf life. For example, breast milk contains leptin (the "satiety hormone"), which regulates feelings of hunger and fullness.[94] In children and adults leptin is a fundamental regulator of appetite and enhances satiety. Breast milk is the main source of leptin in babies in the first six months of life and may help to regulate hunger and satiety during the early weeks and months. We know that babies consuming breast milk that contains higher levels of leptin grow less rapidly during the first few years, which we know is better for their later health (as discussed in Chapter 3).[95]

Other appetite hormones are also present in breast milk, including ghrelin (the "hunger hormone"), which stimulates hunger. These hormones are thought to play a role in the development of the appetite-control centers in a baby's developing brain, as well as the cells that line the gut. They are also thought to speed up gastric emptying (how quickly milk leaves the stomach), which happens more quickly with breast milk compared to formula (hence the more frequent number of poops that you'll see from a breastfed baby compared to a formula-fed one). There may also be behavioral differences between breastfeeding and bottle-feeding that play a role in the development of appetite regulation—these are discussed in detail on pages 156–57.

FOOD PREFERENCES

Breast milk, like amniotic fluid, reflects to some extent the flavors of the mom's diet. Your newborn baby's flavor senses are well developed, which means that breastfed babies are repeatedly exposed to a variety of ever-changing flavors for as long as they receive breast milk. This may influence their food acceptance later on, and it may well be one of the first ways that babies learn which foods are safe to eat. One of the first studies conducted in this area randomized women to drink a glass of carrot juice four times a week during the first two months of breastfeeding or to avoid carrots altogether (and a third group drank carrot juice during only the last trimester of pregnancy).[96] The babies whose moms had had carrots were more receptive to carrot-flavored cereal later on than those whose moms had avoided them altogether. Babies whose moms eat plenty of fruit during breastfeeding are also more likely to enjoy fruit during complementary feeding. Other studies have shown that flavors such as aniseed, garlic, ethanol, mint, vanilla and even blue cheese (!) appear in breast milk one to two hours after a mother has consumed them, and they take six to eight hours to disappear.[97]

Breastfeeding may therefore provide another window of opportunity for "programming" your baby's taste preferences in the long term and might be particularly advantageous when it comes to increasing your baby's acceptance of bitter-tasting vegetables later on. Some research has shown that children who were breastfed versus formula-fed (or breastfed for longer) eat more fruit and vegetables and are more willing to try new foods during childhood and will be less picky.[98] However, all of the research conducted so far has been based on observational or small studies rather than large randomized controlled trials. This means that we can't be completely sure if Mom's diet during breastfeeding really *causes* the baby's food preferences, or if moms who breastfeed also go on to feed their children more fruit and vegetables later (and are more likely to eat them in front of their child), and it is this that accounts for their child's willingness to eat them rather than the flavor of the breast milk.

The early flavor experience of a formula-fed baby is pretty monotonous in comparison to a breastfed baby's. There are, however, differences in the flavors of different formulas, and babies tend to learn to prefer the formula they are fed, and subsequently the foods that contain these flavors.[99] It also means that if your baby doesn't seem to like a particular brand of formula milk, they may prefer another.

Vegetarians and Vegans

Vegetarians and vegans who are breastfeeding have a fantastic opportunity to introduce their baby to all of the wonderful flavors of their own diet if it is rich in vegetables and fruit and varied. But if you don't consume any animal products, the American Dietetic Association recommends that you take an extra vitamin B12 supplement while you are breastfeeding, because vitamin B12 is only found in animal products (primarily meat, fish, milk and milk products and eggs),[100] and exclusively breastfed infants whose moms consume no animal products can have very low levels of vitamin B12 and may become deficient shortly after birth.[101] Vitamin B12 deficiency in an infant can result in permanent and severe brain damage.[102] The recommended daily allowance for vitamin B12 is 2.8 mcg for a breastfeeding mom and 0.4 mcg for a baby up to six months old.[103] Vitamin B12 deficiency can be diagnosed through a blood test.

There are also a couple of other dietary considerations that you will need to plan for, but you won't require a supplement if you can get enough of the necessary micronutrients from food sources. Breastfeeding requires a bit more zinc (12 mcg per day),[104] which you can get from nuts, legumes, and seeds (sesame, pumpkin and sunflower). You will also need about 80 percent more calcium than a non-breastfeeding adult (1,000 to 1,300 mg per day),[105] so eating calcium-rich and calcium-fortified foods is also important, such as calcium-set tofu, Chinese cabbage, figs, kale and broccoli. You will need a bit more iodine, too (290 mcg per day);[106] vegetarians can get this from milk, dairy products and eggs, but it is a bit trickier to source iodine from a vegan diet. Sea vegetables such as seaweed are often rich in iodine, but amounts vary and some products can be too high in iodine (particularly brown seaweed such as kelp); it can sometimes contain other contaminants as well.[107] Taking an iodine supplement is one way to ensure that you get sufficient levels during breastfeeding, but some organizations advise against using a seaweed or kelp supplement because the amount can vary enormously from that on the label and you can end up having far too much.[108] We recommend that you seek advice from your medical doctor or a registered dietician if you are thinking about taking an iodine supplement.

If you are a vegan mom who is breastfeeding, the British charity First Steps Nutrition provides information and recipe ideas to help ensure you get all of the nutrients you need in their booklet *Eating Well for New Mums*. It is free to download from firststepsnutrition.org.

THE BOTTOM LINE

- How you feed your baby is *your decision* and yours alone.

- There is pretty convincing evidence that breastfeeding your baby will help to protect him from infections during the period he is receiving breast milk. It may also reduce his risk of SIDS and boost his intelligence a bit, too. The longer-term benefits are less clear.

- Breastfeeding can be hard, especially in the first few days and weeks. The moms who persevere are the ones who get the help and support they need from health professionals, lactation consultants, friends and family *early*. There is help available, so if things aren't going well and you're struggling to get the hang of it, please ask for help if you want to continue. Be pushy if you have to be!

- Some women are unable to breastfeed no matter how hard they have tried. Like most biological processes, breastfeeding doesn't always work perfectly for everyone. This can feel devastating, and many moms end up feeling guilty, but it is not the end of the world; your child's physical and mental health will not be solely determined by whether or not he is breastfed. There are plenty of opportunities to be a fantastic parent.

CHAPTER 5

Formula-Feeding

Sometimes it isn't possible to breastfeed your baby—some moms are not able to or decide not to, some parents have adopted their baby and some dads or grandparents are responsible for feeding their baby. Some moms have also told us that although they started off breast-feeding, after returning to work it was too difficult to pump enough breast milk to keep up with their baby's appetite. And some felt uncomfortable doing this at work or simply didn't have the time. There are many reasons why parents decide to use formula, and any reason is valid. In these instances, formula offers a vital source of nutrition for your baby.

The decision to formula-feed is purely personal and depends on what is right for you and your family circumstances. Some moms feel guilty about doing this, but it is your decision to make and yours alone, and all moms want the best for their baby. Life with a young baby can be very stressful, and coping with the many competing demands can feel overwhelming. Sometimes the only way to keep your sanity is to take practical decisions to make your life a little bit easier, and, for some, this means using formula. Your own mental health and well-being are hugely important—especially when caring for a young baby—and any feeding decisions that you make should take your own health into account, as well as that of your baby. A well-nourished baby and a happy mom are great goals, however you get there. You have no need to feel guilty, apologize to anyone or justify your decision. And you should feel confident that formula is a safe way to feed your baby.

It is our view that parents need evidence-based information about formula-feeding so that they can make well-informed choices about what formula to use. In this chapter we provide you with sound scientifically based information about infant formula.

Reasons Why Some Parents Choose to Formula-Feed

Some of the parents we spoke to told us about the practical advantages of bottle-feeding or using formula. Here are some of the things they reported (some of these also apply to feeding expressed breast milk through a bottle):

- Other people can feed your baby, which gives you a break.
- It gives other people the opportunity to form a close bond with your baby while feeding.
- You can be certain about how much your baby is drinking.
- Formula has some vitamins and other nutrients that breastfed babies have to get from supplements (vitamin D).
- It avoids any embarrassment that women may feel when breastfeeding in public.

The CDC's National Immunization Surveys 2016 and 2017 reported that of the babies born in 2015, 17 percent had received formula in the first two days of life, 29 percent before three months and 35 percent before six months.[1]

Formula-Feeding Myths

Just as there are myths about breastfeeding (see page 117), there are also a few about formula-feeding.

IT ISN'T POSSIBLE TO BOND WITH YOUR BABY IF YOU BOTTLE-FEED HIM

This is simply not true! There are plenty of ways to bond with your baby, and you can still bond with him if you are bottle-feeding. An important part of feeding your baby is *how* you feed him, not just *what* you feed him. The key is to feed him responsively. You can do this whether you breast- or bottle-feed. We describe exactly how to do this in Chapter 6.

"You can still give your baby some of the benefits of breastfeeding/ nursing if you are using formula. Doing skin-to-skin contact with your baby, especially in the first few weeks of life, has many benefits! Strip your baby down to his diaper and hold/carry him right up against your bare chest. Then cover the both of you with a blanket (making sure you don't cover his head or face). Your body heat will keep your baby warm and save him the work of keeping up his body temperature. Your heartbeat will provide a soothing beat. Skin-to-skin time also increases bonding."

—Dr. Bridget Young, research assistant professor, Department of Pediatrics, Allergy and Immunology, University of Rochester School of Medicine and Dentistry

FORMULA-FEEDING IS EASIER THAN BREASTFEEDING

You may be in for a surprise if you think that formula-feeding is easier than breastfeeding. It has its challenges, as well. The biggest one is the number of steps that you will need to go through in order to prepare a bottle safely. Cleaning all the nipples and bottles is a hassle. If you are not using ready-to-feed formula (like most moms), it takes a while to make a bottle from powder or liquid concentrate. It can be a challenge when your baby is hungry and you need to get him a bottle quickly. We have provided step-by-step instructions on how to do this on page 149.

YOUR BABY WILL SLEEP FOR LONGER AT NIGHT IF YOU GIVE HIM FORMULA

You may be disappointed if you were counting on a full night's sleep by giving your baby formula at night or switching over completely. Research suggests that babies often wake up in the night regardless of whether they are fed formula or breast milk.[2] Your baby may not even want a feeding and may wake up anyway (we provide information about how to check if your baby is really hungry on page 167). The sleep patterns of breastfed and formula-fed babies are discussed in more detail on pages 118–19.

FORMULA IS VIRTUALLY THE SAME AS BREAST MILK

Although formula milk is a perfectly safe alternative source of nutrition for your baby, it is not compositionally the same because it isn't possible to manufacture something that includes all of the properties of breast milk. Human breast milk is thought to contain over 300 components (that we know of so far; there could also be additional unknown ones), compared to about 75 in typical formula. The composition of formula is described in detail below.

Formula Milk Composition

In the US the manufacturing of formulas for infants less than twelve months of age is regulated by the Food and Drug Administration (FDA) under the Infant Formula Act of 1980 (revised in 1986). Manufacturers must be able to prove that the formula they produce supports "normal physical growth" (anything other than weight faltering—see page 78) and that it adheres to nutritional guidelines stipulating the minimum levels of twenty-nine different nutrients (and maximum levels for ten) that must, by law, be in all formula marketed to infants in the first year of life. New formulas don't need to be approved *before* they go on the market, but manufacturers are required to test the nutrient content of the product before it goes out and at the end of its shelf life and test for harmful bacteria (*Salmonella* and *Cronobacter*). The FDA carries out yearly inspections of all facilities that manufacture infant formula and collects and analyzes samples of each product to ensure it is safe. If any product is deemed risky, it is recalled.[3] The FDA's requirement for adding new ingredients to formula is that they are "generally recognized as safe."[4] According to the FDA, this means that the scientific data about the ingredient is widely known, and there is a consensus among "qualified experts" that the ingredient is "safe" for that intended use.[5] However, the FDA doesn't define who the qualified experts need to be or what "safe" means.

THE ESSENTIAL COMPONENTS

Given the dynamic and complex composition of human breast milk (it contains tons of live cells and differs from mom to mom), it isn't possible to manufacture an identical substance, but formula is intended to act as an effective substitute for human milk. As such, every effort has been made to mimic the nutritional profile of human breast milk. Most infant formulas are based on cow's milk, but cow's milk contains higher levels of protein and certain minerals compared to breast milk, so it needs a fair amount of processing to ensure it's suitable for human babies. Then, the nutrients that are lacking, such as vitamins, minerals and certain fats, are added to formula to better approximate the composition to human breast milk and increase its health benefits.

There are big differences in the types of proteins in human milk versus cow's milk. Milk protein comes in two categories: casein and whey. The proportion of these two categories is different: Cow's milk has a much higher casein content; human breast milk has more whey. For this reason, some formula companies (but not all) add additional whey into the formula to make the ratio of whey-to-casein more comparable to breast milk.

Like breast milk, standard formulas contain about the same number of calories (19 to 20 calories per ounce/30 ml), although the calorie content isn't regulated in the US (it is in the European Union). Standard formulas tend also to be largely similar to breast milk in the proportions of fat, protein and carbohydrate, although some are considerably higher in protein.[6] In standard formulas the fats come from vegetable oils, the protein from cow's milk, and the carbohydrate is usually lactose (the sugar found naturally in breast milk). However, in the US there are no regulations for the amount or type of carbohydrate that can be used in formulas, which means that table sugar (sucrose) can be the main ingredient in some products, and corn syrup can be added (although a recent review of twenty common brands found no high-fructose corn syrup[7]). In the EU, neither sucrose nor glucose is permitted in any formula milk based on cow's milk (lactose must be used), and no formula milks can contain fructose. This reflects a concern about the possible risk of childhood obesity and the desired goal to make formula that resembles breast milk as closely as possible, for which the sugar is lactose. Something to be cautious about is the amount of sugar in the formula that you buy, and the relative sweetness of different sugars; lactose tastes much less sweet than sucrose. An investigation by *The New York Times* found that a popular brand of organic formula milk using sucrose rather than lactose was judged as sweet as grape juice or lemonade by a panel of tasters.[8] Early infancy is thought to be a crucial period for the development of taste preferences (see page 124–25), so we would recommend that you choose a formula with a lower sugar content and with lactose as the main sugar, to avoid encouraging your baby to develop a sweet tooth. Lactose is also less damaging to babies' teeth than other types of sugar.

The minimum protein content allowed in the US is 1.8 g per 100 calories (approximately 5 ounces/150 ml), and the maximum is 4.5 g per 100 calories, which is higher than the upper limit allowed in the EU (3.0 g per 100 calories—soon to be reduced to 2.5 g per 100 calories by 2020). There is growing evidence that higher protein content in infant formulas increases a baby's risk of rapid weight gain and obesity in childhood,[9] and as a result most European formulas now have protein levels at the lower end of the stipulated range. So, we would recommend that you opt for a formula milk below 3.0 g per 100 kcal.

The fat content of formula can range from 3.3 to 6 g per 100 kcal in the US. Most formulas are based on skim milk, and the fat comes from vegetable oils, which include sunflower, coconut, palm, safflower and/or soybean. Because babies can't make certain essential fats themselves—such as linoleic acid (LA)—this has to be added to formula.

All US formulas must contain iron, but the possible range is large compared to that permitted under EU law. In the US the minimum allowed is 0.15 mg per 100 kcal (half that stipulated under EU law), and the maximum is 3.0 mg per 100 kcal (more than double the amount allowed in the EU). So, while they all contain iron, some formulas don't contain enough to meet a healthy baby's needs. For this reason the law requires that formulas with different iron contents be labeled clearly; a formula containing more than 1.0 mg per 100 kcal must be labeled "infant formula with iron" (or a similar statement); a formula containing less than 1 mg per 100 kcal must include the label "additional iron may be necessary." Iron is a crucial micronutrient for healthy growth and development of babies, and so, in line with the AAP, we would recommend you opt for a formula with at least 1.0 mg per 100 kcal iron, unless your pediatrician has advised you to use a low-iron formula. But there are almost no "low-iron" formulas on the market now, so this is not a hard recommendation to follow.

Vitamin D has to be in all formulas, but the guidelines for manufacturers range from 40 to 100 IU per 100 kcal. This means that babies who are given a formula with the minimum vitamin D content will need to consume 1.5 liters (about 50 fluid ounces) per day in order to meet their recommended daily intake (400 IU per day). This is far more than most babies should be drinking in a given day. So, we would recommend opting for a formula with a higher vitamin D content, or if you are using a formula with a low vitamin D content, talk to your pediatrician about giving your baby a vitamin D supplement, as well.

THE ADDED EXTRAS

Aside from the twenty-nine nutrients that must be in all formula milks by law, companies often add various other ingredients that tend to be found naturally in breast milk. These added extras are often used as the basis for pretty bold health claims about the superiority of that particular formula over another, and to claim that it is closer in composition to breast milk and therefore better. They also come with a fairly hefty price tag. But substances that are isolated from breast milk and recreated in a lab don't necessarily confer the same health benefits as they do in their natural form, so you can't assume there are any real health benefits to these added substances; this needs to be tested in research. In fact, many of the minimum levels of vitamins and minerals that must be present in formula are far higher than they are in breast milk because it is harder for babies to absorb them from formula. So, the mere presence of a substance in formula that happens to be in breast milk does not necessarily mean it has any real health benefit when added to formula.

Docosahexaenoic acid (DHA) and arachidonic acid (ARA) are long-chain polyunsaturated fatty acids (omega-3 fatty acids) found in high levels in brain and eye tissue and are thought to play a key role in brain and visual development. DHA and ARA must accumulate in the brain in large amounts during the first two years of life, and early studies found that they were higher in the brains of babies who'd been breastfed rather than formula-fed. As a result, since 2002 most formulas have included them. But do they really benefit infants when included in formula? Randomized controlled trials of cognitive or visual development among term infants fed formulas enriched with DHA and ARA have had mixed results, and there is certainly no conclusive evidence for any real benefits beyond infancy.[10] However, there is a lack of studies that have looked over a longer period, and, importantly, no studies have found any evidence of harm from adding DHA and ARA to formula milk.[11] So, on balance, they seem like a reasonable addition to formula milk—they are not harmful and there is *potential* for benefit. For this reason, under new legislation the inclusion of DHAs and ARA will be a mandatory inclusion in all formulas in the EU from 2020. Currently in the US there is no legal requirement for their inclusion, but most formulas do contain them.

Prebiotics and probiotics (and synbiotics, which are a combination of the two) are substances that are thought to promote healthy bacteria in the gut and support immune system development. Probiotics are live microorganisms; these are the "friendly bacteria" that keep the nasty disease-causing bacteria in check and tend to live mainly in the large intestine. Prebiotics are nondigestible carbohydrates (such as oligosaccharides) that make it all the way to the large intestine where they "feed" the friendly bacteria and help them to grow. Human breast milk contains lots of both pre- and probiotics, which are thought to play a role in creating a healthy microbiome in the baby's gut, so companies add them to formula in the hope that they will benefit babies not receiving breast milk. Cow's milk contains oligosaccharides, and it is now also possible to make oligosaccharides that are identical to some of those found in human breast milk. Two of the most common probiotics added to formula are *Bifidobacterium lactis* and *Lactobacillus reuteri*, which are found in breast milk and grow in breastfed babies' intestines. They are usually sourced from food or baby poop (!),[12] and both are safe for babies to consume.[13] Randomized controlled trials have studied the effects of adding prebiotics and probiotics to formula on a large number of health outcomes in babies: growth, diarrhea, respiratory tract infections, colic/fussing, allergies and even poop (regularity and consistency). But a recent high-quality review of the evidence concluded that there is currently insufficient evidence to be able to draw firm conclusions about the benefits of adding prebiotics, probiotics or synbiotics (a combination of the two) to formula.[14] This is probably because the human microbiome is absolutely vast in terms of the variety (and number) of bacteria that reside there, and human milk has a huge number of different prebiotics to feed them, so adding one or two pre- or probiotics to formula is unlikely to have a big impact overall. This is why neither the US nor the EU requires these to be included in commercial formulas. They are certainly unnecessary if you are using formula to supplement breastfeeding, because your baby will already be getting plenty of pro- and prebiotics from your breast milk. Prebiotics in breast milk and formula is a very hot topic in research right now. There is new research emerging and so new products appearing all the time. But we are still a long way away from finding "the perfect mix" of pre- and probiotics that would entice us to universally recommend them.

Nucleotides and nucleosides are molecules used to make DNA (genetic material) and are fundamental to all biological processes. They are found in breast milk, but it isn't clear if they serve a function for the baby or are simply a by-product of milk production. Babies can also make them themselves. Randomized controlled trials have explored if adding nucleotides to formula benefits babies in terms of growth, reduced severity of infections and reduced bouts of diarrhea, but a high-quality review concluded that there was no convincing evidence for any of these outcomes.[15]

As you might expect, these added extras come at a cost and increase the price of formula considerably, but they are often the basis of totally unsubstantiated marketing claims. A recent review of twenty-two products found that half made bold claims, none of which were supported by publicly available scientific evidence.[16] In the US, the FDA does not evaluate the scientific evidence for the marketing claims that are made, because they come under the category of "structural function claims"—claims that describe the relationship between a particular ingredient and a function of the body without actually claiming that the substance affects a *disease*. Classic examples are statements like "probiotics support immunity" or "soy for fussiness." The only requirement for marketing claims in this category is that they must be "truthful and not misleading," which is pretty vague.[17] So, don't feel that your baby's health and development will be better if you give him a formula with these additional ingredients. In fact, when it comes to the composition of infant formula milk, less may actually be more; the European Food and Safety Authority cautions that unnecessary additions in formula put a burden on a baby's metabolism because he has to excrete them.[18]

Which Formula to Choose?

With about a hundred different formulas on the US market, knowing which one to choose can be a challenge. For a start, they come in different forms—ready-to-feed, liquid concentrate and powder—and there are lots of different brands and products. There are different formulas marketed for varying developmental stages, special formulas for "supplementing" breast milk, soy-based versus cow's milk formula, formulas to solve certain problems (such as colic or reflux), organic versus conventional, non-GMO, and specialized formulas for medical conditions (such as cow's milk allergy). The vast majority of babies need only a standard formula. No doubt you will have seen some pretty bold health claims made by standard formulas, but given that all standard formulas (those for babies up to twelve months that are not indicated for special medical purposes) have to adhere to the same formulation regulations, lots of these marketing claims are . . . just marketing. To make your choice, use the information in this chapter to decide what type of protein and carbohydrate you want for your baby. Is standard intact protein fine, or does your baby need a partially hydrolyzed source (discussed below)? What type of carbohydrate is in the formula? Does it include nonlactose sugars? Make your decision based on these ingredient sources.

Dr. Bridget Young says, "Instead of looking at the front of the formula tub, ignore the marketing and bright lettering. Make your decision based on the back of the can—the list of ingredients." She provides up-to-date, independent, evidence-based information about the different types of formula on the US market, and how to choose one, on her website: babyformulaexpert.com.

READY-TO-FEED, CONCENTRATE OR POWDER

Which type of formula preparation you choose simply comes down to practical considerations and cost. Ready-to-feed formula and liquid concentrate are sterile until opened, while powder is not and can contain potentially harmful bacteria such as *Cronobacter* (although this is incredibly rare; see page 138). For this reason the CDC recommends using liquid formula when possible,[19] but you can sterilize powder using hot water before feeding it to your baby to minimize risk (see page 148). Concentrate and powder both need to be mixed with water, but ready-to-feed can be served as is. This, of course, has a practical advantage; some moms prefer to use ready-to-feed formula for night feedings rather than spend time making formula from powder or concentrate at 3 AM. But, other than this, there are no benefits to using one over the other, and the cost difference is enormous. You pay for convenience; ready-to-feed is the most expensive, and concentrate is more expensive than powder because it is a tiny bit easier to mix with water (and is sterile, unlike powder).

FORMULAS FOR DIFFERENT DEVELOPMENTAL STAGES AND FOR SUPPLEMENTING

Infant formula is often marketed for infants at different ages (e.g., newborns to three months), but the regulations are the same for *all* infant formulas up to twelve months of life, so they can't vary that much. Any standard infant formula is safe and appropriate for a healthy baby aged up to twelve months, and you can stick with the same formula throughout the whole of his first year of life if he is doing well on it and it's working for you. Just as you don't need a different formula if your baby is a week old, four months old or nine months old, nor do you need a different formula if you are using it to supplement breastfeeding or to feed your baby exclusively formula. There are either no nutritional differences between the standard versus the supplementing formulas, or they are very small (and with no clear rationale or health benefit). In our view, this is just marketing hype.

ORGANIC AND NON-GMO FORMULAS

There are a few organic and GMO-free formulas on the market. Organic and non-GMO formulas are regulated by the FDA in the same way as standard formulas, but in order to carry the label "organic" they also need to meet the standards of the Organic Foods Production Act. Organic formulas must be produced from cows that were fed organic food and were not given growth hormones or antibiotics, and from plants that were grown with approved pesticides. However, *all* milk is evaluated for antibiotic presence, and there is no difference between organic and nonorganic milks in terms of hormone levels.[20] Importantly, too, there is no difference between organic and nonorganic or GMO and GMO-free formulas in terms of their nutritional content, quality or safety, and no evidence that babies who have them are healthier or do better than babies given standard formulas.[21] They are, however, much more expensive than nonorganic/non-GMO-free equivalents. If these differences in production are important to you and your family, and you can afford the extra cost, then these are perfectly safe. But if you have no real view on the value of organic farming, don't buy them and don't worry about it. Your baby will be fine whichever formula you use.

FORMULAS BY PRICE

The cost of feeding a baby formula over the first twelve months of life can accumulate quickly! Ready-to-feed milks are by far the most expensive, and though they might provide a useful option when there are no facilities to prepare milk safely (and when you are new to bottle-feeding and have a crying baby they will by far feel like the easiest option), you will end up spending considerably more money compared to liquid concentrate or powdered milk. Cheaper does not mean lower quality. For example, store-brand formulas have to adhere to the same regulations as name-brand formulas and are often made in the very same facilities. So, do not hesitate to pick a less-expensive brand of formula for your baby if finances are a factor. You should judge store-brand formulas the same way you judge name-brand formulas—based on the ingredients. Pick whichever type of formula best suits your needs. A Consumer Reports review of formula milks had a few useful tips on minimizing cost (but use these tips only after you have found a formula that you are happy with . . . there is nothing worse than buying a bulk three-month supply of formula and then finding out you need to switch!):[22]

- Shop at mass merchandisers—prices were lowest at mass merchandisers, most expensive at drug stores, and in-between at supermarkets.

- Buy a standard cow's-milk-based formula unless recommended to do otherwise by your pediatrician.

- Buy powder rather than liquid concentrate or ready-to-feed.

- Buy the largest cans you can find because the cost per ounce is less than for smaller cans, but check the use-by date to make sure you'll be able to use it all before it expires.

- Buy a store brand rather than a formula-specific brand.

"GENTLE" OR "COMFORT" FORMULA (PARTIALLY HYDROLYZED FORMULA)

First, the words *gentle* and *comfort* are not regulated, so they can be used on any can of formula. But usually (at the time of this writing) these words are used for formulas advertised for babies with digestive discomfort such as gas, colic or constipation. They are all based on cow's milk but contain partially hydrolyzed proteins—proteins that have been partially broken down into smaller, simpler parts that are easier to digest. Most partially hydrolyzed formulas also have lower lactose content than standard formulas. The claim is that these compositional differences make them easier to digest, and they are marketed as being gentle on the stomach, comforting and for fussiness, colic or crying.

There are very mixed views on the value of partially hydrolyzed proteins in formula for general complaints like gas. A high-quality review of the value of different formulas for symptoms of colic concluded that partially hydrolyzed whey might reduce the duration of crying, but that the current evidence for this was of low quality.[23] Gas, colic, constipation and fussing are common during the first few weeks but tend to improve as the baby matures. There are strategies you can use that don't necessarily involve changing their formula. Offering small feedings more frequently can reduce fussing and distress. But bear in mind that babies cry for all sorts of reasons, and it is not necessarily feeding-related. You can read more about how to deal with a fussing baby on page 171.

There is some evidence that partially hydrolyzed formulas are helpful for preventing and treating eczema (atopic dermatitis).[24] Based on this evidence the AAP suggests the use of these formulas (or fully hydrolyzed formulas—see below), along with breastfeeding, for reducing the risk of allergy-related conditions, such as eczema.[25] However, the 2012 FDA-approved health claim, which allows formula companies to use marketing language about 100 percent whey partially hydrolyzed formula for preventing eczema, is still quite controversial. In 2016, researchers in the UK undertook one of the largest and most thorough reviews of the evidence to date. They concluded that there was no evidence to support the health claim permitted by the FDA that formulas with partially hydrolyzed proteins reduce the risk of eczema; nor did they find any evidence that they prevent allergy to cow's milk.[26] This is still an active area of research, and everyone does seem to agree that more research is needed. If you are worried about eczema or allergies with your baby, then speak to your pediatrician about the most appropriate formula for him. Importantly, because these formulas use cow's milk, they are not suitable for babies with a diagnosed cow's milk allergy.

FORMULA FOR SPIT UP OR REFLUX

Reflux, or "spitting up," is very common in babies during the first few months and will usually have rectified itself by the time your baby turns one. Common symptoms include

- spitting up milk during or after feedings, which can happen several times a day

- feeding difficulties, such as refusing feedings, gagging or choking
- persistent hiccups or coughing
- excessive crying, or crying while feeding
- frequent ear infections.

Reflux happens because the ring of muscle at the bottom of your baby's esophagus (food pipe) that keeps food in the stomach is still developing. This means that some of the stomach contents can leak out and come back up again. But if your baby is gaining weight at a healthy rate and feeding well, there should be no cause for concern. It can still be worrying and stressful for you, though (not to mention all the laundry that has to be done!). But bear in mind that serious reflux that requires medical intervention is rare; and it needs to be diagnosed by your pediatrician. Formulas marketed for reflux or spit up are thickened. In fact, they are about ten times thicker than standard formulas! The thickness increases even more once it makes contact with your baby's stomach acid. A high-quality review of randomized controlled trials found some evidence that they help reduce symptoms such as vomiting (by about one episode per day), regurgitation, irritability and crying.[27] However, these formulas are thickened using rice (or other) starch, which is not in line with the general consensus that infants less than four months old should have no food other than milk. In addition, some researchers have raised concerns about these milks interfering with babies' ability to absorb all of the nutrients.[28] If you are concerned about reflux, speak to your pediatrician before using one of these formulas.

LACTOSE-FREE AND LACTOSE-REDUCED FORMULA

Lactose is the main carbohydrate in breast and cow's milk and an important energy source for babies during the early months and years. Virtually all term babies are born with the ability to digest lactose. Congenital lactase deficiency is an extremely rare inherited condition that causes a baby to have very little or none of the enzyme lactase, which is needed to digest lactose. It can only be diagnosed by a pediatrician. The more common type of lactose intolerance (primary lactase deficiency) develops at older ages when the diet becomes less reliant on milk and lactase production decreases; this is usually after the age of two to three years, and in most cases symptoms don't develop until late adolescence or adulthood.[29] So, it is highly unlikely that your baby has lactose intolerance if he is less than a year old. Babies who are born prematurely at less than thirty-four weeks can have problems with lactose intolerance,[30] which is why formulas for premature babies have reduced lactose. But even premature babies will increase their ability to digest lactose as they grow and mature. If a baby cannot absorb lactose, the symptoms begin shortly after drinking milk that contains lactose and include abdominal pain, severe diarrhea, and flatulence and/or bloating.

For babies with diagnosed lactose intolerance, a lactose-free formula is necessary. Temporary lactose intolerance can also develop following a bout of diarrhea or a bad stomach bug, but it tends to be short-lived, and babies are usually still able to digest and absorb normal amounts of lactose anyhow. Low-lactose and lactose-free formulas are therefore not recommended for most babies with temporary lactose intolerance, and there is no evidence that in developed countries these formulas provide any real benefit over their usual formula.[31] For this reason the AAP does not recommend using a low-lactose or lactose-free formula for temporary lactose intolerance during or following illness.[32]

Low-lactose or lactose-free formulas have replaced the lactose with corn syrup, corn syrup solids, corn maltodextrin (a type of corn sugar), sucrose, glucose syrup and/or brown rice syrup. Some of these sugars are more likely to damage teeth than lactose, especially glucose and sucrose. So, if you use one of these formulas, you need to make sure that you clean your baby's teeth after each feeding. You can do this by wiping his teeth with your finger or a clean washcloth to prevent a layer of sucrose from forming, or using a soft baby toothbrush (but don't use a toothpaste containing fluoride for a baby under two years of age).

The low-lactose and lactose-free formulas are often marketed as "sensitive" formulas and state they are for fussiness, gas and colic. Some even claim that they are for fussiness and gas "due to lactose sensitivity"; this is not a recognized medical condition (like lactose intolerance), so they can make this claim without needing to provide the FDA with conclusive scientific evidence, as they would if they were to make a "health claim." However, a high-quality review found no convincing evidence that lactose-free milks relieve symptoms of colic, and they are not recommended for this use.[33] Lactose intolerance is not the same as an allergy to cow's milk protein, which is also rare but much more serious (see page 145). If you are worried about your baby's symptoms, it is always best to get him checked by your pediatrician, who will be able to give you advice about whether you should change his formula.

SOY-BASED MILK

This plant-based formula uses protein from soybeans instead of cow's milk (no animal protein), and sucrose, corn syrup solids or corn malto-dextrin instead of lactose. Soy protein is rich in phytoestrogens, which mimic female sex hormones such as estrogen, and there is a concern among some organizations that these may affect babies' reproductive development. For example, following a review of the evidence, the UK Committee on Toxicity (COT) of Chemicals in Food, Consumer Products and the Environment cautioned that soy-based formulas pose a potential risk to the future reproductive health of infants.[34] For this reason, the European Society of Paediatric Gastroenterology, Hepatology and Nutrition (ESPGHAN) recommends that soy-based formula milks should *not* be used for babies under six months of age.[35] However, the potential longer-term harm remains a controversial topic on which there has been surprisingly little research. Currently there is *no conclusive evidence* that use of these formulas leads to adverse effects on reproductive health (or anything else) in the longer term.[36] Some organizations therefore take a more lenient view on the use of soy-based formulas in young infants. The AAP is fairly cautious about the use of these milks and recommends them only for babies with very rare medical disorders whereby they cannot tolerate any lactose at all (galactosemia and congenital lactose intolerance, which are tested for at birth), and when the parents are very passionate about a vegan formula source.

There is a common misconception among parents that soy-based formulas are a useful alternative for babies with a cow's milk protein allergy. In fact, there is almost universal agreement that soy-based formula should not be given to babies with cow's milk protein allergy because 10 to 14 percent of these babies are also allergic to soy protein, so this is not a good option for them.[37] Alternative and more appropriate options for these babies are formulas based on extensively hydrolyzed proteins or amino acid preparations (see the following, "Hypoallergenic Formulas"). If you are worried that your baby has a cow's milk protein allergy, you should get him properly assessed by your pediatrician. It is important to note that soy-based formulas are never appropriate for premature infants. This is because the absorption of certain critical minerals is reduced in soy formulas. Premature infants, who have elevated nutrient needs, can develop osteopenia (poor bone formation) when fed soy formulas.[38]

If you feel strongly that you don't want your baby to consume any animal products, a soy-based formula is the only option. But given the question mark over its long-term safety, and the use of sugars other than lactose, we would not recommend that you use a soy-based formula if you have other options available to you.

HYPOALLERGENIC FORMULAS

Hypoallergenic formulas are for babies with a cow's milk protein allergy, which affects between 2 and 7.5 percent of babies,[39] or a soy protein allergy, which is rarer and affects less than 1 percent of babies.[40] Both are serious and need to be diagnosed by a pediatrician, who will advise you on a formula that is right for your baby. Allergic reactions can have immediate or delayed symptoms. Immediate symptoms start right after a formula feeding and can include sickness or diarrhea, a red, itchy rash around your baby's mouth, swelling of his face, red lumps on his body and a very runny nose. Very occasionally symptoms can be more serious (such as breathing problems or losing consciousness), in which case you should call an ambulance. Delayed symptoms include eczema or slow weight gain. It is important to take your baby to the pediatrician if you notice any of these symptoms; don't try to diagnose your baby yourself.

There are two options for babies with a cow's milk or soy protein allergy: extensively hydrolyzed formulas or elemental (amino acid) formulas. Extensively hydrolyzed formulas have had the protein molecules broken down into smaller components (peptides and amino acids) that are much easier to digest and less likely to cause an allergic reaction. This is similar to what happens with partially hydrolyzed formulas, but the protein molecules are broken down into even smaller parts. About 90 percent of babies with soy or cow's milk protein allergy do fine on these formulas.[41] Babies who still have problems can be given an elemental formula. These formulas don't technically contain any proteins—just free amino acids (the building blocks of protein). Because there are no intact proteins left, these formulas cannot cause allergic reactions. They should only be used for babies with severe allergies who continue to have symptoms with an extensively hydrolyzed formula. Both types of hypoallergenic formulas are expensive compared to standard formulas, but elemental formulas are extremely expensive and offer no benefit if your baby tolerates an extensively hydrolyzed formula. While you can buy both of these types of formulas at your local grocery store, they should not be fed to your baby without your doctor's instruction.

PREMATURE FORMULAS

We're not going to provide much detail here on premature nutrition and formulas—your pediatrician is best placed to advise you on this—we will just give you some basic information about why premature babies often need special formula. Premature babies (born at less than thirty-seven weeks' gestation) or those born with a low birth weight (less than 1.5 kg/3.3 pounds) often have specific nutritional needs that differ from those of healthy term babies. His nutritional needs will be taken care of while he is in the hospital. If he is given a special preterm formula while in the hospital, it will differ from standard formula. Preterm hospital formulas contain more calories per ounce (20 to 30 versus 19 to 20) and have higher levels of protein (about 2 g per 100 ml) and other nutrients to support his growth and development.[42] In most products, 40 to 50 percent of the fat used is medium chain triglyceride (MCT) oil (alongside a vegetable oil blend, DHA and ARA) because it's easier for premature babies to absorb. Once he is discharged from the hospital, your pediatrician will advise you about whether he can have a standard formula or needs a special preterm or enriched formula. A preterm formula should only be used under strict medical supervision; you should use it for as long as your pediatrician advises you to, and only switch to a standard formula if they recommend that you do this. It is unclear from research as to whether or not preterm formulas are of value post-discharge,[43] and your pediatrician will make a recommendation based on your baby's specific needs.

FORMULA SUBSTITUTES OR HOMEMADE FORMULAS

There's a growing trend for some parents to make their own formula at home, in the belief that it is healthier for their baby, because they know exactly what goes into it or it's more natural. *This is not a good idea.* Commercially prepared infant formula is the closest thing that we have to human breast milk, and every effort has been made to ensure that it contains the right proportions of fat, protein, carbohydrate and other nutrients that babies need to grow and develop properly during their first year of life. It would be virtually impossible to get this right when making it yourself at home. Aside from the nutritional considerations, you also risk giving your baby a severe bacterial infection. The FDA ensures that the preparation, storage and handling of commercial formula milks meet the highest standards of safety to minimize the risk of contamination and infection. A recent study reported several cases of severe malnutrition (and one death), often requiring hospitalization, among infants less than twelve months of age who had been given nondairy drinks such as almond, chestnut, rice or soy milk in place of breast milk or formula.[44] The main influences on parents were the media (44 percent) and alternative medical professionals—i.e., not medical doctors—(38 percent), and the parents' main reasons for switching from breast milk or formula were suspected cow's milk intolerance and minor digestive or skin problems. If you are worried about your baby's health and development, seek advice from your pediatrician—they are medically qualified to provide advice about what milk your baby should have.

How to Prepare Formula

After scanning the internet and talking to lots of moms and dads, it was clear to us that there is quite a lot of confusion about how to prepare formula safely and why the recommendations are such as they are. We have therefore listed below the key tips and the rationale behind the steps that need to be followed. Good hygiene as well as the correct ratio of water to powder is crucial to ensure that formula is safe for your baby.

PREVENTION OF INFECTION

Your baby's immune system is not yet fully developed, making him more susceptible to infection. Breastfed babies receive some immunity from breast milk, but formula doesn't confer the same protection. This means it's important to make sure you follow some steps to minimize the risk of infection from formula feedings. It is worth noting that the FDA[45] and the AAP[46] take a more lenient stance with regard to preparing formula milk than do other countries and the WHO.[47] The CDC suggests that parents consider taking extra precautions—in line with WHO guidelines—for babies less than three months of age, premature babies and those with a weakened immune system. The WHO recommends always sterilizing bottles and teats before every feeding; the FDA and AAP recommend doing this only before first use and thereafter washing the bottles with soap and water or in a dishwasher (on a hot wash). The WHO also recommends sterilizing the formula powder itself with water that has been boiled and cooled to about 158°F (70°C). This is because formula powder is not sterile and some nasty bugs can find their way in there over time, so formula prepared from powder carries a risk of infection, albeit very small. The main concern is *Cronobacter*, which is incredibly rare—about four to six cases are reported to the CDC each year—but can be deadly in newborns.[48] Given the rarity of infection from formula powder, the FDA considers it safe (in most cases) to use ordinary *cold* tap water that has been boiled for one minute and cooled to room temperature for no longer than thirty minutes to make your formula. The AAP thinks it is unnecessary to boil the tap water first if it is from a safe water source, in which case it can be used straight from the cold tap, but if you are concerned about the safety of your water supply they recommend using bottled water or cold tap water that has been boiled for one minute and cooled for no more than thirty minutes to room temperature. We have followed the AAP's guidance below, but it's a good idea to check with your baby's pediatrician that you don't need to take any additional precautions.

1. Wash your hands thoroughly before preparing a bottle, as you would before preparing any food. Do this *before* you sterilize or clean the bottle and before preparing the formula. This will mean that the germs that you have on your hands are less likely to be passed onto the bottle or formula itself and contaminate it. All other equipment (can opener, mixing cups, spoons, and so on) and the surface on which you prepare the formula need to be clean, too.

2. All bottles and equipment should be sterilized *before first use*. Sterilization means destroying any microorganisms that may cause harm, and boiling water suffices for this—simply put the bottles, nipples and other equipment in a pan of boiling water and keep it on a rolling boil for five minutes. You need to sterilize the bottle the first time you use it whether you are using powdered milk, liquid concentrate or ready-to-feed milk. From then on, you can clean the bottles and equipment before each feeding using hot soapy water or in a dishwasher, unless your pediatrician has advised you otherwise.

3. Prepare feedings one at a time and discard any milk left in the bottle at the end of the feeding. The reason for this recommendation is to prevent infection by bacteria such as salmonella. Bacteria multiply rapidly at room temperature (the optimum temperature being body temperature, 98°F/37°C) and will continue, although at a slower rate, in the fridge. But preparing formula properly is very time-consuming, and one thing parents with a young baby don't have is spare time! So, understandably, many parents would rather not discard a lot of leftover formula that they have just prepared. If you need to store it for a while you can keep a freshly made bottle of formula (if your baby has not drunk from it at all) in the fridge for up to twenty-four hours, and at room temperature for up to two hours, but never reheat it. It is really important to discard any formula left in the bottle within an hour after the end of a feeding; once your baby has been feeding from the bottle, bacteria from his mouth will contaminate the milk and can multiply very quickly (even in the fridge). An open container of

ready-to-feed formula, concentrated formula or formula freshly prepared from concentrated formula should be covered and can be kept in the fridge for up to twenty-four hours.

CORRECT RATIO OF WATER TO POWDER OR CONCENTRATE

Ready-to-feed formula does not need to be mixed with water and should be served as is. But if using powder or concentrate it is crucial to make sure that the amount of water relative to powder or concentrate is exactly right. Some parents dilute formula in order to save money. But too much water relative to formula can result in underfeeding, growth faltering and worse—water intoxication, a life-threatening condition where a baby's kidneys are unable to excrete the water quickly enough, leading to a dangerous imbalance of electrolytes that can cause seizures, a coma and even death. This is also why you should never give your baby water during the first six months, even if it is hot—all he needs during the first six months is milk (either breast milk or properly prepared formula). Too much formula relative to water will make the formula too energy dense (too many calories per ml) and can lead to overfeeding and obesity risk, as well as constipation or dehydration. Here's how to make sure you get it right when you mix water with formula powder or concentrate:

Powder: Pour the correct amount of water into the bottle first and check it to ensure it is the correct volume before adding the powder. Fill the scoop loosely with milk powder and level it off using the back of a clean, dry knife or the leveler provided by the manufacturer. Always use the scoop provided by the particular formula powder you are using because scoop sizes differ between different brands (even when they are made by the same manufacturer). Add the powder to the water in the bottle and shake vigorously. A common mistake is to add the powder to the bottle first and then add the water to the powder. This results in the formula milk being too energy dense (not enough water relative to powder). If you use hot water (about 158°F/70°C) to make up the formula (e.g., if you want to sterilize the powder), it will need to be cooled before giving it to your baby; this can be done by immersing the bottom of the bottle in cold water. Check the temperature of the formula before offering it to your baby by pouring a little bit onto the inside of your wrist; it should be lukewarm or cooler.

Concentrate: Pour the correct amount of formula concentrate into the bottle and add the same volume of water. It doesn't matter whether you add the concentrate or the water to the bottle first. Shake vigorously before giving it to your baby.

If you have prepared formula from cold water (or are taking it out of the fridge) and would like to warm it up before offering it to your baby, the safest way to do this is to stand the bottle in a bowl of warm (not boiling) water or hold it under warm water. Never heat it in a microwave—this can lead to hot spots that can burn your baby's mouth and throat. But bear in mind that formula does not need to be warmed before you offer it to your baby. So, if you are using ready-to-feed formula from the beginning, perhaps refrain from warming it up, because your baby will probably end up preferring it warm, which will make more work for you in the long run!

THE BOTTOM LINE

- If you need to use a formula, choose a *standard* first milk unless you have been advised otherwise by your pediatrician.

- We recommend choosing a standard milk that uses lactose as the main source of carbohydrate (not sucrose or any other sugar), has a protein content of less than 3.0 g per 100 mg, and has a high vitamin D (100 IU per 100 kcal) and iron (at least 1.0 mg per 100 kcal) content.

- Your choice of formula should be driven by the ingredients—ignore the marketing claims. We have given you lots of information about the ingredients so that you and your pediatrician can decide together which ingredient decisions are most important for your baby. Remember that more expensive does not mean better.

- Ready-to-feed milks are much more expensive than powdered milks, but they can be very useful for tired, stressed parents and are a good option in situations where you don't have easy access to clean water.

- You can bond with your baby during feeding, whichever method you decide to use.

CHAPTER 6

Responsive Feeding: The *How* of Milk-Feeding

Once you have decided whether to breast- or formula-feed (or combination-feed), you may be wondering *how* to feed your baby—for example, whether to feed him on a schedule or on demand, or whether or not to use a bottle. The *how* of milk-feeding is largely about understanding what type of feeder your baby is. The bottom line is that young babies are not all the same when it comes to milk. Our research with Gemini has shown that babies respond very differently to milk and the opportunity to feed, right from the beginning of life (see Chapter 1). This is because appetite has a strong genetic basis, so babies are born with different predispositions toward milk and feeding right from the start.[1] Some babies inherit a set of genes that give them a very hearty appetite; these babies are more responsive to milk (they want to feed when they see, smell or taste milk), feed quickly and avidly and need more milk in order to feel satisfied. As you might expect, these babies grow much more quickly during the early weeks and months and are at greater risk of rapid weight gain (see page 76). At the other end of the spectrum are the babies who inherit a set of genes that give them a poorer appetite; these babies have little interest in milk and the opportunity to feed, tend to feed slowly and fill up very easily. These babies grow more slowly in the early weeks and months. This research has implications for you as a parent—it means that your feeding strategies need to take into account your baby's appetite, and the challenges posed to you will be very different if your baby has an avid appetite versus a poor one. In short, babies have different needs.

While genes predispose your baby to have a larger or a smaller appetite, his early experiences with feeding may also shape his appetite regulation. You could think of your baby's genes as setting his appetite potential and his early experiences as acting as the volume control. So, if a baby is born with a genetic predisposition to have a large appetite, certain feeding strategies could increase his appetite even further, making him an even more avid feeder, while other feeding experiences may help to temper it. The same is true for poor feeders—within the right feeding environment a baby with a poor appetite can learn to feed well. But the crucial thing is understanding the type of feeder your baby is and responding using the most appropriate feeding strategies.

How babies are fed (via the breast versus via the bottle, for example), as well as *what* they are fed (breast milk versus formula, for example), may influence a baby's appetite.

Appetite Regulation

Feeding directly from the breast rather than through a bottle is thought to support the development of good appetite regulation, or rather, feeding your baby through a bottle may encourage him to overfeed in some circumstances. We know that babies who are formula-fed consume more milk overall during their first year of life than breastfed babies, and this process begins in the first few days. A review found that on the first day of life, breastfed babies consume only 0.7 ounces (21 ml) milk, in comparison to formula-fed babies, who consume 5.7 ounces (170 ml)—eight times as much. On Day 14 breastfeeding babies are still consuming less—22.8 ounces (674 ml) versus 25.8 ounces (762 ml).[2] Another study showed that these differences in milk intake between breastfed and formula-fed babies persisted at three, six, nine and twelve months of age.[3] By twelve months the breastfed babies were consuming about 450 grams of breast milk per day, while formula fed babies were consuming about 730 grams of formula milk, with no difference in solid food intake between the groups. The assumption is that the amount consumed by breastfeeding babies is the ideal amount, and that formula feeders are consuming too much.

What is going on? Is it that formula milk tastes better than breast milk, or is it just easier to drink milk out of a bottle? The larger volume of milk consumed might be due partly to the fact that babies tend to drink faster out of a bottle than out of a breast. A small study found that two-week-old breastfeeding babies were steadily drinking about 0.25 ounce (8 ml) per minute, while the bottle-feeding babies were drinking 1 ounce (29 ml) per minute.[4] Slower feeding may help babies and toddlers learn to respond to their feelings of fullness—and feeding too quickly can certainly lead to overfeeding because they have consumed too much by the time their satiety signals have had time to take effect. We are all familiar with having eaten something too quickly, only to discover a few minutes later that we have eaten too much and we feel bloated and over-full! Eating or feeding slowly is believed to help prevent this.

Breastfed babies probably consume less milk at each feeding and drink more slowly, because it's just more difficult to get milk out of a breast than a bottle. Breastfeeding requires a lot more work than bottle-feeding; it's not just about sucking—a baby needs to use both their tongue and their jaw to feed from the breast, and there is no help from gravity. This early feeding experience may affect their appetite in the long term. One study found that exclusively breastfed babies fed directly from the breast had better awareness of satiety when they were three to six years old than babies exclusively bottle-fed breast milk.[5] Another study showed that babies fed either breast milk or formula from a bottle gained weight more rapidly from birth to one year than those fed directly from the breast,[6] and they also emptied bottles more often in later infancy.[7] "Bottle-emptying" is a behavior shown by a baby with an avid appetite. However, all of this research has come from observational studies rather than experimental studies (such as randomized controlled trials), which means that we cannot know for sure if *how* a baby is fed causes differences in appetite regulation later, or if actually it is all down to some other factor that wasn't accounted for. Nevertheless, the current research points to the bottle itself promoting overfeeding. This means that if you are expressing your breast milk and feeding it to your baby in a bottle or using formula, be mindful that this makes it easier for him to overfeed.

There are also feeding practices that can encourage overfeeding in *both* breast- and bottle-feeding babies. From as early as six weeks old babies will drink more milk if they are *offered* more. For example, one study asked mothers who were breastfeeding their babies (six to twenty-one weeks old) to express extra breast milk to increase their milk supply, and in response their babies drank more milk and gained more weight.[8] Rapid or excessive infant weight gain (which is common in the US) is linked to poorer health later on in childhood and adulthood (see Chapter 3), so it's something to keep an eye on. In one study, two-month-old babies who were given more milk in a bottle during each feeding also consumed more milk per day (3.8 ounces/114 ml more per day),[9] and the babies fed a larger bottle of milk gained more weight from birth to six months.[10] In fact, exactly the same happens with children and adults when it comes to portion sizes—the more food we are offered, the more we eat, and this is a robust finding that has been replicated over and over again.[11]

However, just as there are factors that might disrupt your baby's appetite, there are also strategies that seem to support good regulation. One key method is responsive feeding, and you can do this whether you are breast- or bottle-feeding.

What Is Responsive Feeding?

Responsive feeding is a method of feeding whereby the parent feeds in response to their baby's hunger and fullness cues. It involves paying close attention to your baby's hunger and fullness signals—feeding only when your baby indicates that he is hungry and stopping as soon as he indicates he is full. This means not encouraging your baby to finish a bottle of milk or continue to feed on the breast if he indicates that he has had enough. This is supposed to teach a baby to recognize when he is hungry and full and to respond by taking only as much milk as he needs. If your baby receives milk promptly after indicating hunger, and milk stops being offered as soon as he indicates he is full, the theory is that he will learn to associate these two feelings with starting and stopping feeding and will regulate his milk intake appropriately (and later on, his food). This means that you do not feed your baby if he is not hungry, and you do not offer milk for any reason other than hunger, such as feeding for comfort—which may lay the groundwork for emotional eating (eating for comfort) later on in life, either as a child or adult.

The prevailing view is that responsive feeding is much easier for breastfeeding babies than those fed with a bottle, the reason being that the breastfed baby is more in charge of feeding. A breastfeeding baby needs to make a concerted effort to get the milk out of the breast and, given the effort required, he's not going to do it unless he wants it. In contrast, drinking milk out of a bottle is much more passive—it requires virtually no effort from the baby, and the milk will even drip into his mouth by itself if the bottle is in the right position. This makes it much easier to coax a baby into having a bit more, even if he's no longer hungry.

Because a mom who is breastfeeding has no idea how much milk her baby has consumed, she has to rely to some extent on her baby's behavioral cues to know when he has had enough (for example, stopping sucking). In contrast to this, parents who are feeding their baby through a bottle can see exactly how much milk the baby has taken and often use this information, rather than their baby's fullness signals, to decide if their baby has finished feeding. In fact, a small study showed that babies were more likely to be cajoled into finishing what's left in the bottle when Mom could clearly see the amount of milk left than if she couldn't (when there was a cover on the bottle).[12] Research has also indicated that for many parents an empty bottle at the end of a feeding is the desired outcome, and 15 to 25 percent will actively encourage it.[13]

In theory this interferes with the baby's ability to respond to his fullness cues, because the parent overrides them. This might mean that the baby is encouraged to continue to feed after he feels full or doesn't have as much milk as he would like to satisfy his hunger. A chronic pattern of continuing to feed your baby after he has indicated he is full may also increase his responsiveness to food later and his risk of developing a tendency to overeat, or reinforce an already eager appetite. Though it can be quite frustrating if your baby doesn't drink all of the formula in his bottle, because it takes time to prepare and costs money, as you begin to learn how much milk your baby will drink, you can avoid waste by making less milk for each feeding.

A recent review concluded that, on the whole, breastfeeding moms do tend to feed more responsively than those feeding through a bottle (whether using formula or breast milk).[14] This may partly account for the higher milk intake of formula-fed babies compared to breastfed babies.

Much less is known about how responsive feeding in early infancy affects appetite regulation. A large study of over 1,000 babies showed that those who were frequently encouraged to empty the bottle during early infancy were less sensitive to satiety at six years of age, insofar as they were twice as likely to eat all the food on their plate compared to those who were rarely encouraged to do so.[15] This study suggests a relationship between responsive feeding and self-regulation. However, while researchers and health professionals pretty much universally believe that responsive feeding is crucial for the development of self-regulation skills, far more research is needed to test if this theory is really true.

RESPONSIVE FEEDING FOR BREASTFED AND BOTTLE-FED BABIES

Breastfeeding may promote good appetite regulation in terms of both the breast milk itself (the *what*) and the very act of feeding from the breast (the *how*), and, as we have seen, responsive feeding is naturally supported by breastfeeding in comparison to bottle-feeding. Nevertheless, breastfed babies are not all the same; babies who are breastfed can and do differ in their appetites. Some have ravenous appetites for breast milk and will feed at any opportunity, possibly even if they are not hungry, while others are more difficult to feed. This means it is still important to make sure that breastfed as well as formula-fed babies are fed only in response to signals of hunger and allowed to stop when they indicate that they are full. It is, of course, important to bond with your baby and to provide physical comfort when needed, but comfort doesn't necessarily need to come in the form of food (see pages 171–73).

WEIGHT GAIN

There haven't been many well-designed studies (trials) of the link between responsive feeding in early infancy and weight gain or later obesity risk. The two most important to date are the INSIGHT (Intervention Nurses Start Infants Growing on Healthy Trajectories) study and the Baby Milk Trial. INSIGHT randomized 145 new US moms of both breastfed and formula-fed babies to a responsive parenting group for one year, in which they were taught to recognize their baby's hunger and satiety cues, to use food *only* for hunger and never as a reward, and not to soothe a distressed but not hungry baby with food.[16] Strategies were also taught for helping babies get to sleep, such as helping them get back to sleep in the night without feeding them, and for feeding solid foods after milk-feeding alongside information about infant emotion regulation and how to monitor growth. A control group of 146 new moms didn't receive any information about responsive feeding. At one year, fewer babies in the responsive-parenting group had gained excessive weight than in the control group, and this was the same regardless of whether the babies were breast- or formula-fed.[17] Less than 6 percent of the babies in the intervention group had overweight at one year compared to 13 percent of the babies in the control group. There were still fewer children with overweight in the intervention group at two years of age (11 versus 21 percent), and at three years of age the children in the intervention group had lower BMIs.[18] What was especially encouraging about this study is that it also had a positive impact on the infants' mental health. At one year of age, babies in the intervention group showed fewer negative emotions, were better at self-comforting when upset and took less time to calm down if they'd been very distressed.[19] This well-designed trial provides convincing preliminary evidence that responsive feeding can prevent overweight early on and improve a baby's general development and well-being, supporting the view that *how* as well as *what* you feed is important.

A second study—the Baby Milk Trial,[20] in Britain—randomized 340 new parents with formula-fed babies to a six-month intervention during which they were given information about responsive feeding, shown how to provide an age-appropriate amount of formula in the bottle (not too much) and taught how to monitor their baby's growth to avoid excessive weight gain. The intervention also supported parents in coping with challenges, such as fussing and crying, and meeting their feeding goals by planning and monitoring their baby's feedings and weight gain. Another 339 babies were randomized to a control group who were given the opportunity to discuss general problems but given no information about responsive feeding. The intervention succeeded in preventing excess milk intake and rapid weight gain during the six-month intervention period.[21] However, although there were slightly fewer babies with rapid weight gain from birth to twelve months in the intervention group versus controls (40 versus 46 percent), this was not a statistically significant difference, meaning it could have been due to chance. These findings suggested that the responsive feeding intervention was successful during the period that parents were being supported but not afterward, highlighting the importance of information and continued support for feeding after the first six months—which we have provided in the subsequent chapters of this book.

The Challenges of Responsive Feeding

One of the questions that still needs to be addressed by research is whether responsive feeding is always the best strategy. Is it really a case of "one size fits all"? One of the main concerns is that responsive feeding could actually lead to overfeeding if parents misinterpret their babies' fussing or crying as hunger cues when in fact the source of their distress is not hunger but some other need. This means it is crucial to understand what hunger cues really look like, as well as satiety cues (see pages 167–68). But there are other complicated issues as well. Responsive feeding assumes that babies have a perfect appetite-control system already in place; it simply needs to be reinforced by their parents through responding appropriately to their hunger and fullness signals. But our research has shown that it isn't as simple as this. Some babies are naturally hungrier than others and therefore demand more feedings. Should parents always respond to their genuine cries for hunger? Or is it acceptable to withhold milk if a baby is gaining excessive amounts of weight? On the other end of the spectrum are those babies who have a poor appetite and are undemanding about feeding. Is it right to wait until they signal hunger before offering milk? Or should you try to coax a picky feeder to take some milk as often as possible to avoid dehydration or weight faltering? These are tricky issues for which science has not yet provided an answer.

In 2013 the National Institutes of Health (NIH) in the US held a meeting to advance understanding of the causes of excessive early weight gain.[22] One of the discussions that took place was whether parents should *not* feed infants every time they signal hunger and on occasion withhold food. The conclusion was that more research needs to be undertaken to test out the pros and cons (and feasibility) of such a stance:

"We need to know how to parent infants with different appetites. It is very difficult to know whether *not* feeding a hungry baby is a practical, feasible or reasonable way of managing their risk of obesity."—Julie Lumeng, professor of pediatrics and communicable diseases, University of Michigan

With this in mind, we have considered the difficulties parents face with babies at each end of the spectrum and have outlined some practical advice on pages 161–63.

In our view, too much blame is placed on parents when it comes to feeding and early growth, especially given what we know about the strong genetic influence on early appetite. Some babies are great feeders, while others are a constant worry. Very little research has been done to examine how parents develop their feeding strategies during the early milk-feeding phase. But in Gemini we looked to see whether the extent to which parents restricted milk (the frequency of feedings or the amount during each feeding) or pressured their baby to feed was related to characteristics of the baby, such as their birth weight and their appetite, or other things more related to Mom, such as her concern about her baby's under- or overweight and feeding method (breast or bottle). Our findings supported the idea that moms develop their feeding strategies in response to the type of baby they have right from the beginning.[23] Moms whose babies were born with a low birth weight, who had a poor appetite and who Mom worried were underweight were more pressuring in relation to milk-feeding; moms whose babies had a hearty appetite were more restrictive. We found no evidence that bottle-feeding moms exerted more pressure than breastfeeding mums, but they were more likely to be restrictive if they had a baby with a hearty appetite. These findings indicate that right from the beginning, moms are sensitive to their babies' needs and develop appropriate feeding strategies in response.

We followed up this research in Gemini by looking at fussy eating in toddlerhood. Along exactly the same lines we found that parents varied their feeding practices when their two twins differed in how fussy they were.[24] This indicated that picky eaters prompt their parents to pressure them more, not that pressuring parents end up with picky eaters. This research helps to combat the pervasive and simplistic view that the way a parent feeds their baby or child causes them to develop certain eating and feeding behaviors.

HUNGRY BABIES

Some babies are born with a larger appetite and will be much more demanding with regard to being fed; we know this is partly due to genetic influence (see pages 22–26). These babies may cry out of hunger more often and need more milk in order to feel satisfied. In this situation, you have two choices as a parent: either feed your hungry baby or withhold milk/food. Given that we do not yet know the long-term consequences of not allowing a hungry baby to feed until they are full, or the consequences for harm in terms of the emotional bond if a parent doesn't respond sensitively to their baby's needs, this may not seem a reasonable option for parents. And many would find this unacceptable, not only because they feel uncomfortable about not responding to their baby's needs, but because it is simply not feasible to withhold a feeding if a baby is hungry.

> "I challenge anyone to resist giving a screaming inconsolable baby a bottle in the night."—**Amy, mom of Grace (eighteen months)**

Another consideration is that restricting the frequency of breastfeeds increases the risk of low milk supply for breastfeeding mums. Responsive feeding may still play an important part in ensuring that a hungry baby doesn't overfeed, without having to deny a hungry baby their food. An eager feeder will happily guzzle milk if it's on offer, even if he is not hungry. For these babies it is important for you to wait until your baby signals to you that he feels hungry *before* offering milk. It is also important to be aware of what hunger cues look like and to be able to distinguish hunger cries from other sources of distress (see pages 167–68).

Feeding should not always be the first "go-to" when your baby is fussing. There are plenty of reasons why babies fuss—it is one of the only ways they can communicate—but crying can indicate many different needs, not just hunger. And inconsolable crying is common during the early period of life (see pages 170–73). Sometimes you will have to use nonfood forms of comfort and make sure that you don't routinely feed your baby to sleep or feed him just to keep him quiet. These babies will also have a tendency to feed past satiety if encouraged. For these babies you may need to pay close attention to fullness signals and stop the feeding as soon as your baby indicates fullness so as not to override his satiety and encourage overfeeding, especially if you use a bottle.

> "Because my baby was hungry all the time, and I was breastfeeding on demand, I got into the habit of just offering him a feeding whenever I heard the slightest whine and he happily guzzled milk pretty much all day and all night."—**Pippa, mom of Sam (five years)**

BABIES WITH A POOR APPETITE

Some babies have a poor appetite and seem disinterested in (or even dislike) feeding. These babies are far less demanding with regard to being fed, take their time over each feeding and may even fall asleep before they finish (although falling asleep on the job is something that all babies tend to do at one time or another!). These babies can be a huge source of anxiety for parents who worry that they aren't getting enough milk. In this case, is it best just to leave it up to your baby to let you know when he is hungry? Some researchers suggest that pressuring a baby or child to eat when he is not hungry or simply doesn't want to feed will lead to problems later on, such as fussiness around food or even food aversion.[25] There is still a strong sense that the way a baby feeds somehow reflects the parents' feeding strategy. However, we know little about the longer-term consequences of pressuring a poor milk feeder, because the research hasn't been done.

For young babies with a poor appetite it would seem reasonable to offer him a feeding at regular intervals even if he has not indicated that he is hungry. If your baby rejects the feeding, leave it for a while and try again a bit later. If you are concerned that your baby may be underfeeding and is not gaining weight (or is losing weight), see your pediatrician.

BARRIERS TO FEEDING RESPONSIVELY

Your baby will bring his own little quirks to the table, and you can only do your best when it comes to feeding. The first few weeks and months with a new baby can be overwhelming, and meeting his every need can feel all-consuming. Though the advice we are providing in this book is based on evidence, we appreciate that when you have a crying baby and are sleep-deprived, following any advice at all may not always seem practical.

Responsive feeding with a newborn baby can be hard; sometimes it can be difficult to judge if your baby is hungry, because you need to take time to get to know him. Not to mention that not all days are the same, and babies can be much fussier on some days than others. There are also growth spurts, during which your baby will seem constantly and unfathomably hungry. But research has shown that it does get much easier to spot your baby's cues as he gets older—so don't worry if you can't seem to figure him out all the time at the beginning.

While there is widespread support for responsive feeding, some parents cannot/do not feed in this way. The Health Promotion Agency in New Zealand commissioned research in 2014 to find out why first-time moms might not do this, so that they could address their concerns.[26] There were two main barriers:

1. A lack of confidence in their ability to read their baby's hunger and satiety cues.

2. A desire to establish a routine as soon as possible and stick to it.

Some moms in the research indicated that their baby never got to the stage of feeling hungry because they were fed so regularly. A few of the moms also did not believe their baby knew when they were full, and some would even continue to eat until they were sick. Most mothers reported feeding their infants and children to a set routine, not based on the baby's or child's hunger cues.

We spoke with one mom who suggested that her baby's feeding cues seemed to diminish as she got older:

> "After I gave birth to Julia in the hospital, midwives told me what feeding cues look like in a newborn baby. I found it easy to spot them, but now when Julia is six weeks she seems to be producing fewer clues or facial/mouth expressions than she used to, so I am feeding her if I feel at least two hours have passed since her last feeding or if she is crying despite having a dry nappy and having just slept."—**Marta, mom of Julia (three months)**

Taking into account these concerns, we have put together a detailed, practical guide based on scientific research on how to feed responsively. This advice is applicable for both breast- and bottle-feeding and for every type of feeder. We know that it can be hard to think about feeding responsively, on top of everything else that is going on in the first few weeks with a newborn. But we hope that this guidance will provide you with clear, practical information that will help you to set your child on the path to a healthy future relationship with food.

How to Feed Responsively

Responsive feeding is providing a prompt and appropriate response to your baby's hunger and satiety cues. This involves

- your baby giving you clear, unambiguous hunger and satiety cues
- your accurate interpretation of those cues
- you responding promptly, providing adequate and appropriate nutrition (milk or withdrawal of milk)
- your baby experiencing a predictable response to his signals to you, which is his gateway to learning.

Recognizing your baby's hunger and fullness signals are the vital first step in feeding responsively. Parents are usually told to "feed on demand," but if you feed whenever your baby cries, this is not necessarily in response to his hunger (crying and soothing are dealt with in detail on pages 170–73). Parents need much more information about when and how to feed. As an aside: If you are breastfeeding, it is important to feed your baby very regularly during the early weeks (especially the first two weeks) to ensure you establish a good milk supply. Once breastfeeding is established, you'll be able to focus on feeding in response to your baby's cues.

> "Many parents are told to feed 'on demand' but what is 'on demand'? Is it when they wake up from sleep, when they fuss, when they cry, when they get squirmy, or only when they are clearly showing signs of hunger? Because a baby will usually feed in response to any of these behaviors, mothers need more precise guidance that feeding 'on demand' should be reserved for hungry babies and not the default response to other normal behaviors."
> —Ian Paul, professor of pediatrics and public health sciences at Penn State College of Medicine, leader of the INSIGHT study on responsive feeding

Research has shown that parents find it much easier to spot their baby's hunger cues than their fullness cues. The typical hunger cues that parents say they recognize are crying and fussing (most importantly) and licking their lips. And the most common fullness cues are pulling away and stopping feeding. We also know that hunger and fullness signals are much easier to interpret as babies and children get older.[27] However, this doesn't mean that responsive feeding isn't possible during the very early weeks and months, and below we provide you with the information you need about how to spot them and how to respond to them. It takes time to learn how to interpret your baby's cues, and this will get easier as you get to know him.

Distinguishing crying for hunger from crying for other reasons is no small task, but there are two concerns about feeding a crying baby who is not hungry:

1. An avid feeder will take the milk anyway and overfeed.

2. A baby may learn to associate distress with being fed, leading to the development of emotional eating later on.

Babies cry for many different reasons. Reasons other than hunger include fear, anger, boredom, tiredness and other discomfort, such as a wet diaper. They also cry for no apparent reason at all. If feeding is the first go-to response, a parent may end up feeding a nonhungry baby, and on quite a frequent basis. The concern is that a nonhungry baby may learn to associate distress with being fed.

Using alternative soothing techniques will help a nonhungry baby to experience being soothed without being fed; in theory this should help him to learn to self-soothe and return to sleep without being comforted by food. It is important for a baby to learn to use healthy behaviors to deal with emotional distress, such as physical comfort. Responsive feeding is about finding other strategies for comfort that work and understanding how a baby's sleep patterns evolve over the first few weeks and months after birth. It is also good to understand a bit about babies' crying behavior in the early months. We have pro-vided information about babies' crying patterns over the first few months on pages 170–73.

In most cases, after the first few weeks you do not need to wake a sleeping baby for a feeding—he will wake up of his own accord when hungry.

"Because most babies lose weight in the first days following birth, pediatricians typically recommend that babies feed eight to twelve times per day (every two to three hours on average day and night). However, once babies regain that weight over the first week or two, pediatricians often omit telling mothers that feeding this frequently or feeding on a schedule is not necessary. I commonly see parents still waking their baby every three hours at age two months, which is completely unnecessary. In truth, once this initial weight loss is regained, the baby, not the parent, should determine when and how often feedings should occur."—Ian Paul

But there are sometimes situations when you *will* need to wake your baby for a feed (for example, if your baby is unwell or taking medications that make him sleepy). Your doctor or medical professional should guide you. Otherwise you can trust your baby to let you know.

SIGNS OF HUNGER AND FULLNESS

Recognizing hunger and fullness signals in very young babies can be tricky, but it is certainly possible to do this, and from a very young age.

Signs of Hunger

There are some pretty universal signs that signal hunger in babies. These are easy to spot once you know what they are, and the signs become clearer as you get to know your baby better. Babies use lots of cues together, or "clustered cues," to indicate their needs. For example, they may bring their hands to their mouth or face, clench their fingers, flex their arms and legs, root, make sucking noises and breathe quickly. All of these behaviors together indicate that a baby is hungry. A single cue does not necessarily indicate hunger. In particular, crying on its own is not a hunger cue but rather a distress signal. Hungry babies might cry, but they will *also* exhibit other hunger cues.

Early hunger signals (tend to be subtle and primarily oral):
- stirring from side to side, opening his mouth and turning his head to the side (the "seeking" or "rooting" reflex)

Active hunger signals (more overt and involve more full-body movements):
- fussing
- stretching
- open-mouth postures and hand-mouth contact
- flexion of the hand
- increased physical movements

Late hunger signals (very overt and tend to be characterized by distress):
- distressed, intense crying
- agitated body movements

- turning red in the face
- sweating

Note: Once your baby is very distressed you will need to soothe him first, before feeding. A baby in a very distressed state is unlikely to feed properly, so it's best to try to calm him down before attempting a feeding. Pediatricians recommend that you hold your baby calmly and even have skin-to-skin contact once he has moved to full-blown crying.[28] (We have provided some detailed tips for how to calm a baby down on pages 171–73.)

Signs of Fullness (Satiety)

Research has shown that parents and caregivers find satiety signals harder to read and are more likely to miss them.[29] But it is also common practice to encourage babies to continue feeding even after their fullness cues have been noticed. It is important to respond to your baby by stopping the feeding.

Early satiety signals:
- slows or decreases sucking
- relaxes/extends arms, legs and fingers

Active satiety signals:
- stops sucking
- releases the nipple
- distracted or pays attention to surroundings more (babies over four months of age)

Late satiety signals:
- pushes/arches away
- turns head away from nipple
- seals lips together (four to seven months of age)
- falls asleep (birth to three months of age)

Tips for Responsive Bottle-Feeding

Given that babies may be more likely to overfeed when bottle-feeding, we have provided some extra tips below for bottle-feeding babies:

- Be cautious about the amount of formula or breast milk that you put into the bottle at each feeding. Do not offer more than is reasonable for a single feeding. If your baby indicates that he is still hungry after he has finished the bottle, you can still offer more. We have provided guidelines on page 181 about the frequency and volume of feedings for babies of different ages.

- If you have a baby who likes to guzzle milk quickly, try using a slower-flowing nipple.

- Invite your baby to take the nipple of the bottle rather than force it into his mouth.

- Never add anything to the formula (for example, cereal or baby rice). This is not recommended; it may interfere with your baby's appetite regulation and lead to overfeeding, and can cause discomfort for babies aged up to four months, who are not developmentally ready for nonmilk foods.

- Don't prop the bottle up (for example, on a pillow or other surface) when babies are not yet able to hold it themselves.

- Do not put your baby to bed with a bottle, as this might make the bottle (and feeding) an emotional comforter, and it can cause tooth decay. Feeding to soothe may lay the groundwork for emotional overeating in childhood. It may also later make it very difficult to put your baby to bed without a bottle.

- Don't pressure or force your baby to finish the bottle if he indicates he has had enough. Healthy babies know if they are hungry and when they are full. Feeding is not about you controlling your baby's milk intake; it's about trusting your baby to decide for himself. If your baby is pulling away from the nipple, crying, closing his lips together and spitting out milk, he is telling you he has had enough.

- Pace the feeding by stopping to burp periodically.

- Try to avoid doing anything that might distract you or your baby while feeding (for example, browsing the internet, texting or watching television). This will allow you to focus on your baby during feeding so that you are able to recognize his feeding cues, and your baby will also be less likely to become distracted. A picky feeder is easily distracted by things that seem more interesting than feeding (such as watching your phone or iPad), while an avid feeder may struggle to pay attention to his feelings of fullness if distracted by something else.

CRYING

The best available evidence suggests that excessive crying or fussing in the early months is, unfortunately, pretty common[30]—about a quarter of parents with perfectly healthy babies report it[31]—so if your baby never seems to stop crying, you are not alone. Dealing with crying is one of the most challenging experiences of being a new parent, and it's good to make sure you know what to expect during the first few months—not only in relation to feeding but also for your own sanity.

The usual pattern is for your baby's crying (which will often be inconsolable) to be highest in the first six weeks of life and then decrease between six and twelve weeks,[32] and it tends to be more common in the late afternoon and evening. *All babies* go through this pattern of crying, but some cry more than others, and for some it can involve prolonged, unsootheable and unpredictable bouts of crying. For you as a parent, this can be frustrating and overwhelming. It has been called the "period of PURPLE crying" by some researchers in the field, which is an acronym for the following features that are typical of this phase and completely normal:[33]

- **P**eak—the crying peaks in the first six weeks.
- **U**nexpected—the crying bouts are unpredictable.
- **R**esists soothing—nothing you do will stop your baby crying.
- **P**ain-like face—your baby may look like he is in pain, but he's not.
- **L**ong-lasting—the crying seems to go on and on and can last for five hours per day (and may feel like twenty-four).
- **E**vening—your baby will tend to have these crying bouts in the late afternoon or evening.

How to Manage It

It is beyond the scope of this book to go into detail about the methods and the research behind crying and soothing. However, research has suggested that there are two things you can do that might reduce your baby's crying by about 50 percent:[34]

1. **Feed your baby promptly in response to his cues of hunger.** This means making sure you get to know your baby's hunger signals and respond to them by offering a feeding before he gets too hungry and gets himself in a tizzy, just as we have described above.

2. **Make sure you have lots of physical contact with your baby.** Ten hours of physical contact per twenty-four-hour period may reduce your baby's overall fussing and crying. And this can be when he is awake or asleep. Skin-to-skin contact is thought to be especially important for your baby during his first few days and weeks—this will help him to feel secure and reassured that you are there. It is also recommended that your baby be in the same room as you (not the same bed, as this can increase the risk of SIDS[35]) when he sleeps for the first six months.

SOOTHING A NONHUNGRY, FUSSING BABY

Your baby will still cry from time to time even if you do these two things. This is completely normal, but it doesn't mean that it's not stressful. As time goes on you will get to know your baby's temperament. Some babies are naturally a bit fussier or crankier than others, and there are times when a baby will be more or less fussy than usual. As you get to know your baby, you'll find it easier to interpret what he needs—whether this is feeding, comfort, a diaper change, entertainment or something else. Some parents claim that over time they get to know what a "hunger cry" sounds like versus crying for some other reason. This is probably the exception rather than the rule, so don't worry if you can't. In one study the parents who reported being able to identify a hunger cry were doing it based on the time of day, not the acoustic characteristics of the cry itself.[36] In fact, research on the acoustics of infant crying has shown that parents are no better than inexperienced adults at distinguishing the emotions behind the cries of babies less than six months old[37]—but it gets easier as they get older.

This means the best way to find out what is wrong is by a process of elimination—test one thing at a time to check for a problem—and only feed your baby if he is signaling that he is hungry.

> "Although responding will often soothe a baby's crying, parents are only partly in charge of this situation. Some bouts of crying in the first few months are difficult or impossible to soothe, but most of these infants are healthy and grow and develop perfectly normally."
> —Ian St. James-Roberts, emeritus professor of child psychology, Institute of Education, University College London

Using a Pacifier

Pacifiers have gone in and out of fashion over the years, but there is enough evidence to suggest that they are worth using to try to calm your baby if he is fussing, and routinely when he is put down for sleep. Pediatricians widely regard sucking as one of the best possible ways to calm a crying baby—it is also a potent pain relief for young babies—and a pacifier may satisfy your baby's need or desire to suck without providing unnecessary milk (through what is called "nonnutritive" sucking).

There is another big benefit, too: The AAP now recommends offering your baby a pacifier during a nap and at bedtime to reduce the risk of SIDS.[38] A review suggested that for every 2,733 babies who are given a pacifier when put to sleep, one SIDS death could be prevented.[39] The risk of SIDS is highest during the first six months, after which pacifier use doesn't really provide much benefit. However, be aware that it may also slightly increase the risk of minor infections (such as ear infections), so weaning your baby off a pacifier after six months is probably wise, and is recommended. It is also recommended that a baby doesn't use a pacifier past two years of age to reduce the risk of developing oral problems.

You may have heard that using a pacifier too early can interfere with breastfeeding, the theory being that sucking on a pacifier is different from sucking on a breast. But a review of four randomized controlled trials found no evidence for this—there was no difference in the breastfeeding rates of babies who were randomized to use a pacifier and those who weren't.[40] So, this is probably a myth. To be on the safe side, we would suggest that you only introduce a pacifier once breastfeeding has been properly established. And do bear in mind that not all babies will respond well to a pacifier, so don't force it if your baby rejects it, but it's worth a try. If you do use one, make sure you offer it consistently at every sleep (day and night) and sterilize it as you would a bottle.

Nighttime Wakings

You don't necessarily have to feed your baby every time he wakes during the night. You only need to feed him if he indicates that he is hungry. This will be a lot of the time when he is really tiny, but less of the time as he gets older. Instead of feeding being your first go-to, try the following:

- Wait for a couple of minutes to see if he will settle on his own (lengthening the wait time as he gets a bit older).

- If not, try soothing techniques besides feeding if he is not indicating any signs of hunger.

- Feed him if he is hungry.

- Make sure that nighttime visits are short and quiet so that he doesn't expect stimulation time in the middle of the night.

The researchers who coined the phrase the "period of purple crying" say one thing is pretty certain when it comes to young babies and crying: "Some things work some of the time, but nothing works all of the time."[41] So, don't feel that you have done something wrong or that you are failing your baby as a parent if you cannot seem to stop him crying no matter what you do. The organization Period of Purple Crying provides evidence-based information to support parents in dealing with excessive infant crying (purplecrying.info).

If, however, you are worried that something is very wrong, then take your baby to your pediatrician. There are a few things that can cause excessive crying that your doctor will be able to rule out, if you are worried. These can include under- and overfeeding (both of which are dealt with below), reflux, allergy and infection. The latter three are thought to only present in about 10 percent of babies who cry excessively.[42]

Underfeeding and Overfeeding

One of the concerns with responsive feeding is how to know whether you are giving your baby enough or too much milk. Underfeeding is when a baby is not consuming sufficient calories for healthy growth, while overfeeding is consuming too many calories, leading to rapid weight gain. One of the biggest concerns of new parents is whether their baby is getting enough milk; few are concerned about overfeeding. Overfeeding is, in fact, more common, but underfeeding is more serious in the short term. Overfeeding is probably more of a problem with bottle-fed babies, but the issue of whether or not it is possible to overfeed a breastfeeding baby is a contentious one. And breastfed babies are thought to commonly experience a form of overfeeding called "functional lactose overload," which we discuss in more detail on pages 176–78.

UNDERFEEDING

Many parents become concerned if their baby does not drink as much milk as expected or as much as they were drinking a few days before. There is some developmental variation in the amount of milk a baby needs, and so a reduction in milk intake can simply be a reflection of the growth process. For example, at around four to five months of age there is a drop in the amount of energy needed (compared to three months) as a baby's rate of growth slows down. Nevertheless, there are some clear signs that point to underfeeding:

- There are fewer than five to six wet diapers in twenty-four hours (for babies older than five days).
- The baby is restless, unsettled, irritable and wakeful.
- Extremely undernourished babies can become excessively sleepy and nondemanding (lethargic, limp and difficult to wake up).
- There is poor (or no) weight gain over several days or weeks.

And here are some causes of underfeeding:

- poor appetite (high satiety sensitivity, low food responsiveness, slow feeding, low enjoyment of feeding)
- rigid feeding schedules rather than feeding in response to a baby's hunger cues
- low or no milk supply if breastfeeding (see pages 110–11)
- premature birth or illness affecting sucking ability
- congenital birth defects that affect ability to suck effectively (for example, tongue tie, cerebral palsy, cleft palate)
- incorrect preparation of formula (too much water to powder)
- giving a baby too much water (before six months babies should not have any water)
- sleep deprivation that causes a baby to be too exhausted to demand feedings, feed effectively or wake during the night for feedings.

What to do:

- Make an appointment with your pediatrician to have your baby assessed for a physical cause.
- If you have done this and there is no clear physical cause, ensure that you pay close attention to your baby's hunger cues. If he is not providing obvious hunger cues, then offer feedings at regular three- to four-hour intervals during the day to see if he will take one.
- Make sure you also still respond appropriately to his fullness cues and stop the feeding as soon as he indicates that he wants to stop. Don't try to force your baby to finish a feeding, even if you are worried about his weight gain, as this can lead to a feeding aversion.
- Make sure he is getting sufficient sleep.

OVERFEEDING

Overfeeding (or "overnutrition") is a common problem, especially for bottle-fed newborn babies (birth to three months old). It is a problem that is overlooked because of the emphasis that is still placed on babies gaining sufficient weight, even if weight gain is excessive. Though it is easier for bottle-fed than breastfed babies to overfeed, it is still possible for a breastfed baby to overfeed of his own accord if he has a voracious appetite for milk. The main symptom of appetite-based overfeeding is rapid weight gain (see pages 76–77).

Causes of overfeeding:

- Baby has an avid appetite and the parent offers feedings too frequently and not simply in response to hunger cues.
- Baby has an avid appetite and the parent offers too much milk in the bottle during feedings (for example, more than he needs/is recommended—see Table 1 on page 181).
- The parent doesn't recognize satiety cues.
- The parent actively encourages baby to feed past satiety.

What to do:

- Feed responsively—only feed when your baby indicates he is hungry and stop when he indicates he is full.
- Don't offer too much milk in the bottle at each feeding (see Table 1 for how much milk to feed).
- Check he isn't feeding too quickly. If necessary, slow down feedings by stopping and taking regular burping breaks, or use a slower-flowing nipple if bottle-feeding. If your baby drinks very quickly, tip the bottle down or remove it for a minute to slow down his drinking pace.

Functional Lactose Overload

Another form of overfeeding that is less well known and under-researched is called functional lactose overload—a common problem related to breast milk oversupply syndrome and overfeeding in formula-fed infants.[43] The Australian Breastfeeding Association estimates that as many as two thirds of breastfed babies experience episodic symptoms associated with this form of overfeeding in the first three months, with a small percentage being affected up to six months.[44] It can also occur in bottle-fed babies, but we don't know how common it is. Functional lactose overload (not to be confused with lactose *intolerance*, which is rare) is thought to occur when babies consume a large amount of lactose and are unable to digest it properly. In formula-fed babies, this can happen from simply consuming too much formula milk and becoming overloaded with the sheer amount of lactose consumed. In breastfeeding babies, researchers have proposed that it occurs when they don't get enough fat from the breast milk. The fat content of breast milk changes over the course of a feeding, with the milk at the end of the feeding containing more fat than the milk at the beginning (see pages 121–22). This creamier "hind" milk slows down the transit speed of the milk through the intestine, allowing the lactose to be absorbed and stimulating the release of a satiety hormone called cholecystokinin, which makes the baby feel full. If a mom has an oversupply of milk or she switches her baby onto the other breast too soon, her baby won't get enough of the creamier hindmilk. A recent paper on this topic suggested that some common breastfeeding practices may be contributing to functional lactose overload:[45]

- *Limiting feedings to a defined period and not allowing for cluster feeding*
  Cluster feeding is when a baby feeds every thirty to sixty minutes, usually during the evening. The milk your baby takes during these feedings tends to be low in volume and high in fat.

- *Always offering the fuller side first*
  This means that your baby will always get a lot of the high-volume and low-fat milk.

- *Always feeding from both sides*
  Although this is very important in the early days and weeks to get your milk supply up, it can mean that your baby doesn't get as much of the creamy, high-fat hindmilk, which he enjoys if he is able to finish all of the milk in one breast.

- *Expressing milk and feeding it through a bottle*
  A breast pump may not be all that great at getting the hindmilk out.

If the milk goes through your baby's intestine too quickly, he won't feel properly sated and the lactose won't be fully digested; instead it will ferment in his colon.[46] Babies with functional lactose overload cry and fuss a lot more, which isn't in the least bit surprising when you read the list of symptoms! Functional lactose overload can lead to excessive weight gain, but not always, because the excess nutrients are not always digested and are sometimes excreted. This, according to these researchers, can lead to symptoms arising from fermentation of undigested lactose in the baby's large intestine (hence why overfeeding is often called "lactose overload") including

- poor satiety and wanting to feed frequently
- crying
- milk regurgitation
- belching due to swallowing a lot of air while feeding too quickly
- frequent sloppy, foul-smelling bowel movements if formula-fed; watery, explosive bowel movements if breastfed
- extreme flatulence
- bloating and cramps leading to fussing, crying and irritability
- sleep disturbance.

Ironically, a mom with oversupply syndrome may think she has an undersupply, because her baby always wants to feed. But, according to the theory, repeated low-fat feeds will only aggravate the problem. Researchers in this field suggest that functional lactose overload is entirely rectifiable through breastfeeding-management techniques—it doesn't signal an inherent problem with Mom's milk, nor does it indicate any type of lactose intolerance in the baby. Functional lactose overload is a poorly recognized problem among health professionals and one that is often missed or overlooked when there are feeding problems.[47] The Australian Breastfeeding Association has some tips on its website for feeding strategies that can be introduced to resolve it,[48] but it is best to seek advice from an international board-certified lactation consultant if you are concerned about this, because there is unlikely to be a "one size fits all" solution. Tailored advice for you and your baby will be much more effective. Do bear in mind, though, that lots of these symptoms are common and will happen from time to time anyway. But lots of them together, and for several days or weeks continually, is a sign that there might be a problem. Also be aware that the science around this is sparse.

How Much and How Often Babies Need to Feed

How much and how often your baby needs feeding during the first six months will depend on age, sex, size (body weight) and individual appetite. Newborn babies have a tiny stomach (it holds about 0.7 ounce [20 ml][49]) and are growing very quickly so need small feedings very frequently. As they mature, they are able to take larger feedings and their growth rate slows down slightly, as well; this means they don't need to feed quite as often. Boys tend to be born slightly heavier than girls and this weight difference remains, so on average boys need a little more milk than girls. Babies born slightly heavier have higher energy requirements than smaller babies so need more milk both to maintain their weight and to grow.

In 2005 the NAM provided recommended calorie intakes per day for babies during their first year of life: Between birth and six months of age, girls should have 520 calories per day and boys should have 570 calories per day; from seven to twelve months of age, girls should have 676 calories per day and boys should have 743 calories per day).[50] However, these are just guidelines, not hard and fast rules, as all babies are different. The key advice is to trust your baby and feed responsively. These recommendations are due to be updated in 2020.

In reality it is impossible to know how many calories your baby is consuming if he is breastfed, even if you are expressing, because breast milk varies in calories over the course of a feeding and from one feeding to the next. Once breastfeeding is properly established, each breast contains about 6 ounces (180 ml) of milk, which is far more than most young babies would consume during a single feeding.[51] But the storage capacity of a breast does vary from woman to woman (from about 2.5 to 13 ounces/75 to 380 ml). So, while it is important to keep an eye on the number of feedings your baby is taking, making sure your baby is gaining weight at an optimal rate is the best indication that feeding is going well (along with diaper checks!). Weight gain is discussed in detail in Chapter 3.

For formula-fed babies, it is possible, in theory, to work out how much milk to feed your baby each day. But translating energy requirements for babies of different ages into the right number of feedings per day, the amount of milk per feeding and the total amount of milk per day is a tricky business. For a start, the guidelines provided by manufacturers vary from one brand to another. On top of this, different brands don't always describe the same ages, making it difficult to compare.

The AAP provides rough guidelines for *how much* milk at each feeding formula-fed babies should be consuming during the first six months.[52] These are shown in Table 1. The guidance on how much and how often to feed takes into account the smaller amount of milk required during the first two weeks. As babies mature over the first few months, they are able to take more milk at each feeding and therefore require fewer feedings. As a rough guide, babies need about 2.5 ounces (75 ml) per day for every pound (453 g) of body weight. According to the AAP, your baby shouldn't be consuming more than 32 ounces (960 ml) over twenty-four hours, so if your baby seems to want more than this regularly, speak to your pediatrician.

These guidelines on the number and size of feedings may differ slightly from those provided by the formula product, as manufacturer guidelines are not always completely in line with best practices. In the UK, for example, manufacturers suggest *too few* feedings (with a larger volume per feeding) during the first few weeks, and the suggested volumes at each age fit bottle size rather than the energy requirements of the baby.[53] Offering very young babies too large a volume of milk at each feeding can be problematic on two counts:

1. The baby consumes too much milk (more than is needed) at each feeding, leading to overfeeding and risk of excessive weight gain (see pages 175–76).

2. The baby can't manage the larger volume of milk offered (and shouldn't necessarily be consuming that much all in one go), and parents feel anxious.

So, we recommend going with the AAP's guidance. However, bear in mind that these are *just guidelines*. The appetites of different babies can vary and change over time. On some days your baby will be more or less hungry than usual. This is completely normal, as babies' appetites can change a bit from day to day, especially if they are having a growth spurt or their growth rate slows down. It is important not to become fixated on exact amounts and numbers of feedings, as long as your baby is growing and developing well. *How* you feed, and feeding responsively, is as important as *what* and *how much* you feed.

TABLE 1: FORMULA FEEDING GUIDANCE FROM BIRTH TO SIX MONTHS[54]

Age	Amount of milk	Number of feeds per 24 hours
First two days	10–15 ml (0.3–0.5 ounces) per feeding	8–12 feeds
Three to four days, to two weeks	30–60 ml (1–2 ounces) per feeding	7–8 feeds
Two weeks	Increasing to 60–90 ml (2–3 ounces) per feeding	6–7 feeds
One month	At least 120 ml (4 ounces) per feeding	6–7 feeds
Two months	120–150 ml (4–5 ounces) per feeding	5–6 feeds
Four months	125–180 ml (4–6 ounces) per feeding	5 feeds
Six months	180–240 ml (6–8 ounces) per feeding	4–5 feeds

The AAP does not provide guidance on number of feeds per day, so this should only be used as a guide. By feeding responsively, feeding frequency will be led by your child.

Use a baby-tracking app or keep a little diary—on your phone or on a pad of paper—of your baby's feeding patterns, sleeping patterns and behaviors such as crying. This will help you to spot patterns in his behavior and will help you to get to know your baby. It might take some time, but you will learn what his feeding and sleeping patterns are, and you can respond accordingly. No one will know your baby better than you do.

THE BOTTOM LINE

- Not all babies are the same when it comes to milk—some will happily guzzle milk whenever it is offered; others don't seem to want it at all.

- *How* to feed is about understanding what type of feeder your baby is and feeding him appropriately, using responsive feeding strategies.

- This means getting to know your baby and his feeding styles right from the beginning.

- Never encourage or force your baby to carry on feeding when he has indicated that he is full—this can lead to overfeeding for an avid feeder, and food aversion for a baby with a poor appetite.

- It is easier to overfeed a baby through a bottle than from your breast, but it is still possible to overfeed a breastfeeding baby.

- Crying a lot is very common during the first three months—it can be incredibly stressful if excessive, but most of the time it doesn't mean there is anything wrong with your baby, and it doesn't necessarily mean he is hungry.

- Don't use feeding as your go-to strategy to soothe your baby if he is crying—only offer him milk if you think he is hungry.

Introducing Solid Foods

NTRODUCING SOLID FOODS (known as complementary feeding) after you have been feeding your baby only milk can seem like a daunting task. There is a lot of information out there—when to start, which foods to start with and how to do it—and this can be confusing. We want to help you navigate what can be a tricky topic, bringing to bear the research we have done ourselves and the studies we have read. In Part 3 we will provide you with advice on solids—*when, what* and *how* to introduce them, based on what the science says.

Being introduced to solid foods can be an exciting time for a baby—his diet finally deviates from the monotony of milk, and he begins to experience a whole range of new textures and flavors. But it can be stressful for some parents, especially when things don't go as planned—for example, when your baby refuses to try certain foods or doesn't seem to be eating anything at all. We will guide you through every aspect of the complementary feeding process and will offer practical advice that we hope will reduce the chance of your baby becoming excessively fussy, maximize his preference for nutrient-dense foods such as vegetables, and enable him to develop a varied diet that will set him up for many years to come.

Our aim is to ensure that you meet your baby's changing nutritional needs and support him in developing his ability to self-regulate his food intake, helping him to grow up healthy, happy and with a good relationship with food.

CHAPTER 7

When to Introduce
Solid Foods

omplementary feeding is the term used to describe the introduction of solid foods and other drinks alongside breast milk or formula. The optimal age at which to introduce solid foods is one of the most debated topics in infant nutrition. Countries (and even organizations within the same country) often have different views, which can make it confusing for parents. It is generally agreed that introducing solid food *before seventeen weeks of age* (less than four months) can be harmful to your baby: He doesn't yet have the ability to swallow food safely (even if puréed); his digestive system and kidneys are not mature enough to be able to handle anything other than breast milk or formula; and there may also be an increased risk of infection, some allergies and later obesity.[1] But what is less clear is whether it is best to wait until six months for all babies, or to introduce solid food between four months (seventeen weeks) and six months, depending on a baby's particular needs or readiness.

In line with the World Health Organization (WHO), the American Academy of Pediatrics (AAP) recommends exclusive breastfeeding for approximately six months, followed by continued breastfeeding for at least one year as complementary foods are introduced (the WHO recommends continuing to breastfeed for two years or beyond).[2] The AAP also provides a general recommendation to introduce solid foods at about six months for all infants, which includes those who are formula-fed.[3] Other countries such as the UK also recommend waiting until your baby is about six months old. But several organizations consider any time between seventeen weeks (four months) and six months to be safe and acceptable, including the European Society for Paediatric Gastroenterology, Hepatology and Nutrition (ESPGHAN), the European Food Safety Authority, the British Dietetic Association, the European Academy of Allergy and Clinical Immunology, and the American Academy of Allergy, Asthma and Immunology. So why do organizations take a different view, and what is the best age to introduce your baby to solid foods?

There is general agreement that babies' iron stores start to deplete at around four to six months of age, which introduces concerns about iron deficiency (anemia), especially for exclusively breastfed infants, because breast milk is low in iron (although iron is absorbed more easily from breast milk than from formula), and this is around the time that a baby needs to start sourcing his iron from food.[4] Iron is crucial for healthy growth and development in infancy, and deficiency can result in cognitive and psychomotor problems, suggesting that some infants may need iron from other food sources earlier than six months. On the other hand, introducing solid foods before six months displaces breast milk, which provides some protection against infection, and introducing solid food earlier than six months may increase the risk of infection. The crux of the timing issue is sometimes referred to as the "weanling's dilemma"—timing of introduction to solids must weigh the benefits of breast milk against the possibility that milk alone is insufficient to satisfy a baby's energy and nutrient requirements beyond four months of age.

These issues are unlikely to be relevant for babies who are predominantly fed formula, because formula doesn't protect against infection and is nutritionally complete with iron and other necessary nutrients to support a baby up to six months. But, although there is very little evidence about the optimal age at which to introduce solid food to formula-fed babies, they are treated like breastfed babies for the purpose of the guidelines. So, if your baby is on formula, do you still need to wait until six months to move him on to solid food? This applies to a large number of babies in the US: 29 percent have received formula before three months and 35 percent before six months; in fact, only 25 percent of babies are *exclusively* breastfed to six months.[5] And what about parents of exclusively breastfed babies who think their baby is ready for food earlier than six months? A national survey in the US found that 55 percent of parents had offered solid foods before their baby was six months old.[6] The US Department of Agriculture's Special Supplemental Nutrition Program for Women, Infants, and Children (WIC) began its Infant and Toddler Feeding and Practices Study in 2013 and found that 20 percent of low-income infants were introduced to infant cereals, fruits, vegetables or meats before four months of age.[7]

What Does the Evidence Say?

The recommendation by the WHO to wait until six months to introduce solid foods (and subsequently adopted by many countries globally, such as the US) is based almost entirely on a review first commissioned by the WHO in 2002[8] and updated in 2012.[9] The review examined whether there were differences in short- and long-term health outcomes for babies who were exclusively breastfed for six months compared to those exclusively breastfed for three to four months (with solid foods introduced thereafter and breastfeeding continued alongside to six months). The health outcomes of moms were studied, too, and evidence was examined separately for twelve high and eleven low- and middle-income countries. All of the studies undertaken in high-income countries that were included in the review were observational; there were no randomized controlled trials at the time, which means that the quality of the evidence in the review isn't very high for high-income countries. But there have been trials undertaken in Iceland and the UK since the review was published, and this adds important information about the optimal timing of introduction to solids for infants in high-income countries. Two high-quality trials in low-income countries were included in the review (both conducted in Honduras). Bear in mind that this review only compared babies who were all exclusively breastfed for at least three to four months; it did not compare breastfed and formula-fed babies, and there is very little research into the best time to introduce solid foods for babies fed formula milk. The recommendation to wait until six months for all babies is based solely on research on breastfed babies.

WHAT ARE THE BENEFITS OF WAITING UNTIL SIX MONTHS TO INTRODUCE SOLID FOODS?

Of the studies undertaken in higher-income countries, the review from 2012 reported that in the largest study done in Belarus, slightly fewer babies who were breastfed exclusively for six months had one or more gastrointestinal infections in the first year of life than those who were breastfed for only three to four months (5 percent versus 7.4 percent). None of the studies indicated any differences in early growth, and the largest study in Belarus showed no differences in height, weight, body mass index, tooth decay, cognitive ability or behavior later on in childhood. In addition, studies from Finland, Australia and Belarus showed no difference in risk of allergies (including eczema, asthma and other allergic diseases). As far as the moms were concerned, the benefits of breastfeeding for six months rather than three to four were seen only among women in low-income countries (Honduras, Bangladesh and Senegal), of whom a slightly larger proportion were still not having periods at six months, and women in Honduras had lost slightly more weight at four to six months after giving birth (but the amount was trivial—about 1 pound/0.4 kg).

So, the review suggested that in higher-income countries exclusive breastfeeding for six months has a slight benefit over three to four in terms of reduced gastrointestinal infection risk for the baby (in Belarus), but nothing else. However, since this review was published, a recent high-quality study of more than 70,000 infants (including 22,000 sibling pairs) from Norway found no difference in infection rates between breastfed infants introduced to solid foods at four to six months versus after six months, indicating that introduction to solid foods at four to six months does not necessarily increase the risk of infection in high-income countries with relatively low infection rates.[10]

ARE THERE ANY DOWNSIDES TO WAITING UNTIL SIX MONTHS TO INTRODUCE SOLID FOODS?

A review of the trials from Honduras and Iceland found that breastfed babies introduced to solids at six months had lower iron levels than those introduced to solids at four months,[11] suggesting that babies may benefit from being introduced to iron-rich foods alongside breastfeeding from four months, even in high-income countries with low risk of deficiency. More recently, and since the WHO-commissioned review was published, new evidence has also been emerging that early introduction to certain allergenic foods may reduce the risk of developing an allergy to those foods. In particular, the introduction of peanuts between four and eleven months and cooked egg between four and six months significantly reduces the risk of allergies to both.[12] However, there is insufficient evidence that babies benefit from having these foods introduced *before* six months rather than *at* six months, because few studies have compared introduction at four versus six months (allergies are discussed in more detail on pages 221–22).

WHAT AGE SHOULD YOU GO WITH?

The evidence suggests that babies who are breastfed exclusively for six months compared to three to four may experience slightly fewer gastrointestinal infections, without any real detriment in growth or other outcomes, although it's not entirely clear if babies in all high-income countries necessarily benefit to the same extent. The downside of waiting until six months to introduce solids is that iron levels are compromised slightly. However, the AAP recommends that babies be given iron supplementation from four months of age, making this less of a concern for US babies who follow this guidance.[13] So, weighing the pros and cons, it makes sense to wait until six months to introduce solid foods if you are exclusively breastfeeding your baby, he is growing and developing well and it is working well for you. But babies can differ in their needs, so the best way to make sure that waiting until six months is best for your baby is to take him for his regular well-child care visits during the first six months and discuss this with your pediatrician.

Although there is virtually no research to draw on to provide any helpful guidance for the best time to introduce solid foods to babies who are mainly formula-fed, they don't seem to need to be introduced to solid foods before six months. This is because they receive adequate nutrition from formula until then. But again, babies may differ in their needs, and when to start your baby on solid foods if he is formula-fed will depend on his health and development, which your pediatrician will be able to advise you on.

Can Solids Be Introduced Too Late?

In short, yes. Just as introducing solids too early (before seventeen weeks) can be detrimental to your baby, it is also important not to leave it too late. Although there are no specific guidelines on this in the US, the ESPGHAN committee on nutrition recommends that complementary foods can be introduced from seventeen weeks and should be introduced *no later than six months*.[14] Nutritionally, exclusively breast-fed babies need iron and other micronutrients such as zinc from six months, and introducing solids allows you the opportunity to provide him with iron-rich foods. But there are other important reasons, too. Learning to chew and swallow are crucial parts of your baby's development. The way that the muscles of the mouth and tongue are used to drink milk differs greatly from the processes required to eat solid food, even when it is puréed. Introducing solid food at the right time (approximately six months) therefore helps your baby develop his mouth and tongue muscles to learn how to eat. In addition, the training that your baby undergoes when learning to eat solid foods also helps him to develop the necessary muscles for speech. If you leave it too late, you risk the chance of your child having impaired oral development. Research also suggests that babies who are introduced to solid foods after one year are less accepting of new textures.[15] This is thought to have a long-lasting impact and points to the importance of introducing texture by twelve months at the very latest. If your baby is six months old and not yet showing signs that he is ready (see pages 191–92), seek advice from your pediatrician.

Some researchers have also suggested that there may be a period during which babies are more accepting of new *tastes* (between four and seven months of age). For example, one study conducted in the UK examined whether the age solid foods were introduced (either before five and a half months of age or after) influenced acceptance of vegetables in a group of sixty babies.[16] Over a period of nine days, half the babies in each age group were given either a variety of vegetables (zucchini, parsnip and sweet potato) or a single vegetable (carrot) and then their acceptance of a new vegetable (pea) was assessed. The babies who were given the variety of vegetables after five and a half months ate more pea purée than those given a single vegetable, but the younger infants were accepting of the new vegetables regardless of exposure to either variety or a single vegetable. This suggested two things:

1. There may be a window for the acceptance of new tastes or flavors.

2. Babies who move on to solid foods at six months or later might benefit from being given a variety of tastes rapidly.

However, this was a very small study, and far more research is needed to confirm the idea that there is a window for taste preferences.

Although the guidance is to introduce solid foods at about six months, every baby is unique, and some babies vary in their readiness. We feel that age is not the only factor that should determine when you start introducing solids. It is also important to look out for signs that your baby is ready for solid food.

Key Signs Your Baby Is Ready for Solids

Generally there are three key signs that you can look out for to help you decide whether your baby might be ready to move on from milk to solid food:

1. He can sit upright and hold his head up. This is important to ensure he can swallow food.

2. He has good hand-eye coordination so he can look at food, pick it up and put it in his own mouth.

3. He can swallow food. If your baby is not ready, he will use his tongue to push the food back out of his mouth (this is known as the tongue thrust reflex).

If your baby is showing all of the above signs and is six months old, then you can feel confident that he is ready to start solids.

MYTH BUSTING

These three signs are the most common ways to tell that your baby is ready to start solid foods. There are some things that are often mistaken as signs a baby is ready, including

- Chewing fists: To eat food, your baby needs to be able to move his tongue to the back of his mouth and swallow. If your baby is chewing on his fist, this does not tell you he is able to swallow; he might just be teething or playing with his hands.

- Reaching for food: It is normal for babies to be interested in new things, and this on its own does not tell you that your baby is ready to eat what you are eating.

- Waking in the night when he used to sleep through: Research suggests that parents will offer solid foods before six months because they believe it will help their baby sleep longer. A CDC study, for example, found that 46.4 percent of almost 1,500 mothers did so for this reason.[17] Until recently there had been virtually no research into whether introducing solid foods before six months helps babies to sleep for longer, but a few small studies indicated that it didn't.[18] But very recently the first large trial of 1,300 British breastfed babies explored whether introducing allergenic solid foods from three versus six months affected babies' sleep.[19] Results showed that babies in the early introduction group slept longer and woke less often than infants in the standard introduction group, but the effect was small. The findings need replicating before we can be clear about whether introducing solids really aids infant sleep. It is best to start your baby on solid foods because he is developmentally ready, not as a means to get him to sleep for longer.

- Wanting extra milk feeds: This means that your baby is hungry or thirsty, but it does not necessarily mean that he needs more than just milk.

These are normal baby behaviors and, unless they are occurring with the three key signs listed in the box on page 191, your baby is not necessarily ready to move on from milk. What's important is that your baby's digestive system is ready for solid foods and that he is able to swallow them, not necessarily how big or small he is.

WHEN TO INTRODUCE LUMPS AND TEXTURES

Unfortunately, there have been very few studies of the age of introduction of lumps and the acceptance of food later. However, a large study of over 8,000 British babies, called the Avon Longitudinal Study of Parents and Children, showed that children who were introduced to foods with lumps between six and nine months had a more varied diet at fifteen months and seven years of age and fewer feeding difficulties (not eating enough, refusing food, being choosy with food, overeating and having difficulty getting into a feeding routine) at seven years than children who were introduced to lumps after ten months.[20]

The problem with this study is that it was observational rather than experimental (such as a randomized controlled trial). This means that it could have been some other unmeasured factor that caused the feeding difficulties in the children introduced to lumps later, rather than the timing of the introduction of lumpy food per se. For example, parents whose babies were genetically predisposed to have a poorer appetite and be picky eaters may have delayed offering them lumpy foods until after ten months, but these babies were more likely to grow into picky eaters with poorer appetites anyhow, by virtue of their genetic endowment. Nevertheless, given that there is no harm in introducing your baby to lumpy foods from six months of age, it is probably a good idea to move your baby on to lumps as soon as he indicates he is ready and not to leave it too late. Parents who use "baby-led weaning" introduce lumps and textures right from the start, and this is perfectly fine (see pages 196–97).

Premature Babies

Compared to term babies, premature babies are sometimes delayed in reaching developmental milestones. Some have difficulty managing lumpy foods, and it is thought that introducing solid food to premature babies too early may contribute to the development of food fussiness. If your baby was premature, we would recommend speaking with your pediatrician before introducing solid foods, to make sure that he is developmentally ready.

THE BOTTOM LINE

- Introducing solid food is a crucial period for establishing acceptance of tastes and textures and speech development.

- Introducing solids before seventeen weeks (four months) could be harmful.

- Evidence suggests that exclusively breastfeeding your baby for six months may provide him with some protection against infection.

- Do not delay the introduction of solids beyond six months of age if your baby is healthy.

- Breastfeeding along with solid foods will ensure that your baby continues to receive the benefits of breast milk.

- Look out for signs your baby is ready for solid food. If this is before six months, speak to your pediatrician.

CHAPTER 8

How to Introduce Solid Foods

As well as having to think about *when* to introduce solid food, another decision is *how* you're going to do it. The two main methods used are spoon-feeding your baby (puréed or mashed food) and baby-led weaning (BLW), a term that originated in the UK to describe the method of introducing complementary foods whereby the baby feeds himself handheld foods instead of being spoon-fed by an adult. In this chapter we describe the two methods, including the evidence for each, so you can make an informed decision on which is best for you and your baby.

Spoon-Feeding

This traditional method of introducing solids involves gradually moving a baby from milk to solid food by puréeing foods and feeding them to him with a soft spoon. Babies are then moved on to thicker textures (mashed foods rather than purées), and this way they gradually learn how to move food around in their mouth and swallow it. Eventually they are able to chew food into smaller pieces and can be given soft finger foods. Advocates of this approach suggest it is a smooth transition from liquid to solid foods and the baby develops the oral skills necessary for safer eating.

Spoon-feeding allows you to see how much your baby is eating and means that you know he is getting energy and nutrients, which can be reassuring. However, it can be time-consuming preparing purées from scratch and costly if you buy ready-made ones. In addition, it has been suggested that it is possible to overfeed your baby if you control the spoon. But just as is the case with milk-feeding, this depends on *how* you feed your baby. In Chapter 6 we covered some of the ways to tell if your baby is full or if he is hungry when he is milk-feeding. The same principles apply with solid food—it is crucial to feed *responsively*, whichever method you decide to use. Feed your baby promptly when he indicates that he is hungry and pay close attention to his satiety signals so that you stop feeding when he is full. This will help your baby to develop good appetite regulation when he moves on to solid food. We will explain how to do this in detail beginning at page 201.

Baby-Led Weaning

Baby-led weaning (BLW) has become quite popular in the US in recent years, and it does what it says—the baby takes the lead in the feeding process when they move on to solid food (alongside breast milk or formula). The term was originally coined by Gill Rapley in 2001, a former midwife in the UK. The basis of this method is that you decide *what* to offer, but your baby feeds himself. In theory, this means that your baby decides whether or not to eat the food at all, how much of the food to eat and how quickly to eat it. Parents often provide chunks of soft food or finger food and their baby explores the food by touching it, putting it in his mouth and feeding himself. It is therefore recommended that you wait until six months of age if you decide to do BLW, by which age most babies are able to do this. BLW advocates suggest this approach promotes greater participation in family meals, which is a great way for babies to imitate healthy eating behaviors and learn how adults eat. It is thought to provide babies with exposure to family foods and helps a child become independent—developing skills such as hand-eye coordination—and learn by themselves when they are hungry and full. In addition, it has been suggested that babies may accept textures more readily, as proper fully formed foods (with all their textures and lumps), rather than purées, are introduced immediately.

This method is less time-consuming than preparing purées from scratch, but it is messier and it is not always possible to see how much your baby has actually eaten. Be prepared for a lot of the food to end up on the floor! It is also important to keep in mind that it can be unsafe to provide your baby with finger foods if he isn't yet ready. So, it is important to consider his readiness cues, as opposed to his age, in order to introduce solid foods safely (see page 191). Babies who are developmentally delayed with motor skills, such as crawling or walking, might struggle with BLW, as their hand-eye coordination may also be delayed. Some health professionals also worry that babies may not be able to eat enough if feeding themselves, especially when they are very young, and there have been particular concerns about babies getting sufficient iron intake because the consistency of foods rich in iron can make them challenging for babies to self-feed. Foods that are easy for babies to hold themselves—such as fruits and steamed or cooked vegetables—are most commonly offered, but these are generally low in both iron and calories. Some parents are also concerned about the possibility of their baby choking with BLW, though there is currently no evidence to suggest that choking is more likely with BLW than with spoon-feeding.[1] However, as with spoon-feeding, it is important to ensure your baby is sitting upright and is supervised at all times while eating.

Top Tips to Avoid Choking

Whichever method you choose, it is important to know the difference between choking and gagging. When babies are introduced to solid foods, they will often gag, usually because the food is cold, they have too much of it in their mouth or they don't like what they are eating. Gagging is a very natural reflex in babies, designed to bring up whatever is in their throat, and will involve the child coughing and spluttering. It can be quite frightening for parents, but it is nothing to worry about and, crucially, it is very different from choking. Choking is when something is stuck in the back of the baby's throat, blocking their airway and stopping them from breathing. If your child is choking, there will be no sound, your child may begin to turn blue, they will look frightened and they may put their arms out to you looking for help. The CDC provides guidance on how to help a choking baby, and the AAP (healthychildren.org) has a useful short film ("Choking Hazards Parents of Young Children Should Know About").

1. Always supervise your child when he is feeding.

2. Ensure your child is sitting upright in a high chair when feeding.

3. Be aware of problematic foods such as cherry tomatoes and grapes—these should be cut in quarters, to avoid the risk of choking.

4. Whole nuts, including peanuts, should not be given to children under the age of five because of the risk of choking.

5. Know the difference between choking and gagging: Choking is life-threatening, while gagging is a normal part of experiencing foods for the first time.

Which Method of Complementary Feeding to Choose?

There have been very few well-designed studies comparing BLW and spoon-feeding. So, in spite of its growing popularity, the benefits that advocates of the BLW approach promote are based largely on intuition, not evidence. A major problem with the few (mostly small) studies that have been conducted in the past is that moms who choose BLW often differ in important ways to the general population who use traditional spoon-feeding—on average they breastfeed for longer, are wealthier, more educated, older, more likely to be married and more confident.[2] This means that we can't know what the impact of BLW really is on the baby, because all of these other factors probably influence the baby's development as well.

However, a large, well-designed randomized controlled trial was published recently that looked at whether BLW really results in a lower risk of overweight than spoon-feeding, whether it affected appetite regulation and whether or not babies are more likely to choke.[3] This two-year trial, called BLISS (Baby-Led Introduction to Solids), randomized 105 women to receive routine care and another 101 to receive additional support on BLW from pregnancy to nine months of age. Those women receiving additional support were given three contacts with a trained researcher who advised them on offering foods that are easy to pick up and eat from six months onward, responsive feeding (such as paying attention to hunger and satiety cues), and providing high-iron and high-energy foods at mealtimes. They were also given very detailed resources on how to feed in a baby-led manner, food ideas and recipe books for each age, and also information about choking. The study looked at how many babies had overweight or obesity at twelve and twenty-four months of age to see if there were differences according to whether they were weaned using BLW or spoon-feeding. There were no meaningful differences by group; at twenty-four months there were slightly more infants with overweight in the BLW group (10.3 percent) than in the spoon-fed group (6.4 percent), but this was not a statistically significant difference, which means it may have been due to chance.

However, the study suggested that BLW has an impact on appetite regulation, but not in the expected way. Babies who were weaned using BLW had more avid appetites insofar as they had *lower* satiety responsiveness (they were *less* sensitive to their fullness) and *greater* enjoyment of food at twenty-four months. This contradicts the idea that BLW may help children learn how to self-regulate, as these aspects of appetite put children at greater risk of obesity. A thoughtful commentary about this trial by experts in child feeding suggested that giving babies complete autonomy over how much they eat at such a young age provides the opportunity for those with an already avid appetite to overeat, as there are fewer parental boundaries in place to ensure they do not overeat, if they are that way inclined.[4] In light of this, it may still be important to be mindful about the portion sizes and types of finger foods that you offer when using this approach, so as to make sure babies with hearty appetites are not encouraged to overeat. While there were no big impacts on rates of overweight or obesity at twelve or twenty-four months, the impact on future weight is unknown and more research is needed.

On the plus side, the babies in the BLW group were less fussy about food and were no more likely to have a serious choking event, although they gagged more frequently at six months but not at eight months. Importantly, too, there was no difference in intakes of iron at either seven or twelve months of age, nor were there any differences in the babies' own iron levels at twelve months of age.[5] However, the parents in the study were specifically instructed to provide the babies with high iron foods, so if you are using a BLW approach it is important to do this (see page 226 for iron-rich foods). The babies in the BLW group did, however, consume more salt[6]—probably because they were eating more family foods, which are not all suitable for young infants. High salt intake can be harmful for babies, so it is important to be mindful about not giving your baby family foods with high levels of salt if using this approach (see pages 254–55 for more about how to limit salt intake). This important trial indicates that the method used to introduce solid food does not appear to impact importantly on weight gain or nutrition, but it does seem to increase appetite. The advantages of BLW are that it may help with preventing fussy eating and appears to be safe. Much more research is needed in this area to really know if one method offers significant benefits over the other. The European Society for Paediatric Gastroenterology, Hepatology and Nutrition committee on nutrition came to the same conclusion, following a recent review of the benefits of traditional spoon-feeding versus BLW, as did a recent independent review of the evidence.[7]

So, which method to go with? We recommend that you try to combine both approaches to give him the "best of both worlds." You can start by offering your baby spoon-fed puréed or mashed iron-rich foods (see page 226 for examples), but allow him to spoon-feed himself or control the spoon if he is able to. This will help ensure the development of the oral motor skills (tongue control, strength and stamina) necessary for chewing solid food, while giving him some autonomy over how much and how quickly he would like to eat. It will also encourage the intake of iron, important for cognitive development and the development of tissues, as puréed or mashed food is more likely to be ingested. This is especially important for breastfed babies given that breast milk is low in iron. But we would also recommend giving your baby something to hold and chew in between mouthfuls of spoon-fed food as well. This way your baby will not only obtain essential nutrients via puréed or mashed foods but will also take some control of his eating. It will help him to become familiar with the textures and appearances of different foods, too. But in the absence of any strong evidence for the superiority of one method over the other, you should feel free to choose whichever method you prefer.

Smooth foods, such as puréed broccoli, can be prepared by cooking or steaming them well and then using a blender to purée them.

Mashed foods are raw or cooked foods that are mashed, such as avocado mashed with a fork, so that they are slightly lumpy.

Finger foods are pieces of food that your baby can easily pick up, hold and feed himself. Ideally, finger foods are soft and easy to bite—for example, parboiled carrot or strips of banana. Take care not to offer finger foods with the seeds remaining, such as cherries, as they can be a choking hazard.

Responsive Feeding During Complementary Feeding

Whichever method you choose for introducing solid food, it is still important to feed your baby responsively—feed him when he indicates to you that he is hungry and stop when he indicates to you that he is full. This is just as important when it comes to food as it was when your baby was being fed only milk (we described how to feed responsively during milk-feeding in Chapter 6). Responsive feeding is thought to support babies and children in developing good appetite regulation.

Responsive feeding with solid foods has the same principles as it does with milk-feeding, except that there are a few more things to consider as your baby gets older and starts to move from a solely milk-based diet to other food. In other words, things get a bit more complicated! From decades of research, we know that there are four important components of responsive feeding that are thought to support your baby in developing good appetite regulation and a healthy relationship with food:[8]

1. **Let your child decide how much he wants to eat—don't pressure him.**

   A crucial part of responsive feeding is allowing him to eat only as much as he wants to satisfy his hunger. Never pressure him to eat more than he wants to. Examples of pressuring your child to eat are making him clear his plate even though he has had enough; refusing to let the meal finish until he has eaten certain foods, such as his vegetables; coercing him to eat a bit more than he wants to; punishment; and emotional blackmail (for example, "Mommy will be really upset if you don't eat your carrots"). Pressuring your child to eat can have detrimental consequences. For a child with a poor appetite it can lead to anxiety around food, food refusal and increasingly stressful mealtimes.[9] In fact, there is a reasonable amount of evidence to suggest that children whose parents pressure them excessively can have poorer weight gain over time and become even fussier than they were before.[10] So, although it can be frustrating when your child doesn't want to eat as much as you'd like him to, exerting large amounts of pressure on him is unlikely to help and can even make matters worse. It's best just to leave it up to him to decide. There are plenty of positive strategies you can use with your child if he has a poor appetite and is very fussy—these are discussed in detail in Chapter 10.

   On the flip side, it is also possible that pressuring a child to finish everything on the plate could potentially encourage him to ignore his hunger and satiety signals and *overeat*. Although the evidence for this theory is lacking, probably because parents only tend to pressure their child to eat if he has a poor appetite or is a picky eater—they don't tend to pressure the eager feeders simply because they don't need to! What we do know is that parental feeding strategies and child appetite is a two-way street: Children who are gaining weight too slowly and/or have poorer appetites are pressured by their parents more, but also children who are pressured more by their parents seem to become poorer eaters as time goes on, and their weight gain slows even more.[11] So, this is not a good strategy to use with poor feeders. Allowing your child to decide when he has had enough is a fundamental part of the BLW approach, but it is also possible to make sure you feed your child in a responsive way if he is being spoon-fed.

2. **Use covert rather than overt ways to restrict your child's intake of unhealthy food.**

As any parent will know, given the food environment that we live in today it is important to limit the amount of high-fat and high-sugar foods your child eats, to some extent. If you don't, and your child has a hearty appetite and a penchant for these foods, he may overeat, given the chance, and will be at risk of developing overweight. If your child has a poor appetite, the temptation might be to give him his favorite foods that are high in sugar and/or fat to make sure he eats something, but this can mean that he will fill up on less-nutritious foods and have an even poorer appetite for the more nutritious foods, such as vegetables, and certainly less interest in them. Whether restricting food is a good thing, a bad thing or totally pointless in terms of a child's appetite and weight gain is something that has been hotly debated for years. One large ongoing study showed that restriction seemed to protect young children from gaining excessive amounts of weight or developing overweight, but that it didn't work for older children (over ten years).[12] And lots of other studies haven't found any effect at all of parental restriction on children's weight gain, suggesting it doesn't work.[13] In fact, some imaginative early experimental research with a small number of children showed that restriction could even be a bad thing.[14] When young children's access to a particular fruit-bar cookie that they really liked was restricted (and placed in a transparent jar in front of them), their liking for it increased and they ate more of it when they were finally given access to it. This method of restriction is what researchers call "overt"—the child is completely aware of the food that they are not allowed, because they can see it. This study suggested that *overtly restricting* what a child is allowed to eat could actually backfire, because the children develop an even greater desire for the restricted food and will eat more of it when it is then freely available simply because they haven't been allowed it. This has been called the "forbidden-fruit effect"—we all want what we can't have, and children are no different in this respect.

So, what is the deal when it comes to restricting children—should you do it or not? The mixed findings in research probably reflect the fact that there are *different ways* to restrict your child's access to unhealthy food, and some ways may be better than others for your child's appetite and weight in the long run. *Overt* restriction—such as having a transparent jar of cookies on show in the kitchen that your child will ogle but isn't allowed access to—may have a detrimental effect. But *covert* restriction—restriction that your child cannot see and is unaware of (for example, not keeping chocolate bars in the house or not walking home from school via the bakery)—is probably a better way to restrict his access to foods (and drinks) high in sugar and fat, without increasing his desire for them. But restriction should never be excessive, and it doesn't have to mean that you always decide what he eats. Children also need to learn how to interact with these foods in a healthy way and that eating an appropriate amount of them from time to time is fine. A good strategy is to make sure that you give your baby a range of healthy food choices—for example, offering a choice of vegetables with his meal. This will help him to feel in control and have options to choose from, but you are able to make sure that there are boundaries to his active choices.

Although restriction might not seem important when your baby is still very young, it is something to be mindful of as soon as your baby starts to eat solid food, as he will become increasingly aware of the foods that are around him—in the house and out—and certainly of the foods that you are eating. An effective way of restricting foods high in sugar and fat and increasing your child's intake of nutritious foods is for you to lead by example—your child will do what you do, and we call this modeling. This is described in more detail on page 233.

3. **Offer him age-appropriate portion sizes.**
Regardless of the type of food that you offer your baby when starting on solids, it is important to make sure that you offer him a portion that is appropriate for his age (see page 260 for portion size guidance) and his appetite. Babies can still overeat on nutritious food. A baby with a big appetite—one who is less sensitive to his fullness and more responsive to food cues—will tend to eat more if it is there because it is harder for him to know when he is full, and because he enjoys eating. He will be guided more by the opportunity to eat than his internal feelings of hunger and fullness. Ensuring that the portion of food that you offer your baby is an appropriate size for his age (not too much) will help him to learn to eat only as much as he needs, and not more than he needs. If your baby indicates to you that he is still hungry after he has finished his food, you can offer him a small amount more. On the other hand, when it comes to a baby with a poor appetite, offering too much food can be overwhelming and even anxiety-provoking. For these babies, it is better to offer an amount that looks manageable. Again, once he has eaten it you can introduce a

little bit more food if he indicates that he is still hungry, but leave it to him to let you know.

4. **Offer food only in response to his hunger, not for any other reason.**

A fundamental part of responsive feeding is making sure that you only offer your child food because he is hungry or it is a meal- or snack-time, not for any other reason, such as comfort, entertainment or to control his behavior. If your baby is upset, irritable or just bored, the temptation is to offer him his favorite food to cheer him up, calm him down or keep him quiet. The problem is that research has suggested this lays the groundwork for learning to emotionally overeat—a habit that's difficult to break, and something that many older children and adults struggle with. Gemini—which was the first twin study into the origins of emotional eating in childhood—showed that emotional eating already starts to emerge during the early toddlerhood years and that it is entirely learned, not inherited (genes are unimportant in shaping a young toddler's tendency to do this).[15] With researchers from Norway, we used a large ongoing study of 1,000 families to show that offering a young child food in order to soothe him when he is upset teaches him to turn to food to control his emotions later on.[16] Emotional feeding tends to work best with toddlers who love their food (toddlers with no interest in food find little comfort in it being offered), but they are already at higher risk of developing overweight, so it is particularly important to not use this strategy with babies who are very food responsive. Using food to deal with negative emotions isn't only a concern in relation to overweight; it also means that children won't learn positive strategies for coping with unpleasant feelings. It is important to find nonfood strategies to comfort your baby if he is upset, such as giving him a cuddle or talking to him calmly and openly about how he is feeling.

Parents often use food for entertainment as well—we can all remember being given chocolate or candy as children to keep us quiet during a long car journey or at a wedding or other important event. But again, this can teach your baby to use food for entertainment and could lead to boredom eating. Instead, try giving him a toy or game to keep him occupied.

Lastly, never use your child's favorite food as a bribe to get him to eat a nutritious food that he dislikes (such as vegetables). Although this might seem like a good strategy (and it might work the first couple of times), research has shown that it may serve to increase his dislike of the nutritious food (he may conclude that vegetables are so awful that he needs to be given ice cream to compensate for eating them) and increase his desire for his favorite food, which now takes on the lofty status of a reward.[17] This is particularly problematic with very fussy children, who don't need much encouragement to reject nutritious foods such as vegetables and opt for the more-palatable foods instead. The best way to get your baby to eat something that you want him to eat is to eat it yourself in front of him. This and other strategies are described in more detail on pages 231–34.

FEEDING A HUNGRY BABY

Just as some babies are eager feeders and poor feeders during milk-feeding, not all babies will respond in the same way to solid food. The four principles of responsive feeding are important to follow, whatever type of feeder you have.

If you have a baby with a big appetite, the following tips are important:

- **Don't pressure him to eat past the point at which he feels full.**
  If he has low satiety, he is more likely to eat more than he needs if encouraged to, because it is more difficult for him to recognize when he is full. Supporting him to learn to recognize his feelings of fullness is important.

- **Try to think of covert ways to restrict his intake of high-fat and high-sugar foods.**
  The best way to do this is to not bring too many of these foods into the house in the first place. If he sees them, he will want them, and if he knows they are there, he will want them. Offering your baby a choice of nutritious food options is a useful strategy to make him feel that he has some control over what food he eats, and that you are not always just saying no but offering him alternative options.

- **Make sure you offer him an appropriate portion size of food.**
  Only offer him as much as he needs, not more, at mealtimes. If he has low satiety sensitivity, then he will eat more than he needs if there is more food available. If he is food responsive, he will continue to eat the tastier foods until he has finished them simply because it is a pleasurable thing to do, not because he is

hungry. You can always offer him more if he indicates to you that he is still hungry.

- **Don't offer him food for any reason other than hunger.**
  If you have a very food-responsive baby who loves eating, he will probably respond well to bribery—for example, "If you sit quietly you can have a cookie"—and the temptation is to use this strategy to control his emotions or his behavior. But it won't help him to develop a healthy relationship with food in the long run. He needs to learn to think of food as providing nourishment, not as a source of comfort or entertainment or as a reward.

FEEDING A BABY WITH A POOR APPETITE

If you have a baby with a poor appetite for solid food, it can be anxiety-provoking (more so than having an enthusiastic feeder), but the same tips are just as important for different reasons:

- **Don't pressure him to eat past the point at which he feels full.**
  If he is very sensitive to his internal feelings of satiety, continuing to eat past satiety is an unpleasant feeling. Pressuring him to continue to eat will make him feel stressed or even anxious. In unusual cases (with high amounts of pressure) it can even lead to food aversion. You are unlikely to get anywhere with this strategy, so it's not a fruitful endeavor. Your baby will let you know when he has had enough and, once he has indicated this to you, trust him and let him finish eating at this point.

- **Try to think of covert ways to restrict his intake of high-fat and high-sugar foods.**
  If you have more enticing foods in the house than the nutritious ones that your baby won't eat, he will want them instead, if he knows they are there. This can make it challenging to get him to even try the foods that he is automatically suspicious of. Having those nutritious foods around and in sight will help him to feel familiar with them and that these are the options available. We discuss food fussiness and strategies to deal with it in much more detail on pages 279–87.

- **Make sure you offer him an appropriate portion size of food.**
  Only provide your baby with as much as he can manage, not more. Offering a large plate of food to a child with high satiety sensitivity may overwhelm him and create anxiety.

- **Don't offer him food for any reason other than hunger.**
  Babies with a poor appetite are often fussy eaters, who are more likely to reject vegetables and opt for the foods they know and like already. Offering him these foods as a reward for eating the foods he doesn't like will do you no favors in the long run—it may make him even more suspicious of the foods he doesn't like and even more likely to refuse to eat them. There are far better ways to get him to eat his greens, such as modeling (described on pages 233–34).

UNDERSTANDING YOUR BABY'S HUNGER AND SATIETY CUES DURING COMPLEMENTARY FEEDING

It is clear from research that it is important to feed your baby responsively. This means that you need to be able to read his hunger and fullness cues for food, just as you did for milk. The good news is that this is a bit easier now your baby is older. An evidence-based coding tool—the Responsiveness to Child Feeding Cues Scale—has recently been developed to provide a description of cues that babies provide to indicate when they are hungry and full during complementary feeding.[18]

Hunger cues
If your baby is hungry and wants food or is willing to eat, he will

- lean forward
- reach for the spoon or food
- point to food
- get excited when you present him with food
- put the spoon or food voluntarily into his own mouth
- accept food quickly
- open his mouth when the spoon or food is a distance from his mouth.

Satiety cues
Avoidance or an unwillingness to eat can be recognized if your baby

- slows down his eating
- turns his head away
- looks away or looks down
- pulls his body away
- arches his back

- becomes fussy or cries
- pushes the spoon or the food away
- clenches his mouth shut
- becomes playful
- becomes distracted or more interested in what's going on around him.

How Much Food Does My Baby Need?

Young babies are exploring food, and starting solid foods is less about calorie intake and more about engaging with and tasting a variety of foods. The idea is not for your baby to be eating three meals a day just yet, and, although you do want him to be absorbing nutrients such as iron, at this stage the key is for him to get used to different flavors and textures. You should prepare for a lot of the food you offer your baby to end up on the floor, which can be a source of worry because many parents fear that their baby is not getting enough to eat.

MILK-FEEDING DURING COMPLEMENTARY FEEDING

You should continue to give your baby breast or formula milk as your baby moves on to solid foods. Whole (full-fat) cow's milk can be given as the main milk source *from twelve months of age* but not before, as it doesn't contain the right balance of nutrients; it has insufficient iron and vitamin E and too much sodium and potassium compared to breast or formula milk. It is also considerably higher in protein, which is linked with an increased risk of obesity in infancy (see page 244–45). And it is a lot harder for a baby to digest. In fact, several studies have shown that babies who consume a lot of whole cow's milk before they are twelve months old are more likely to be deficient in iron, because cow's milk is low in iron, it can interfere with iron absorption from other foods and it can lead to blood loss in their intestines.[19] Babies drinking high amounts of cow's milk before twelve months tend also to consume more calories, fat and protein overall and grow more rapidly.[20] For this reason it shouldn't be the main drink before twelve months of age, though small amounts can be added to complementary foods or used in cooking (for example, your baby can have it in oatmeal).

The US doesn't provide any clear guidance on the amount of milk that infants should be consuming during the first two years of life during the period of complementary feeding; guidelines are currently being developed and will be released in 2020. The British charity First Steps Nutrition has provided a helpful guide for the amount of milk required from six months to two years for babies drinking formula or cow's milk (see Table 2), based on babies' changing calorie requirements.[21] First Steps Nutrition advises breastfeeding mothers to feed responsively.

TABLE 2: MILK-FEEDING GUIDANCE FROM SIX MONTHS TO TWO YEARS FOR INFANTS CONSUMING FORMULA AND COW'S MILK

Age	Feeding guidance	Suggested intake per day
Seven to nine months	Infant formula could be offered at breakfast (150 ml/5 ounces), lunch (150 ml/5 ounces), dinner (150 ml/5 ounces) and before bed (150 ml/5 ounces).	About 600 ml (20 ounces) per day
Ten to twelve months	Infant formula could be offered at breakfast (100 ml/3.5 ounces), dinner (100 ml/3.5 ounces) and before bed (200 ml or 6.75 ounces).	About 400 ml (13.5 ounces) per day
One to two years	Full-fat cow's milk could be offered at snack times twice a day (100 ml/3.5 ounces x 2), and as a drink before bed (200 ml or 6.75 ounces).	About 350 to 400 ml (12 to 13.5 ounces) per day of whole cow's milk or another suitable milk drink

Which Milk to Choose?

In the US there are many different formulas on the market, but most formula-fed babies only need a standard "infant" formula (marketed for babies aged up to twelve months). The exception is if your baby has an allergy, in which case he may then be prescribed an alternative formula by your pediatrician. But infant milks are suitable for the majority of babies *up to one year of age*. After this your baby can move on to cow's milk or an appropriate alternative. Any whole (full-fat) milk (cow's, goat's or sheep's milk) is suitable as a main drink for babies from one year providing it is pasteurized. Unsweetened calcium-fortified soy milk, oat milk or coconut milk can also be given from one year of age. (See chapter 5 for guidance on choosing milks during the first year of life.)

We do not advocate using formula milks that are marketed for young children (often called "toddler milks"), which are targeted at infants beyond twelve months of age. The WHO states that these milks are not needed,[22] and, compared with standard infant milks (up to twelve months) or cow's milk (over twelve months), they have been found to have no nutritional benefit, are far more expensive, and are high in sugar. Given that solid foods should be introduced at around six months of age, most babies will obtain all the nutrients they need once they start on solid food. Infant milks are closer in composition to breast milk than the milks marketed at children older than twelve months, so these should be used for the first year of life if a baby is not being breastfed.

A relatively recent product to enter the market is PediaSure Grow & Gain. Worryingly, this is targeted at children up to thirteen years of age who are "behind on growth." It claims to be "a source of complete, balanced nutrition especially designed for children 1 to 13 years of age" and suitable as "the sole source of nutrition or as a supplement," as per the product information.[23] It is extraordinary that a single shake could claim that it is nutritionally complete for both a toddler and an adolescent, given how much nutritional needs change with development. It is available to buy in the baby and toddler snack aisle in leading pharmacies. We strongly discourage the use of such shakes (unless they have been prescribed by your pediatrician)—in our view they will not help your child to develop healthy eating habits and have a varied, balanced diet (see Chapter 9 for more on key nutrients and their impact on health). Children need to be encouraged to taste food and learn how to eat proper food; a shake is no substitute for a balanced diet. See pages 279–83 for tips on how to feed a fussy eater.

THE BOTTOM LINE

- The method you choose for introducing solid food is a personal choice: There is no evidence that one is better than the other.

- Baby-led weaning is safe insofar as there is no convincing evidence that babies are more likely to choke.

- If you begin with puréed foods, gradually introduce mashed textures and finger foods as soon as your baby indicates that he is ready, and offer finger foods alongside.

- Only offer your baby food if he is hungry and let him stop eating as soon as he is full.

- Never pressure your baby to eat if he doesn't want to.

- Provide a portion of food that is appropriate for your baby's age.

- Never use food to manage his emotions or provide entertainment.

- Never reward food with food.

- Continue with breast milk or standard formula (infant milks) alongside solid food.

- Toddler milks and food replacement shakes are not needed or recommended.

CHAPTER 9

First Foods

Complementary feeding is a crucial period for establishing healthy eating habits, largely because during this process your baby will develop taste preferences that may stay with him for many years. Research shows that food preferences can be "programmed" in early life.[1] This means that tastes and foods that your baby is exposed to during complementary feeding may shape what he likes as an older child and even as an adult. It's therefore a great opportunity to introduce your baby to foods that you would like him to eat in order to reap the benefits for years to come.

Many new parents choose to use baby rice cereal as the very first food, but we would strongly advise you *not* to do this. Rice cereal is incredibly bland in flavor. Introducing solid foods is about developing your baby's taste preferences and openness to new textures, not simply about calories and nutrition, and it is the perfect opportunity for your baby to try new flavors. Rice cereal or other bland food will not achieve this.

Vegetables First

We are all born with an innate preference for sweet foods and a dislike of bitter foods. Historically, a sweet preference meant we readily stored up energy to protect us against starvation when food became scarce, and an aversion to bitter tastes protected us from eating poisonous foods. Today our taste biases mean we have a tendency to eat too much of the readily available and cheap, high-calorie foods (for example, chocolate) and too little of the low-calorie foods that taste bitter but are nutritionally dense (for example, vegetables such as spinach). The upshot of this is that traditional, plant-based diets rich in vegetables have been replaced with diets high in fat and sugar. Vegetables are nutrient-dense (they contain many vitamins, minerals and fiber) and have a low energy density (a low number of calories per gram) because they are low in sugar and fat. For example, there are just 23 kcal in 100 g (3.5 ounces) spinach, but milk chocolate has 535 kcal per 100 g (3.5 ounces). This means we can eat large quantities of vegetables without eating too many calories and will obtain essential nutrients from them.

The benefits of eating vegetables are clear, but trying to get children to eat them can often be challenging. Vegetables are the type of food most commonly disliked by children,[2] and many parents struggle to get them to eat enough, especially when it comes to the more bitter vegetables, such as broccoli or cabbage. However, even though humans have an innate tendency to dislike bitter foods and prefer sweet foods, much of what we like is learned through experience. This means that it is possible to teach a child to learn to like and eat vegetables and other nutritious foods. The very early years offer a window of opportunity for "setting" your child's liking for vegetables, which will maximize the likelihood that he will eat and enjoy a wide variety of vegetables during childhood and later on in adulthood. Although this process may start as early as pregnancy and possibly continues during breastfeeding, complementary feeding probably plays a more important role. Research suggests that starting with vegetables is a good way to help your child learn to like vegetables, and he will be more accepting of future vegetables and eat a wider variety of them later in life.[3] The theory is that things can only get better for them in the taste stakes. If something sweet (for example, apple) is their first taste, what is the advantage of eating broccoli when they know other foods taste much sweeter? It makes sense that they will reject the broccoli, and who can blame them? However, it would be fair to say that there isn't a lot of high-quality research into the long-term effect of introducing vegetables first. Most studies have been observational, which means we can't be sure that introducing vegetables first *really caused* babies to increase their liking for them and eat more of them later, because other factors that weren't measured could have been more important.

However, researchers from our group at University College London conducted one of the few well-designed randomized controlled trials in this area; this study was able to show that introducing a vegetable as the first food had lasting positive effects on taste preferences, and this was probably due to using a vegetable as the first food.[4] In the TASTE study researchers randomly assigned sixty British mothers who were about to start weaning their four-to-six-month-old babies to either an intervention group or a control group. The intervention group was visited by researchers at home and offered advice on introducing five different varieties of vegetables (on their own, not disguised with fruit) for the first fifteen days of complementary feeding; the control group was visited at home but not given advice on starting with vegetables. After one month, the researchers assessed how much of an unfamiliar vegetable and fruit the babies ate. Babies in the intervention group ate double the amount of an unfamiliar vegetable than infants in the control group (33 versus 16 g), and the researchers and mothers also rated them as *liking* the vegetable more. What was interesting was that there was no difference between the groups in their liking or intake of the fruit. This suggests that introducing vegetables instead of fruit as first foods is a great way of improving acceptance of vegetables. On the other hand, starting with fruit might be a lost opportunity because babies tend to be accepting of fruit anyway.

Currently in the US, few new parents offer vegetables as a first food. The Feeding Infants and Toddlers Study 2008 found that the most common first foods given were grains such as infant cereal (52 percent) followed by vegetables (25 percent) and fruit and fruit juices (22 percent).[5] We would recommend offering a "rainbow" of different varieties of vegetables early on, including lots of dark green vegetables, and avoiding sticking to things like sweet potato, parsnips or carrots, because they are naturally quite sweet. Start with a range of different single vegetables including the least sweet varieties (for example, broccoli and spinach). If your baby doesn't seem to like something, don't give up; offer it again another day. Exposure to a variety of flavors during complementary feeding is important for fostering healthy food preferences. A more varied diet during complementary feeding has been linked with eating a greater variety of foods later in childhood and children being more accepting of novel foods.[6] Evidence also suggests that offering *different* vegetables each day is more successful in increasing acceptance of novel foods during the complementary feeding stage than giving the same vegetable for multiple consecutive days. In Chapter 10 we offer a step-by-step guide on how to introduce vegetables as first foods, and we explain the science behind the benefits.

FRUIT

There is no disputing that fruit is good for us; it is full of nutrients and fiber, and is unprocessed. It does, however, also contain a reasonable amount of sugar (hence the sweet taste), which is why babies tend to like it. It is highly unlikely that your baby will turn his nose up at banana, pear or apple. But if you try to give him vegetables once he has tried fruit, you may be disappointed. We would therefore recommend that the first foods that are introduced to your baby are vegetables. There are some fruits, such as plums or cherries, that can be quite sour so may initially be rejected by your baby, and we recommend introducing these earlier than the sweet fruits.

Fruit Juice

Five ounces (150 ml) of pure unsweetened orange juice (a standard serving) contains about 20 g sugar[7] (more sugar than you would find in four bags of animal crackers), and a child would need to eat several oranges to get the same amount of juice! There are currently no specific recommendations on sugar intake for infants under twelve months of age in the US, but the *2015–2020 Dietary Guidelines for Americans* recommends that children one to three years of age should consume less than 10 percent of their calories from "added" sugar (see pages 245–46 for more on added sugars).[8] Sweet drinks are particularly problematic not only because they can lead children to develop a sweet tooth, but they can also lead to tooth decay. Another, less well-known problem is that sweet drinks are not recognized by the brain's satiety center in the same way as solid food. This means that the calories are not compensated for (they don't make us feel any fuller), and it is easy to consume excess calories in the form of drinks (this doesn't apply to milk).

We recommend not giving your baby fruit juice; he only needs water or milk, especially during the complementary feeding period. The AAP also recommends not giving babies younger than twelve months fruit juice.[9] If you do choose to offer fruit juice or smoothies to your baby, always dilute them with water (one part fruit juice to ten parts water) and offer them with a meal, not on their own. If you offer fruit juice after your baby is twelve months old, the AAP recommends not giving more than 4 ounces (118 ml) of 100 percent fruit juice per day. Fizzy drinks (sodas) have no nutritional value at all and should be avoided.

Juice and fizzy drinks (sodas) should not be given to your baby in a bottle, as this is bad for his teeth, so do not use bottles for anything other than water, breast milk or formula. The AAP suggests that your baby should have transitioned from a bottle to a cup by eighteen months at the latest.[10] In fact, this would be considered late in the UK, where the guidance is to introduce a cup rather than a bottle from six months of age and to have stopped using bottles with nipples by twelve months, as babies can end up using these as a comforter.[11] We would recommend that from twelve months you try using an open cup or sippy cup so that your baby learns how to sip rather than suck. Sucking from a bottle or spout means the drink is in contact with your baby's teeth for longer and can lead to tooth decay.

MIXED MESSAGES

Many parents look to family, internet forums, websites, pediatricians, government sources, friends and parenting groups for support on infant feeding. Health professionals and other organizations often suggest dry infant rice cereal as the first food[12] followed by fruit and vegetables, so rather than the focus being on taste development and building healthy eating habits, it tends to be on the mechanics of eating and starting with something plain (although cereal is also high in iron, which is an important consideration—see page 226).

The internet is a minefield when it comes to introducing solid foods, and if you search online for guidance, you are bound to come across advice from baby-food "experts" that contradicts the scientific evidence. A quick glance at what's out there showed us that parents are being given advice to offer "root vegetables and ripe fruit" as first foods because "they are naturally sweet and can be easily puréed to a smooth texture." There is very little guidance provided on how to encourage babies to accept vegetables. This is not in line with the best scientific research to date on which we are basing our guidance.

A similar issue is that you will find lots of recipes for starting solids online, but many of them contain fruit or they mix fruit and vegetables together. We found recipes such as "Celery, Carrot and Apple," "Banana and Avocado," and "Kiwi and Avocado." There are two main problems here. Firstly, mixing fruit and vegetables prevents babies from being able to identify the vegetables because the flavor is masked with the sweetness of the fruit. Secondly, in real life adults do not tend to have fruit mixed in with vegetables. Children need to learn to eat how adults eat—not many of us would mix kiwi and avocado together for ourselves, so why do it for our babies?

Baby Foods

In 2016, the North American baby food market was valued at approximately $21.18 billion.[13] The 2008 Feeding Infants and Toddlers Study reported that more than 50 percent of babies aged six to nine months had consumed commercial baby foods.[14] Many ready-made baby foods on the market are great, and it can be very helpful to use good-quality products when you are pushed for time. But many also contain a lot of sugar, and foods with added sugar should be avoided in the first twelve months of your baby's life (see pages 245–46). In particular, many processed baby foods, regardless of whether they are organic or not, often use fruit, such as apple or pear, as the basis—for example, mixing broccoli and peas with pears. If you try some of this food, you may be quite surprised by how sweet it tastes. A recent review of baby foods in the US found that fruits were listed as the first ingredients (meaning most of the product is fruit) more commonly than all vegetables, and that dark green vegetables were rarely listed first. In particular, less than 10 percent of the 548 vegetable products contained single vegetables.[15] So few baby foods contain simple, individual vegetable flavors, and those that do usually have sweet vegetables, such as carrot or sweet potato, as the main ingredient, which babies are more likely to accept. Less readily accepted vegetables, such as broccoli, spinach or cauliflower, are often not included and are usually not the dominant flavor.

In addition, jars and pouches of baby food often go through high-heat processing, which may remove some of their nutritional goodness, and the quantities of iron or vitamin D in fish or meat products are likely to be much lower than a home-prepared alternative. Often these products also contain a lot more water than foods made at home, which reduces the energy density (number of calories per gram) of the food and means that a baby needs to eat greater quantities of it to obtain the same nutrients. There is the possibility this may interfere with a child's ability to respond to their feelings of fullness, if they learn to eat larger portions from a very young age. Overall the portions of jars and pouches are very big for the start of complementary feeding, and once opened they can only be stored for limited periods of time, which can lead to overfeeding or lots of waste.

Aside from the nutritional benefits of preparing food at home, there are also cost benefits; it is far more expensive to purchase ready-made baby foods. The cost difference is the packaging and obviously the convenience—it does take time to prepare, boil and purée your own vegetables, but it is far more cost-effective, and it can actually be very quick and easy, especially if you create a large batch and freeze portions to give to your baby at a later date (see page 230).

By preparing your baby's food at home, you can be sure that you only include the ingredients that you want him to have, and a smaller portion would probably be needed to achieve the same nutrient content. Not only is home-prepared food more cost-effective, there is also a difference in appearance and texture, as the supermarket versions are highly processed and often less textured (e.g., fewer lumps).

However, many working parents don't have time to make all their children's food from scratch, and commercial baby foods offer a time-saving alternative. If you purchase jars and pouches, our advice would be to start with those that contain only individual vegetables, although there are not many of these available on the market so you may need to look around. Try to avoid jars and pouches that mix fruit and vegetables together, and delay giving ones that contain only fruit until later in the process. Also, purées in a pouch should be transferred to a spoon before being fed to your child. If you allow your child to squeeze the food straight into his mouth he may miss out on key oral development that is learned through taking food from a spoon, not to mention he may end up eating far too quickly.

Foods to Avoid

Babies can be offered most foods, but there are a few things they shouldn't be given:[16]

- honey, until one year of age, as it can contain spores of a bacterium called *Clostridium botulinum*, which can cause infant botulism, a rare but potentially fatal illness of the digestive system[17]

- cow's milk as a drink, until twelve months of age (from twelve months whole cow's milk can be given, but reduced-fat milk should not be given until at least two years of age); cow's milk can be used in small amounts in food and cooking from six months of age (see page 209)

- any foods that require chewing or that can be a choking hazard, such as seeds or whole nuts (including peanuts or chunks of peanut butter—these should not be given to children under the age of five, but babies can be given small amounts of nut paste or smooth nut butter); hot dogs (including meat sticks or baby food "hot dogs"); chunks of meat or cheese; whole grapes; popcorn; raw vegetables; whole fruit chunks (such as apple chunks); hard, gooey or sticky candy; and gum

- processed foods made for adults and older children, because they can be high in salt and other preservatives.

Allergenic Foods

Food allergies in the US have increased over the last few years: The CDC estimated that in 2011, 5.4 percent of people were affected, compared to just 3.4 percent in 1997;[18] currently, 6.2 percent of children are affected.[19] US law lists the following eight foods as the most common major allergens, which together account for about 90 percent of all allergic reactions to food: milk, eggs, fish (e.g., cod, bass, flounder), crustacean shellfish (e.g., shrimp, lobster, crab), tree nuts (e.g., almonds, walnuts, pecans), peanuts, wheat and soybeans.[20] Given the increasing prevalence of food allergies and their seriousness, there has been a lot of research into how to prevent them. Evidence is mounting that introducing your baby to peanuts and eggs early during complementary feeding is a good strategy to prevent allergies to these foods, especially for babies at high risk. A recent high-quality review of the evidence concluded that introducing cooked or heated eggs (not raw egg, which can cause severe allergic reactions) between four and six months reduced the risk of egg allergy by 44 percent in all infants, including those at normal or very high risk of developing an allergy; introducing peanuts between four and eleven months also reduced the risk of peanut allergy by 71 percent.[21] There was no strong evidence that early introduction to other allergenic foods prevented allergies, but early introduction did not increase the risk of developing allergies, either. Research therefore indicates that there is no reason to delay introduction to any allergenic foods, even if your baby is at high risk (for example, a family history or severe eczema).

In response to the strong evidence that early introduction to peanuts prevents allergies, the US National Institute of Allergy and Infectious Diseases developed three guidelines for introducing peanuts to infants at various levels of risk:[22]

1. Infants with severe eczema, egg allergy, or both should have introduction of age-appropriate peanut-containing food as early as four to six months of age to reduce the risk of peanut allergy. However, parents are recommended to have their child evaluated for peanut sensitivity by their physician before offering peanut.

2. Infants with mild to moderate eczema should have introduction of age-appropriate peanut-containing food around six months of age.

3. Infants without eczema or any food allergy should have age-appropriate peanut-containing foods freely introduced in the diet, together with other solid foods, at a time when it suits the family.

The American Academy of Allergy, Asthma and Immunology recommends not delaying the introduction of any other allergenic foods and reassures parents that they can all be introduced between four and six months.[23] They suggest introducing allergenic foods:

- after other solid foods have been introduced and tolerated

- at home, rather than out at a restaurant, in case an allergic reaction occurs

- one at a time and in small amounts, every three to five days, to ensure that if a reaction occurs, you have an idea as to which food caused it.

Mixed foods containing allergenic foods should not be given unless tolerance to each item has been tested. If your baby is at high risk of having an allergic reaction to one of these foods (for example, he already has one food allergy, moderate to severe eczema or a family member with a severe food allergy), they suggest that you ask your pediatrician to evaluate him properly before introducing any allergenic foods.

SALT

Your baby's first foods do not need any salt. Babies have never experienced salt, and it only masks the flavor of foods, which is not helpful when your baby is trying to develop taste preferences. Too much salt is also dangerous for babies because their kidneys are not able to deal with it and it may increase a baby's risk of developing several health problems in later life, including high blood pressure and obesity. There are no guidelines for how much salt babies less than twelve months old should have—they need very little, and the amount already present in breast milk or formula is sufficient. For children one to three years of age, the National Academy of Medicine (NAM) set the "adequate intake" level of salt at 2.5 g per day;[24] this is the sufficient amount for most children, so they don't need more than this (the upper safe limit for children this age is 3.75 g of salt per day[25]). The required amount is not a lot—approximately two slices of unbuttered bread. Stock cubes, gravy, sauces, some cheeses and processed foods all contain a lot of salt, so we advise you do not use these during the complementary feeding process. Research has shown that children can develop a preference for salty foods if they are introduced to them early in life. One such study involved offering babies aged two months and six months either salty water or fruit and then assessing their preference for salty foods at three to four years of age.[26] The babies who had been exposed to the salty water preferred salty foods, to the point where they were more likely to lick salt from the surface of foods at preschool age and more likely to eat plain salt!

SUGAR

Introducing sugary foods and drinks early on may enhance your child's preference for sweetness. This is not only bad news in terms of tooth decay but also for risk of overweight and type 2 diabetes. In the US there are no guidelines for sugar intake for babies less than twelve months of age (children one to three years of age should consume less than 10 percent of their calories from added sugar; see pages 245–46 for more on added sugar), but there is no need to add sugar to your baby's food during complementary feeding. Where possible offer your baby fresh fruit rather than dried. Dried fruit has had the water removed from it, which concentrates the natural sugars: 170 g (6 ounces) of *fresh* cranberries contains 2 g sugar, while 170 g (6 ounces) of *dried* cranberries contains 37 g sugar (more than a standard-sized can of cola). Dried fruit also sticks to your child's teeth, which increases the risk of tooth decay. If you offer your child dried fruit, include it in a meal; don't offer it on its own. This can help prevent damage to his teeth.

Essential Nutrients

Complementary feeding provides the perfect opportunity to expose your baby to essential nutrients, such as vitamin D and iron. However, research has shown that many young children are not consuming enough of some important nutrients and consuming too many of others. In both Gemini and the National Diet and Nutrition survey (NDNS)[27]—an annual survey to collect dietary information from individuals eighteen months or older in Britain[28]—we found that toddlers were consuming far too little vitamin D and iron. This is also the case in the US.[29]

VITAMIN D

Vitamin D is essential for the formation of strong bones and teeth and keeps muscles healthy. It is also important for a range of other functions, including immunity. The main source is sunlight, but in the US, dietary vitamin D is often obtained from fortified foods, especially milk and yogurts. Some other foods such as breakfast cereals, margarine and orange juice are also commonly fortified with vitamin D. Low intakes of vitamin D in infancy and childhood have been linked to health conditions such as rickets, a bone condition that can result in bone pain, poor growth and deformities of bones, such as bowed legs and curved spine. Rickets is more common among children with darker skin because they need more sunlight to get enough vitamin D.

Few natural foods contain vitamin D, and although many foods in the US are fortified with it, it can be difficult to get sufficient vitamin D from diet alone—sunlight is by far the best source. Also, vitamin D tends to be found naturally in foods that young children are not keen on eating, such as liver. It is for this reason that the American Academy of Pediatrics (AAP) recommends that exclusively and partially breast-fed infants receive supplements of 400 IU per day of vitamin D shortly after birth and continue to receive these supplements until they move on to complementary foods and consume at least 1 quart (1 L) per day of vitamin D–fortified formula or whole milk. Similarly, all non-breastfed infants ingesting less than 1 quart (1 L) per day of vitamin D–fortified formula or milk should receive a vitamin D supplement of 400 IU per day.[30] We would recommend that you give your baby vitamin D supplements but also introduce your baby to vitamin D–rich foods from an early age. The following are good animal and vegetable sources of vitamin D.[31]

Animal Sources	Vegetable Sources
salmon	vegetable-fat spread
egg yolk	fortified breakfast cereals
fresh trout	fortified nondairy milks (almond, soy)
liver*	fortified orange juice
mackerel	
fortified dairy products	

VITAMINS C AND A

Vitamin A is important for immunity, vision and skin health, and red blood cell circulation. Severe deficiency is the leading cause of preventable childhood blindness and increases the risk of infection and night blindness (difficulty seeing in dim light). Vitamin C is needed for the growth and repair of tissues including skin, bones and cartilage. Severe deficiency can lead to scurvy, which causes fatigue, inflammation of the gums, joint pain and poor wound healing, but deficiency in either vitamin A or C is extremely rare in the US.[32]

High levels of vitamin A (intakes above 600 mcg/2,000 IU per day) can be harmful for infants and children up to three years of age and are not recommended,[33] so foods that are very rich in vitamin A (for example, liver) should be limited to once per week. See pages 47–48 for other food sources of vitamin A and C.

IRON

Iron is a vital micronutrient for your baby's health and development and supports growth, production of some hormones, and cell and tissue formation, among other things. Low intakes of iron have been linked

---

* Liver contains a high quantity of vitamin A. This can be harmful in large amounts, so do not offer this to your baby more than once per week.

to anemia, a condition where the body has fewer red blood cells to transport oxygen in the blood. This keeps organs and tissue from getting the oxygen they need and can affect your baby's development. Iron found in animal foods (heme iron) is a key source of iron, as it is absorbed at a greater rate by the body than iron found in plant foods (nonheme iron), so animal sources are the best source of iron for your baby. The recommended daily intake for babies aged seven to twelve months is 11 mg (see page 248 for iron supplementation and information on iron requirements after one year).[34] It is estimated that about 12 percent of babies aged six to eleven months in the US don't consume enough iron.[35] Listed below are good animal and vegetable sources of iron.[36] It is important to introduce a range of these foods early on in complementary feeding.

Animal Sources	Vegetable Sources
lamb	broccoli
beef	kale
salmon	spinach
kidney	white beans
tuna (canned)	kidney beans
beef liver[*]	chickpeas
eggs	tofu
	lentils
	soybeans
	fortified breakfast cereals or breads

ZINC

Zinc helps to form a baby's organs, skeleton, nerves and circulatory system and is important for the immune system—it is vital for healthy growth and development. Babies need to consume it daily to ensure a steady amount for development because the body has no way to store it. Zinc is found in meat, eggs, dairy products, pulses, whole grains, nuts, certain types of seafood (e.g., crab) and most cereals. Beans and peas such as kidney beans, pinto beans, black beans, chickpeas, split

---

[*] Liver contains a high quantity of vitamin A. This can be harmful in large amounts, so do not offer this to your baby more than once per week.

peas, and lentils are great sources. The NAM recommends a daily intake of 2 mg for infants from birth to six months (breast milk provides sufficient zinc for the first four to six months of life), and 3 mg per day for children aged seven months to three years.[37] Breast milk does not provide sufficient zinc for infants older than six months, so beyond this age children must consume age-appropriate foods or drinks containing zinc.

THE BOTTOM LINE

- Start with vegetables, preferably bitter-tasting ones that are also high in iron (for example, spinach).

- Introduce a variety of individual vegetables; don't mix vegetables together, and don't mix them with fruit.

- Early on, try to include a range of iron-rich foods such as beef and green leafy vegetables, especially if breastfeeding, as breast milk is low in iron.

- Introduce fruit later in the complementary feeding process and begin with sour fruits—for example, cherries (with pits removed) or plums.

- Avoid teething rusks or baby rice cereal as first foods, as they are bland in flavor: Starting solids is about encouraging your baby to develop taste preferences.

- Be cautious of online advice that recommends introducing vegetable/fruit combinations.

- Avoid salt and sugar: Be wary of sauces and gravies that may contain salt, and do not add salt or sugar to first foods.

- Try to offer only water and milk as drinks for your baby—fruit juices contain a lot of sugar, and sodas have no nutritional value.

- Starting solids is not so much about calorie intake (most of your baby's energy will still be coming from milk). It is more about experiencing food and flavors—don't worry if most of it ends up on the floor.

CHAPTER 10

Your Guide to Introducing Solids

This chapter provides you with some essential tips on how to introduce your baby to solids to give him the best possible chance of
developing healthy eating habits that will endure for many years. If
your baby is exclusively or partially breastfed, we recommend that you
follow the American Academy of Pediatrics' recommendation to give
him a liquid iron supplement until he is eating enough iron-rich foods
to get all he needs from food.[1] Your pediatrician will be able to advise
you on the dose and when you can stop doing this.

Stage 1: A Variety of Individual Vegetables (Days 1 to 15)

We recommend starting with a *variety* of *individual* vegetables, as this
will introduce your baby to a wide range of flavors. A landmark experimental study of 147 babies from Germany and France[2] found that
babies who were randomized to be given a high variety of vegetables
at the beginning of complementary feeding (carrot purée, followed by
artichoke purée, green beans, then pumpkin, rotated for eight days)
were more accepting of new vegetables one month later than children
who were randomized to have no or low variety. But, importantly, the
effect was still observed at six years of age; they were also more accepting of familiar vegetables, too. This study indicated that giving babies
a high variety of vegetables during this important transition might have
lasting effects on your baby's food preferences. We recommend introducing one vegetable at a time to begin with—this will help your baby
to learn the flavor of that vegetable. That way, when you start combining

foods together, he can still identify the individual vegetable and will be more likely to accept what you are offering. This applies whether you are spoon-feeding or doing baby-led weaning (BLW).

We recommend offering a new, individual vegetable every day for five days and then rotating this twice more so that your child gets three tastes of each vegetable over fifteen days. Start with iron-rich, non-sweet vegetables (including some bitter-tasting ones, such as spinach) and introduce each of these in between milk feedings so that your baby is not too hungry or too full. This can be at any time of day. An ice-cube-sized portion is enough for the first few days, as most of your baby's energy will be coming from milk, and this stage is really about getting him used to new flavors. Gradually you can increase the portions as your baby's milk intake decreases. The vegetables we have suggested are by no means intended to be prescriptive; they are simply an example, using iron-rich, non-sweet vegetables. Introduce whatever vegetables you wish to and at a time of the day that suits you and your baby. If you are starting your baby on solids at six months and he seems enthusiastic and hungry, you can offer him two different vegetables on each day instead of one; for example, one around midday and another midafternoon. In general, just try to stick to three principles:

1. *Daily changes:* Don't give him the same vegetable for two consecutive days; mix it up.

2. *Repetition:* Make sure that you rotate the vegetables every five days so that he gets repeated exposure (three times) during the first two weeks.

3. *Variety:* During the first few weeks of complementary feeding, try to introduce him to as many different vegetables as you can.

Making Purées

Steam your chosen vegetable (or fruit) until tender (steaming will preserve more of the nutrients than boiling). Once cooked, purée in a blender or with a handheld blender, or just mash it with a fork. Adjust the texture with your baby's usual milk or with boiled water if you wish. Leave to cool before spoon-feeding to your baby.

Remember that there is no need to add salt, sauces or other flavors—the aim is for your baby to try the individual flavors of the vegetables and learn to like them so that going forward he can detect the flavors in food and enjoy them.

Freezing Purées

A great way to avoid spending a huge amount of time preparing purées from scratch every day is to make a large batch and freeze them. You just need ice cube trays, plastic wrap and freezer bags. Make up a large batch of one or more purées and allow it to cool down.

Once cooled, fill the ice cube trays and wrap in a layer of plastic wrap to keep them covered. Place in the freezer (-0.4°F/-18°C) and, once frozen, pop the cubes into freezer bags. Make sure you date the bags so that you know when the purées were made and use them within three months. Defrost each portion as you need it by placing it in the fridge for ten to twelve hours. Reheat the purée if you wish in a saucepan or microwave. If using the microwave, make sure you stir thoroughly to avoid hot spots and test the temperature yourself before feeding to your baby. Do not refreeze the purée once it has been defrosted.

FIRST FOODS TIMETABLE

Day 1	Day 2	Day 3	Day 4	Day 5
broccoli	spinach	peas	kale	asparagus
Day 6	Day 7	Day 8	Day 9	Day 10
broccoli	spinach	peas	kale	asparagus
Day 11	Day 12	Day 13	Day 14	Day 15
broccoli	spinach	peas	kale	asparagus

INTRODUCING LUMPS AND TEXTURES

It is entirely up to you to decide whether you start with puréed smooth foods, mashed foods or finger foods. We would recommend that you use a mixture. For example, if you purée or mash some foods and spoon-feed them, give your baby some finger foods to try by himself, as well. This way he will get the best of both worlds. If you start off with puréed foods, it is probably a good idea to move him on to lumps and textures as quickly as possible, as soon as he is showing signs that he is ready. This tends to be when he uses his tongue to push the food around his mouth, almost like chewing. This helps develop muscles important for speech. Every child is different, and as a parent you are likely to know if your child seems able to cope with lumps or if you need to wait a bit longer. It can sometimes be a bit disconcerting for new parents when they feed their baby lumps for the first time, as often babies will gag and parents worry they are choking. But gagging is very different from choking (see pages 197–98). Don't worry too much if he doesn't seem very keen on lumps at first; just as babies vary in the timing of their developmental milestones (such sitting or crawling), some babies take a bit longer to get used to lumps and textures than others. It's not a race, and he will get there eventually, so try not to worry if it takes a while for him to get used to lumpy and textured food.

PERSEVERANCE IS KEY

A baby's expression of interest or surprise in response to a new food is often misinterpreted as disgust, and what tends to happen is that the parents then stop offering that food. Try to focus on your baby's willingness to continue eating rather than his facial expressions. You might indeed find that your baby does not like some of the vegetables you offer him at first, and that is fine and totally normal. It is not unusual for babies to reject vegetables when they first try them, as the flavors are new to them.

It is important not to give up the first time your baby turns away or spits the food out. Repeated experience with a taste has been shown to increase acceptance of it.[3] So, if you want to increase your baby's acceptance of vegetables, you need to give him lots of opportunities to try them. It can be very difficult, and you may lose motivation to keep offering your child a food that he seems to clearly dislike, but perseverance is the key. The scientific evidence suggests that repeatedly exposing babies to the same vegetable eventually leads to most babies accepting and liking that vegetable. In one study, forty-nine mothers identified a vegetable purée that their infant (aged seven months) disliked and offered that vegetable on alternate days for sixteen days (eight exposures).[4] On the other days they offered a liked vegetable (carrot purée). They found that on first exposure, the babies ate 39 g of the disliked vegetable, on average, and 164 g of the liked one. Over the following days, intake of the disliked vegetable increased, and by the eighth exposure they ate 174 g, about the same amount as the liked vegetable (186 g). But what was most encouraging was that most children were still eating and liking the initially disliked vegetable many years later, at three (73 percent of children) and six years of age (57 percent of children).[5] This shows that if your baby initially dislikes a vegetable, the key is to persevere—and it may well pay off in the long term. It might be necessary to offer your child the vegetable as many as fifteen times (especially with older babies), which may feel like a lot, and each time your child rejects it you might be very tempted to give up, but keep trying and it should pay off.

A very recent review of the scientific literature on complementary feeding highlighted that introducing vegetables first, frequently and in variety, can increase acceptance of vegetables during this period and into childhood.[6] The UK Scientific Advisory Committee on Nutrition also carried out a comprehensive review of infant feeding during the first twelve months and concluded that evidence supports repeated exposure as a proven method for enhancing babies' acceptance of new foods.[7] Our suggested timetable offers a new vegetable every day for five days and then repeats twice for another ten days (so your baby will get three exposures to each vegetable). Be sure to offer the individual vegetable each time and repeat any that your baby seems to dislike. A "taste" can be as small as a teaspoonful, because the idea is for your baby to do just that—have a taste.

FOOD FUSSINESS

It is important to add that some children are just less likely to accept vegetables than others. Vegetable liking seems to be influenced strongly by genes, but just because some children have a genetic tendency to dislike vegetables does not mean that preferences cannot be changed.

Genes alone do not tell the whole story, which means there is room for change. Following our guidance will help your child to become more accepting of foods and less fussy. We cover more on fussy eating in Chapter 12 (pages 280–83).

PRAISE, PRAISE, PRAISE

Praising your child's good behavior helps him to learn that what he is doing pleases you, and the praise acts as a reward. As psychologists, we call this positive reinforcement—if something rewarding follows a behavior, it is more likely that the behavior will occur again in the future. This technique is deceptively simple but is a very effective method for managing a child's behavior, including eating. If you offer a new or disliked vegetable to your baby and praise him for trying it, he will quickly realize that eating the vegetable makes you happy, and he will be more likely to eat it again. Looking happy when you are feeding your baby achieves the same thing—lots of smiles and encouragement will help to show your child that these vegetables are to be enjoyed.

MODELING

Babies and children learn what is safe to eat vicariously by observing other people, and it's no different with food. Your baby is looking to you to let him know that a food is safe to eat—he wants you to "test-drive" it for him. This means that if you want your child to eat something, the best way to do this is to eat it and enjoy it with him or in front of him. If there is a vegetable you don't like—a good example is probably the commonly disliked brussels sprout—try to hide your dislike from your child. If he sees you grimacing when you feed him or when you eat them yourself, he will pick up on that. He will quickly learn that brussels sprouts are unpleasant or unsafe and to be avoided; this will make him much more likely to reject these foods. If it is going to be too difficult to eat something you dislike and pretend to like it, don't let this stop you from offering it to your child. They will never learn to like it if they never try it, and you might find that they actually enjoy it.

You are a model to your child—if you don't like or eat vegetables, you can expect your child to follow suit. If you want your child to eat vegetables, you must eat them, too. Aim to eat *with* your child as often as you can, even if it is not every mealtime, and show him that vegetables are nutritious as well as delicious. Your baby can be included in family meals right from the start, and this can help with modeling, as he will learn how to eat by watching you and others around him at the table. It is important to always bear that in mind. We will cover more on the influence of modeling healthy eating behavior and the importance of family mealtimes in Chapter 12.

Stage 2: Offer Multiple Vegetables and Introduce Other Foods

When you have introduced individual vegetable tastes for the first fifteen days, you can begin offering your baby two or three familiar vegetables from Stage 1 at the same time, for example spinach and broccoli. But ensure that they are not mixed together, as you want your baby to taste the individual flavors. As with Stage 1, the key is to keep trying if your baby rejects them. Start introducing new vegetables, too—for example, green beans, celery, cauliflower, leeks, red pepper, green pepper and fava beans (although the fava bean is one vegetable that Hayley has never learned to love!). At this stage you can begin introducing sweet vegetables as well, such as parsnip, carrots, sweet potato, butternut squash and rutabaga.

Other age-appropriate foods should also be introduced at this stage—and it's especially important to offer as many iron-rich foods as you can, such as red meat. You may find that your baby will more readily accept some of these other foods than vegetables—especially fruits, because they are sweeter. Be very careful that you do not offer some fruits (such as grapes or cherries) whole to babies, as they are a choking hazard. Many fruits, such as apples and pears, will need to be cooked first to soften them, and we would recommend peeling them, as the skin can be a bit tough. Try starting with less sweet fruits, such as cherry or kiwi, as your baby is more likely to accept these at this stage. We would not recommend combining fruit with vegetables, as the sweetness will disguise the vegetable flavor (see page 285). If you are going to offer fruit, just offer it on its own. It's really important that your baby becomes familiar with the individual flavors of many different vegetables and fruit. During this stage, repeat any foods your child seems to dislike, just as you did with the vegetables during Stage 1.

It is important that other new foods, such as meat, fish, beans, pasta, rice, egg and dairy foods like yogurt, are also introduced to your baby during complementary feeding to ensure he consumes a balanced diet and is getting all the nutrients he requires (although there are some foods that should be avoided while your baby is still very young; see page 220). While introducing solids to your baby you are preparing him for the types of foods we as adults eat, so it is great for him to experience as many different food groups as possible during this stage. Your baby will be learning to chew, so a range of textures is important for his oral motor development. A varied diet is also essential for providing him with a range of nutrients needed to support healthy development. It's an opportunity to introduce items that are less commonly eaten by young children, such as oily fish. Here are some great examples of foods you could introduce in Stage 2.

- Fish without bones (for example, salmon)
- Hard-boiled eggs
- Meat (for example, beef or chicken)
- Dairy products made from whole milk (for example, unsweetened yogurt)
- Starchy foods (for example, sweet potato or pasta)
- Pulses (for example, lentils or beans)

Oily Fish

Oily fish, such as salmon, is a fantastic source of polyunsaturated fats that are important for brain development, among other things. But oily fish contains low levels of mercury that can build up in the body, and high levels can harm a young child's developing nervous system. To be on the safe side, the AAP recommends avoiding oily fish with very high levels, including tilefish, swordfish, shark, marlin, king mackerel, orange roughy, and bigeye and bluefin tuna.[8] But babies and children can have as much white fish as they want to.

> Good oily fish options include salmon, trout and herring. Other great white fish and seafood options include cod, pollock, catfish, sole, lobster and shrimp.

Where at all possible, offer your child foods that you are already preparing for yourself. For example, if you are making lasagna, keep aside some of the ground meat for your baby. This will make less work for you in terms of preparation and help your child get used to eating family foods, but remember not to add salt to the dish during cooking.

FINGER FOOD IDEAS

Offering your baby finger foods will encourage coordination and help him to develop the skills he needs to bite, chew and swallow. Finger foods can be introduced from the start if you are doing BLW or as your child is getting used to lumpier textures if spoon-feeding. They need to be easy to pick up and hold and free from seeds, pits or bones. Here are some ideas for finger foods.

- Steamed broccoli/cauliflower florets
- Ripe avocado
- Steamed carrot or parsnip sticks
- Steamed green beans or snow peas
- Cooked potato or pasta
- Melon with the skin removed
- Mango
- Banana
- Toast or bread fingers

ALLERGIES

Allergic reactions occur more commonly with dairy foods but can occur with other types of foods, as well (such as eggs, nuts, seeds, wheat, soybeans, fish and shellfish—see pages 221–22 for more detail on allergenic foods). If you notice any of the following after your baby eats a new food, please consult your pediatrician immediately:

- diarrhea or vomiting
- a cough
- wheezing or shortness of breath
- itchy skin
- a rash
- swollen lips or throat
- runny or blocked nose
- sore, red and itchy eyes.

Rarely, an allergic reaction is severe and life-threatening (in cases of severe anaphylactic reaction). If you think your baby is having a severe allergic reaction, call emergency services immediately and ask for an ambulance. If your child does have an allergy, there are plenty of food options out there for him—for example, dairy-free cheese or wheat-free bread. Your pediatrician will be able to assist you with this.

Stage 3: Family Food

Once you have introduced new food groups, it is time for your child to start eating a modified version of the family diet. By about seven to nine months he should be offered three meals a day in addition to breast milk or formula (see Table 2, page 210, for guidance on how much milk babies should be consuming from six months to two years). By the time your baby is ten to twelve months food does not need to be mashed; it can be minced or chopped instead. It is important to keep offering as wide a range of flavors, textures and food groups as possible in the transition to the family diet. By twelve months your baby should be eating roughly five times a day (three meals and two snacks). There are still some things you need to be mindful of, such as not introducing cow's milk as a drink until twelve months (it is fine in cooking from six months of age) and limiting the amount of salt (avoid adding gravy and sauces to his food), but overall there is not much stopping your baby from eating the same foods as the rest of the family. Restaurants often serve "kids' meals," and many parents will spend time preparing a different meal from the rest of the family for their young child, but this is not necessary and we wouldn't recommend it. Your baby is still learning textures at this age, and he will not have a full set of teeth yet, so you may need to modify his food slightly—for example, break a slice of toast into smaller pieces or mash roast potatoes with a fork. However, most of the foods that you eat he can eat, too.

An important part of learning to eat is the social context—watching others and establishing how to eat. To help with this, aim to offer your child the same meal as the rest of the family and try to sit down together as a family. As much as possible avoid eating in front of the television, as this may prevent children from responding to their feelings of fullness. We cover more on this in Chapter 12 (pages 274–75).

THE BOTTOM LINE

- Give a different single vegetable each day for five consecutive days and then repeat this twice. This will ensure your baby has three exposures to five different vegetables over the first two weeks of complementary feeding.

- Keep trying: Your baby might need several tastes before accepting certain foods.

- Don't disguise or hide vegetables with other flavors, such as mixing them with fruit or covering them with a sauce.

- Try to introduce your baby to lumps and different textures as soon as he indicates he is ready; don't leave it too long.

- Make sure you offer your baby as wide a variety of foods as you can during the first few weeks and months after introducing solid foods.

- Make sure you offer your baby plenty of iron-rich foods.

- Praise your baby and give lots of smiles and enthusiasm when he tries a new vegetable or a food he seems to dislike.

- You are a role model: If you want your child to eat vegetables, then you must, as well, in front of him.

- Toward the end of the first year of life, babies can eat most of the foods adults eat—there is no need for "kids' menus."

PART 4

Early Childhood

F ROM ONE YEAR OF AGE, CHILDREN gain more independence with eating as they become more communicative. For parents, there are lots of opportunities to make a real difference to *what* and *how* your child eats now and in the future. As your child grows, some things get easier, while some get a bit harder, especially if your child becomes excessively fussy about what he will eat. And, unfortunately, fussiness becomes fairly common in the toddler years, so you can expect some of this. Making sure that you establish healthy eating habits in the first 1,000 days is more important than ever, given the high levels of overweight and obesity among preschool children in the US.

Data from the National Health and Nutrition Examination Survey (NHANES) 2015–2016 estimated that 14 percent of children aged two to five years had developed obesity.[1] Although the health risks of obesity don't usually make an appearance until well into adult life, the problem is that once a child has developed overweight or obesity they are likely to stay that way as an older child, and then as an adult. We know from a review of over 200,000 people that most children with overweight continue to have overweight as adolescents and as adults.[2] In particular, a large study of more than 50,000 children showed that nearly 90 percent of three-year-old children with obesity continued to have obesity or overweight in adolescence (ages fifteen to eighteen), and rapid weight gain during the preschool years was a key risk factor for obesity in adolescence.[3] Helping your child to maintain a healthy weight in the first 1,000 days of his life is therefore crucial.

The psychological and health consequences for children with overweight can be far-reaching and enduring. Psychological consequences for children can include poorer health-related quality of life, emotional and behavioral disorders (such as depression and anxiety) and worse academic performance.[4] The longer-term consequences for children with obesity can include raised risk of type 2 diabetes, coronary heart disease and a range of cancers in adulthood.[5]

Toddlerhood provides a great opportunity to set your child on a healthy weight trajectory. Optimal nutrition (*what* your child eats) during these early years will pave the way for lifelong health and ensure that he thrives now and well into adulthood. But it is also the time when eating habits are formed, which can set him up for life. Based on the largest study of the diets and eating habits of toddlers in the UK (Gemini), the tips and advice in the final part of this book will help you to ensure that your child is on the right track to optimal nutrition (*what* he eats—Chapter 11) and support him in developing healthy eating habits (*how* he eats—Chapter 12).

CHAPTER 11

The Importance of a Healthy Diet

A healthy, balanced diet is crucial for your toddler's health and development. But it can be difficult to know just what a healthy diet is, especially when foods can be marketed for children as "healthy" when in fact they are not. Part of this involves knowing the dietary requirements for your toddler, but it also means taking time to read food labels—which can be very confusing. This chapter will equip you with the knowledge to understand better the US guidelines on energy and nutrient intakes and portion sizes, and how they apply to your child. We will guide you toward choosing foods that contain essential nutrients and advise on portion sizes that are appropriate for toddlers. However, be aware that dietary guidelines specifically for infants and children up to two years of age in the US are in the process of being developed and will be published in 2020.

A Typical Toddler's Diet in the US

So, how many toddlers in the US actually manage to eat a healthy diet? The short answer to this question is: not very many. Large surveys of US children have highlighted some concerning shortcomings of toddlers' diets. In fact, the problems are largely the same as the ones we see in the UK, although we didn't know much about British toddlers' diets until Gemini. In the UK, we recognized that a large study of the eating habits of contemporary toddlers was needed to assess whether they are meeting dietary recommendations and, if not, where the problems are. With Gemini, we therefore conducted a large-scale dietary survey of over 2,000 UK children at about two years of age. Parents completed three-day diet diaries and used portion guides to record every single thing each child ate and drank, as well as the amount. The diaries were able to tell us about the average calorie and nutrient intake for the whole sample of children.[1] The important insights that this study gave us into young children's eating behaviors have fueled our passion for this area of research and were an impetus for writing this book. The study has paved the way for us to give parents much-needed guidance on how and what to feed their children during the toddler years. Below we highlight the major areas of concern for the diets of toddlers in both the US and the UK.

ENERGY INTAKE

In the US, the National Academy of Medicine (NAM) states that babies aged one to two years require about 1,000 calories per day.[2] The *2015–2020 Dietary Guidelines for Americans* recommend that children aged two consume about 1,000 calories per day and those aged three consume about 1,000 calories if they are sedentary, and between 1,200 and 1,400 calories per day if moderately active or active.[3] The Feeding Infants and Toddler Study (FITS) in 2008 found that the average daily energy intake for children aged two to three years was 1,249 calories,[4] but by 2016 this had increased to 1,379 calories per day.[5] These values are at the higher end of the recommended range of energy intakes (those that only apply to three-year-old children who are fairly active).

In Gemini we found that UK toddlers exceeded recommended intakes by about 70 calories per day. Though this may seem relatively small, it adds up over time, and if this is sustained day after day during childhood, it can eventually lead to overweight for some children. With an excess of 70 calories per day, within just two months children would consume about 4,000 extra calories (about four whole days' worth of extra eating). It is easy to see how a small amount of additional calories each day can lead to excess weight gain over time in young children. However, over a third of the children in the sample consumed less energy per day than recommended, so it is not the case that all children were eating too much—all children are different.

It is virtually impossible to know the calorie content of every single piece of food your child eats throughout the day, and we would never suggest that you count calories obsessively for your child, but being *calorie aware* is useful (this means taking time to read nutrition labels). However, healthy eating is not just about calories—it's about making sure your child has a balanced and varied diet and is offered age-appropriate portion sizes.

PROTEIN

The *2015–2020 Dietary Guidelines for Americans* recommends that children aged one to three years of age need 13 g of protein per day for healthy development, and protein should account for between 5 to 20 percent of their total daily calories (i.e., 50 to 200 calories per day from protein if consuming 1,000 calories per day).[6] So, how much protein do most US toddlers consume? In FITS 2016, children one to two years old were consuming 46 g per day (15 percent of their energy from protein), and children two to three years of age were consuming 52 g per day (16 percent).[7] So, US toddlers are consuming more than three times the amount they need and are at the higher end of the recommended range. While there is popular belief that a high-protein diet is a good way to maintain a healthy weight (or lose weight) as an adult, research actually shows that high-protein intake in infancy and early childhood is linked to obesity. For example, one study demonstrated that babies and toddlers consuming higher amounts of protein between twelve and twenty-four months of age had higher body mass index (BMI) and a higher percentage of body fat when they were seven years old.[8] The current consensus among researchers is that high levels of protein stimulate the production of insulin, which encourages sugar in the blood to be stored as fat. It also seems to stimulate the production of something called insulin-like growth factor 1, which promotes faster growth (and may also "program" for obesity in adulthood and related diseases such as type 2 diabetes and cardiovascular disease).[9]

In Gemini we also found that toddlers were consuming high amounts of protein—on average 40 g per day, which is nearly three times the recommended amount in the UK (15 g). What's more, the toddlers who were eating more protein also gained more weight between two and five years of age.[10] We know that protein from dairy (such as milk and cheese) rather than other animal-based protein (such as meat or fish) or plant-based protein (such as pumpkin seeds and lentils) was driving the increases in weight gain seen in Gemini, in line with other studies, too.[11] In fact, almost a quarter of the energy intake was consumed from milk, and many Gemini children (13 percent) were still consuming formula at two years of age.[12] This suggests they were consuming too much milk, which contributed to the excess protein and the excess daily energy intake. It is therefore a good idea to keep an eye on how much protein your toddler is getting each day. It can easily creep up if he is drinking a lot of milk, which also displaces other vital nutrients such as iron. See our guidance on page 181 on recommended quantities of milk for infants and toddlers if you feel your child is consuming too much milk.

CARBOHYDRATES AND SUGAR

Children aged one to three years in the US need 130 g of carbohydrates per day to thrive and are recommended to consume 45 to 65 percent of their calories from carbohydrates (i.e., 450 to 650 calories per day from carbohydrates if consuming 1,000 calories per day).[13] FITS 2016 found that one- to two-year-olds consumed 51 percent (152 g per day) and two- to three-year-olds consumed 53 percent (188 g per day) of their calories from carbohydrates, so this is in line with recommendations but at the higher end.[14] Good sources include pasta, rice, cereal and other starchy foods (see pages 252–53 on achieving a balanced diet).

Children aged one to three years should also be consuming *less than* 10 percent of their total calories from added sugar (i.e., less than 100 calories per day if consuming 1,000 calories per day). This equates to about 25 g a day, which isn't a lot. To give you an idea of how much this is, a standard-sized can of cola (12 ounces) contains 39 g of sugar. Other drinks that contain a lot of sugar include all sugar-sweetened fizzy drinks (sodas), energy drinks, most fruit smoothies and fruit juices, and milkshakes. Foods that contain a lot of sugar include cookies, candy, cakes, chocolate, sugared breakfast cereals and ice cream. It's difficult for children to get all of the nutrients they need while staying within their daily calorie recommendations if they consume more than 10 percent of their calories from added sugar. In order to keep below this limit, we would recommend that your child doesn't have any sugar-sweetened drinks and only occasionally has food with sugar added to it.

FAT

In the US, children one to three years of age are recommended to consume between 30 and 40 percent of their energy intake from fat.[15] So, for a child eating 1,000 calories a day this equates to between 300 and 400 calories per day. Fats are an essential part of your child's diet but shouldn't be consumed to excess because fat is very energy dense—it contains a large number of calories even in very small amounts. To put this into context, 1 g fat contains 9 calories, but 1 g protein or carbohydrates contains only 4 calories (so fat has more than twice the number of calories for the equivalent quantity). Once your child is two years old, as long as he is growing well and is healthy, you can offer him lower-fat foods over full-fat ones—for example, reduced-fat (2 percent) or low-fat (1 percent) milk instead of full-fat (whole) milk; but the American Academy of Pediatrics (AAP) recommends transitioning him from full-fat to reduced-fat to low-fat over a few weeks.[16] Fats also come in different forms; some are good for you, whereas others are less good for you and so need to be limited.

Saturated Fat and Trans Fat

Children aged one to three should get less than 10 percent of their calories from saturated fat (i.e., only 100 calories if consuming 1,000 calories per day). The best way to ensure this is to make sure your child doesn't eat too many nonessential foods that are high in saturated fat. These tend to be processed foods such as chips, pastries, pies, ice cream, chocolate, cookies and cakes. The NAM recommends that everyone have as little trans fat (partially hydrogenated vegetable oil) as possible in their diet, and we would recommend that you read nutrition labels and ingredients lists to make sure you avoid these fats for your child as much as possible.

Unsaturated Fats

Unsaturated fats are the "good" fats and there are two main types: monounsaturated fats and polyunsaturated fats. Polyunsaturated fats are *essential* fats, which means that they are necessary for various functions in the body and you can't make them, so it's important that your child gets these from his diet. There are several types, and children aged one to three are recommended to have 7 g per day of an omega-3 fatty acid called linoleic acid (LA) and 0.7 g per day of an omega-6 fatty acid called alpha-linolenic acid (ALA).[17] These are found in some nuts and seeds (such as walnuts and flaxseeds) and their oils (flaxseed oil and walnut oil), oily fish (such as salmon, tuna and herring), and eggs (opt for the omega-3-enriched ones). Foods high in monounsaturated fats include olive oil, peanut oil, avocados and most nuts, but there is no recommended intake for these.

FIBER

In the US, children aged one to three years of age are recommended to have a minimum of 14 g per day of fiber (if they are consuming 1,000 calories per day).[18] Recent data from the Feeding Infants and Toddler Study in 2016 showed that the average intake of fiber fell short of recommendations for both one- to two-year-olds (at 10 g per day) and two- to three-year-olds (at 12 g per day).[19] In 2019, the WHO commissioned the largest review ever undertaken into fiber and health; it found that eating lots of fiber and whole grain foods reduced the risk of premature death from any cause, as well as coronary heart disease, stroke, type 2 diabetes and colorectal cancer. It was also linked with lower weight, blood pressure and cholesterol levels.[20] As we mentioned on page 44, there are two types of fiber: soluble (found in bananas, baked beans or carrots) and insoluble fiber (found in high-fiber breakfast cereals, whole grain bread or brown rice).

VITAMIN D AND IRON

The AAP recommends that all children in the US consume a minimum of 10 mcg (400 IU) of vitamin D per day, and the *2015–2020 Dietary Guidelines for Americans* recommends a higher daily intake of 15 mcg (600 IU) for children aged one to three.[21] Low vitamin D intake is relatively common among young children within the US, and sufficient intakes of vitamin D are difficult (if not impossible) to achieve through diet alone. In NHANES the average intake of vitamin D from food, drinks and supplements fell short of recommendations, at 7 mcg per day for one- to four-year-olds.[22] We would strongly recommend following the AAP's guidance to offer your child a vitamin D supplement each day of at least 10 mcg.

The recommended iron intake for US children aged one to three years is 7 mg per day.[23] Average intakes among children one to four years of age in NHANES were between 10 to 13 mg per day and therefore met recommendations.[24] See pages 224–26 for good sources of vitamin D and iron. Offering your child a varied diet with the recommended amount of vitamin D–fortified milk and a decent amount of oily fish and meat, as well as foods that have been fortified with vitamin D and iron, can all help to ensure that he gets enough of these important nutrients.

SALT

Salt (sodium) increases the risk of raised blood pressure and heart disease in adulthood. The NAM has set "adequate intake" levels of salt for US children aged one to three years at 2.5 g per day (1,000 mg sodium); this is the amount that is needed to meet the needs of healthy and moderately active children.[25] The *Dietary Guidelines* have set the maximum safe level for children this age at 3.75 g of salt per day (1,500 mg sodium).[26]

In NHANES in 2009 to 2012, 39 percent of children aged one to two years and 70 percent of children aged two to three years exceeded the maximum safe level of salt consumption.[27] Aside from the detrimental impact that this may have on their health, another study has shown that this may set taste preferences for the future—preschool children (three to four years of age) who had been exposed to starchy table foods (a source of salt) at six months of age preferred salty solutions, were more likely to lick salt from the surface of foods and were more likely to eat plain salt.[28] It is therefore really important not to add salt to any food you prepare for your child and to be mindful of processed foods (which have been altered in some way during preparation), such as ready meals, cheese, chips, ham, bacon and sausages, as these often contain a lot of salt. The AAP's healthychildren.org is a website for parents that provides evidence-based guidance on various aspects of child health, including early-life feeding. Their webpage "We Don't Need to Add Salt to Food" provides examples of prepackaged foods containing high levels of salt, with the salt content listed. It's worth a look; you may be quite surprised by just how much salt is in some of those foods.

How to Achieve a Healthy Diet

How do you make sure your toddler gets optimal nutrition? It's not easy, but it's about offering him more of the nutrient-rich foods and less of the foods that are high in sugar, salt and/or unnecessary fat. Offering healthy snacks as well as healthy meals, and ensuring that portion sizes of meals and snacks are age-appropriate, is crucial, too. An important part of this is familiarizing yourself with food labels, so you can spot foods that are good choices and those that should be limited.

UNDERSTANDING FOOD LABELS

Food labels contain a lot of information, and it can be very difficult to know what you are supposed to be looking for and what it all means. Learning how to read food labels is essential to know what we are eating. It empowers us to make informed, healthy choices. The FDA stipulates that most prepackaged foods have a label *on the back or side of the packaging* with nutritional information, called Nutrition Facts (very few foods are allowed not to have one). In fact, this label is simpler now than it was several years ago—in 2016 the FDA updated the nutrition information included on the label because many people in the US couldn't understand it.[29] The new label should make it easier for people to make better informed food choices (it has to be implemented by all food companies by January 2021).[30]

The following key pieces of nutritional information are on the Nutrition Facts label:

1. **Calories and serving size**

   Calories tell you the total energy in one serving of the food. It's a good idea to know which foods tend to be far higher in calories than you expect, so that you can make sure your child doesn't have too many of these, if they are nonessential. The serving size on the new label will be based on the amount that people *typically* consume of that type of product (e.g., ice cream), not on how much they should consume (and the percent daily values are worked out based on this serving size). The serving size allows you to understand how much of a nutrient you are eating, to compare the nutritional content of two similar food products and to compare the serving size to the amount you eat. If your child eats the serving size listed on the package, he will get the amount of energy and nutrients that are listed. But if it is a much smaller amount than your child usually eats, he will end up consuming more of the calories and nutrients that are listed "per serving." Also bear in mind that food labels and nutritional information are based on adult serving sizes, so you would need to check the appropriate-sized portion for your child.

2. **Fats**

   Total fat, saturated fat and trans fat are all listed on the food label. There is no requirement for nutrition labels to include any information about unsaturated fats.

3. **Cholesterol**

   The amount of cholesterol in a food product is shown on the food label. Many foods high in cholesterol also tend to be high in saturated fat, so try to limit your child's intake of these foods.

4. **Sodium**

   The sodium level indicates the amount of salt in the food. Sodium is a mineral and one of the chemical elements in salt (sodium chloride). You can calculate the salt content of the product by multiplying the amount of sodium in grams on the label by 2.5 and dividing by 1,000—for example, 500 mg of sodium = (500 x 2.5) / 1,000 = 1.25 g salt.

5. **Carbohydrates**

   The food label will list total carbohydrates and then break this down further into fiber and sugars. There are two types of sugar:

   - naturally occurring sugar, such as the lactose in milk or natural sugars found in whole fruit and vegetables

   - added sugars, which include sugar that is added to food by individuals (e.g., sugar added to tea) or manufacturers in processing (e.g., candy, cookies, cakes, sugar-sweetened sodas), as well as the sugars naturally present in honey and syrups. Added sugar is a new addition to the Nutrition Facts label.

   Many of the foods and drinks containing "added" sugars tend to have a lot of calories but few other nutrients.

6. **Protein**

   The Nutrition Facts label will list total protein in the food.

7. **Vitamins and minerals**

   Vitamin D, potassium, calcium and iron are also listed on the Nutrition Facts label; many Americans don't get enough of these, so this information helps people to keep an eye on their intake. Vitamins A and C are no longer required, since deficiencies of these vitamins are rare today.

8. **Percent daily value**

   Percent daily value (DV) shows how much a nutrient in a serving of the food contributes to the daily recommended amount. Use the percent DV to determine if a serving of the food is high or low in an individual nutrient. The values listed on most foods will be for adults, so they won't be relevant to your child. As a general guide, 5 percent DV or less of a nutrient per serving is considered low, and 20 percent DV or more of a nutrient per serving is considered high.

Ingredients List

Food labels also have an ingredients list, which can also be used to help you decide how healthy a food is. Ingredients are listed by weight, starting with the ingredient that weighs the most and ending with the ingredient that weighs the least. Those that appear first in the list make up a bigger share of the food product, so if these are high in saturated fat or sugar, such as butter, cream or sugar, the product is usually less healthy.

ACHIEVING A BALANCED DIET

The trick to achieving a balanced diet for your toddler is to know the different types and proportions of foods that he should be eating each day. MyPlate (at choosemyplate.gov) was developed in 2011 by the US Department of Agriculture (USDA) Center for Nutrition Policy and Promotion. It is an infographic that makes it easy to see which foods, and how much of each type, people should be eating. There are five food groups (fruits, vegetables, grains, protein foods and dairy), with specific recommendations for daily intakes for all ages. Below are the recommended daily intakes for children aged two to three who are consuming about 1,000 calories per day (daily intakes of all food groups are higher for children whose recommended calorie intakes are higher).

1. **Fruits:** Any fruit or 100 percent fruit juice counts as part of this group. Children two to three years old are recommended to have one of the following per day: one cup of raw, cooked or canned fruit (for example, half a large apple; one large orange, peach or banana; or one medium pear); half a cup of dried fruit; or one cup of 100 percent fruit juice. Although fruit juice and dried fruit are included in this group, given the high sugar content, we would recommend that you opt for whole fruit instead.

2. **Vegetables:** Any vegetable or 100 percent vegetable juice counts as a member of this group. Based on their nutrient content, vegetables are organized into five subgroups: dark-green vegetables, starchy vegetables, red and orange vegetables, beans and peas, and other vegetables. Children two to three years old are recommended to have one of the following per day: one cup of raw, cooked or canned vegetables; two cups of leafy salad greens; or one cup of 100 percent vegetable juice. Although vegetable juice is included in this group, given the low fiber content, we recommend that you opt for whole vegetables instead.

3. **Grains:** Any food made from wheat, rice, oats, cornmeal, barley or another cereal grain is a grain product. Bread, pasta, oatmeal, breakfast cereals, tortillas and grits are examples of grain products. Grains are divided into two subgroups: whole grains and refined grains. Whole grains contain the entire grain kernel—the bran, germ and endosperm. Examples of whole grains include whole wheat flour, bulgur (cracked wheat), oatmeal, whole cornmeal and brown rice. Refined grains have been milled, a process that removes the bran and germ. This is done to give grains a finer texture and improve their shelf life, but it also removes dietary fiber, iron and many B vitamins. Some examples of refined grain products are white flour, degermed cornmeal, white bread and white rice. Most refined grains are enriched. This means certain B vitamins (thiamin, riboflavin, niacin, folic acid) and iron are added back after processing. Check the ingredient list on refined grain products to make sure that the word *enriched* is included in the grain name. Some food products are made from mixtures of whole grains and refined grains. Children two to three years old are recommended to have three 1-ounce servings of grains per day. A single 1-ounce serving includes 1 slice of bread; 1 ounce of ready-to-eat cereal; or half a cup of cooked rice, pasta or cereal. Half of all grains should be whole grains (for example, whole grain bread).

4. **Protein Foods:** All foods made from meat, poultry, seafood, beans and peas, eggs, processed soy products, nuts and seeds are part of this group. Meat and poultry choices should be lean or low-fat. Children two to three years old are recommended to have two 1-ounce servings of protein foods per day. A single 1-ounce serving includes 1 ounce of cooked or canned lean meat (beef or lamb), poultry (chicken or turkey without the skin), fish or seafood; one egg; 1 ounce of nuts; 1 tablespoon of peanut butter; a quarter of a cup of cooked beans, tofu, chickpeas or lentils; or 0.5 ounce of ground nuts or seeds (these cannot be given whole to children less than five years of age because of the risk of choking).

5. **Dairy:** All food and drinks made from milk are considered part of this food group. Foods made from milk that retain their calcium content are part of the group, but foods made from milk that have little to no calcium, such as cream cheese, cream and butter, are not. Calcium-fortified soy milk is also part of the dairy group. The recommendation is that these should be low-fat or fat-free. Children

two to three years old are recommended to have two cups of dairy per day. One cup of dairy includes one cup of milk; one cup of yogurt (8 fluid ounces); one cup of fortified soy milk; 1.5 ounces of natural cheese such as cheddar; or 2 ounces of processed cheese.

LIMIT UNHEALTHY FOODS AND SNACKS

Try to check food labels and limit the amount of processed high-fat, high-sugar foods, such as pastries, candy, chocolate and chips, that you have in the house. This is probably the easiest way to help your child eat healthily. To cut down on the amount of sugar you give to your child, we recommend offering him water for the majority of drinks, not fruit juice. We would not recommend simply replacing sugar with artificial sweeteners, because this could still encourage your child to develop a preference for sweet flavors. If you have sugar in your tea, you will probably think that tea without sugar tastes terrible, because you have become used to it tasting sweet. It's best not to create or encourage these preferences for sweeter flavors in the first place, to avoid encouraging a "sweet tooth" in your child. Try to avoid purchasing too many processed foods, as many of them have more sugar than you would add if you were to make them at home.

It is also surprising how easily children can consume too much salt. For example, if your child is two years old and has a 0.7-ounce (20 g) bowl of cornflakes for breakfast (0.37 g salt), half a cheese sandwich for lunch made up of one slice of whole grain bread (0.4 g salt) and 1 ounce (30 g) cheese (0.5 g salt), half a small bag of chips as a snack (0.17 g salt) and an evening meal of two fish sticks (0.23 g salt) and vegetables, they will be close to the recommended limit of 2.5 g per day. These are common everyday foods for many children, and you would probably not consider some of them to be particularly high in salt, but processed cereals, bread and cheese are foods that have a surprising amount of salt in them. Here are other foods that are high in salt.

- Bacon
- Gravy granules and stock cubes
- Soy sauce

- Sausages
- Smoked meats and fish
- Coated chicken
- Ham

One good way of reducing the salt in your child's diet is to prepare food yourself rather than buying ready-made foods. You can add flavor using other ingredients, such as fresh herbs, black pepper, tomato paste (no salt added), garlic, balsamic vinegar and lemon juice, and you could purchase low-salt stock cubes. Roasting vegetables is a great way to bring out their flavor rather than adding salt to the pot when boiling.

Small changes can make a big difference to your child's diet, without him feeling shortchanged or hungry. Healthy swaps include

- carrot sticks and hummus instead of a bag of chips
- a whole piece of fruit instead of dried fruit
- a frozen banana instead of ice cream (this is a great snack and kids love it!)
- boiled or poached eggs instead of fried eggs
- fruit bread instead of cakes and cookies
- low-sugar breakfast cereals (for example, plain shredded wheat or oatmeal) instead of those coated in honey or sugar
- low-salt stock cubes instead of standard stock cubes.

HEALTHY SNACKS

Many parents are unsure what constitutes a healthy snack. A lot of the snack foods available for children are high in sugar or fat, but they are marketed in such a way as to make them appear healthy. Busy lives often mean there is limited time to prepare all of your child's food from scratch, so it's a good idea to have foods available at home that require no preparation, such as fresh fruit and vegetables. There is such a wide variety of fruit and vegetables to choose from, vibrant in color so they will look appealing to young children. A wealth of research has shown that having fruit in a bowl in the house attracts children and leads to them eating more of it.[31] We would recommend that you only offer your chid whole fruit and give him water to drink if he is thirsty. He can be offered milk to drink as a snack.

Your child will, of course, occasionally have snack foods that are high in fat and/or sugar, such as chocolate and chips. This is perfectly OK. Simply try to be careful about how often you give these and how much you offer to your child, because too many are bad for his teeth as well as his health.

Healthy Snack Ideas

When thinking about snacks for your child, it's a good idea to combine at least two different food groups to make sure he gets lots of nutritional variety. It's also a great opportunity to get him to eat more fruit and vegetables.

- ½ cup yogurt with ½ cup fruit (strawberries, blueberries, banana, pear or orange)
- ½ mini bagel with ½ tablespoon hummus
- 2 snack slices of rye bread with ½ cup cottage cheese
- ½ cup vegetable sticks (carrot, cucumber or bell pepper) with ½ cup yogurt
- 1 rye crisp bread with ½ tablespoon peanut or almond butter
- ½ small piece of corn bread with ½ tablespoon guacamole

Snacks that require no preparation are great if time is limited, but if you do have a bit of time it is a good idea to get your toddler involved in preparing food with you, as it will familiarize him with different foods and may make him more likely to try new ones.

NUTRITIONAL SUPPORT FOR LOW-INCOME FAMILIES

The Special Supplemental Nutrition Program for Women, Infants, and Children (WIC) provides federal grants to states for foods; referrals to health, welfare and social services; and nutrition education and counseling for low-income pregnant, breastfeeding and non-breastfeeding women (up to six months after birth) and babies and children up to age five who would benefit from nutritional support. If you are struggling to afford to feed yourself and your child, it is worth getting in touch with your local WIC agency to find out if they can support you.

Portion Size

It is sometimes difficult to know whether your child is eating enough or eating too much, but parents tend to worry much more about their child undereating than overeating. Children all differ in their appetites, and how often and how much food your child eats will vary depending on his appetite (as well as other things, such as how fast he is growing at that particular time).

Many parents struggle to know what an appropriate portion size is for babies and toddlers. Large portions are problematic because research has shown very consistently that children (and adults) will eat more food if they are served more.[32] We all have a tendency to eat a bit more *if it is there*, simply because we can—this is known as the "portion size effect." One study involved thirty-five children aged three to five years old being served snacks differing in portion size.[33] The amounts eaten during the snack and a subsequent lunch were measured, and, regardless of age, the children who had been served larger snacks ate more overall. Another study that looked at the daily food intake of sixteen children aged four to six years old found that the most powerful influence on the amount children ate was the amount served to them.[34] These particular studies were small, but this effect has been observed over and over again in all sorts of other studies, and with older children and adults as well. This tendency to eat more when served more was probably helpful many thousands of years ago, when food was less plentiful and it was wise to eat every last scrap when you came across it. But in the current food environment, where there is virtually no limit to food for most people in the Western world, this tendency can quickly lead to excessive weight gain. And children who are less sensitive to their fullness and more responsive to food cues are more susceptible to overeating in response to larger portions.

Now this might sound obvious, but there are two ways to eat more calories during a meal: a large volume of food is eaten, or a small volume of food is eaten but it is higher in energy density (more calories per gram). Therefore, another important consideration when thinking about the portion size of foods you serve your child is the energy density of that particular food.

Energy Density

Energy density is the amount of energy (calories) per gram of food. Lower energy-density foods, such as soups, stews, fruit and vegetables, tend to have a higher water content, so they provide fewer calories per gram of food. High energy-density foods, such as cookies, cakes, chips, peanuts and cheese, tend to be high in fat and have a low water content.

In theory, if a food is high in energy density, your child should naturally eat *less* of it through the process of self-regulation, but this doesn't seem to happen (at least not for every child). In the study of four- to six-year-olds mentioned above, the children did not adjust the amount they ate based on the energy density of the food. If the children were served more, they ate more. There is also a perception among researchers that children should eat less following a snack before a meal; so if you go for a meal and your child has an appetizer, he should eat less of his main course to compensate. But again, research has shown that not all children do this.

Studies such as these provide evidence that some children, like adults, can be influenced by certain aspects of their eating environment (for example, portion sizes and energy density) rather than their internal feelings of fullness. Even babies as young as six weeks old have shown this tendency—mothers of eighteen breastfed infants aged six to twenty-one weeks old expressed extra breast milk as a means of increasing milk production, and, as a result of the increased supply of milk, their babies drank more and had a greater energy intake.[33] This suggests that serving large portions interferes with our ability to regulate our intake, even for very young babies. A review of the evidence for the impact of portion sizes on the consumption of food and drinks was conducted in 2015.[35] Fifty-eight studies involving a total of 6,603 participants were assessed, and it was concluded that exposure to larger portion sizes increased quantities of food consumed among children and adults. The authors suggested that if portion sizes were reduced across the whole diet, average daily energy intake could be reduced by 144 to 228 kcal. Another review estimated that if you double the portion size, people eat 35 percent more on average.[36] This is a lot and highlights that age-appropriate portion sizes could make the difference between maintaining a healthy weight and developing overweight for some children. What is particularly concerning is that according to large national surveys in the US, the portion sizes of a whole range of foods served to children both at home and outside the home have increased markedly from the late 1970s to the 2000s, and this is particularly pronounced for "fast food."[37] Another problem with the increase in portion sizes over time is that larger portions have become "normal"—called "portion distortion"—and what we now expect.

WEIGHT GAIN

In a large national sample of British babies and toddlers, we looked at whether those who consumed larger portions were more likely to develop overweight.[38] We found that all children ate, on average, five times per day (three meals and two snacks), but the children who had developed overweight ate larger portions at each meal or snack. In Gemini we looked at how portion size affected the children's rate of weight gain from two to five years of age.[39] We found that children who consumed larger average portions gained weight at a faster rate than those who consumed a smaller portion each time. Our research suggests that, in toddlerhood, overweight is strongly linked to eating larger portions during each meal/snack, highlighting the need to be vigilant about the portion sizes that you offer to your child. Early childhood is also a great opportunity to shape your child's expectations about what portion sizes are appropriate.

PORTION SIZE GUIDANCE

Many parents of young children are not sure where to go for portion-size guidance. The MyPlate website provides detailed information on age-appropriate portion sizes for different types of food within each food group, as well as ideas for meals and snacks. We recommend that you have a look and familiarize yourself with the portion sizes of the foods that your child commonly consumes. In general, younger children should be eating slightly less than older children, but it also depends on their level of activity—if your child spends most of the day running around, he'll need more calories to grow. But we suggest that, as well as having a rough idea of your child's nutritional needs, an important part of judging how much food he needs is to know what type of eater he is and respond accordingly. (See the next chapter for more on this.) As was the case with milk-feeding your baby and starting solid food, the principle that we would suggest you follow is *responsive feeding*.

THE BOTTOM LINE

- Familiarize yourself with your child's dietary requirements.
- Use choosemyplate.gov to provide a balanced diet for your child.
- Read food labels to inform your food choices.
- A few healthy swaps can make a big difference to your child's diet.
- Be mindful of portion sizes. Large portions have been shown to influence weight gain in young children.
- Children will eat more when served more, so they need child-sized portions.
- Portion sizes are not an exact science—the amount your child needs will depend on his weight and level of activity (and his appetite—discussed in the next chapter).

CHAPTER 12

Responsive Feeding in the Toddler Years

The first 1,000 days provides a unique window of opportunity for you to lay the foundations for your toddler's eating habits that will (hopefully!) endure for many years. *What* he eats during this period is important, but *how* he eats matters, too. During toddlerhood, the way you feed your child and the routines you establish can help to optimize his appetite regulation and encourage him to like a wide variety of foods, not to hanker after less-nutritious foods and to be open to trying new ones. You have the opportunity to help him foster a good relationship with food so that he views it as nourishment rather than comfort, entertainment, a reward or even something to be feared.

You will now be well versed in the principles of responsive feeding—recognizing what type of eater your child is and using appropriate feeding strategies that support his particular eating styles. You should continue to use this approach now that he is becoming a more integrated member of family meals. But ensuring that he develops good eating habits goes further than responsive feeding now that he is older. It will also involve establishing structured mealtime routines and including him in the preparation of meals and shopping for food. All of this will pave the way for him to make good choices when the time comes for him to start making decisions about food on his own.

What the Evidence Says

Systematic reviews of responsive feeding, weight gain and appetite regulation in toddlerhood and childhood have highlighted that responsive feeding is linked to better appetite regulation and healthier weight gain.[1] But the vast majority of studies haven't been designed in such a way that it is possible to know if unresponsive feeding is really the cause of poor appetite regulation and risk of overweight, or whether parents tend to use less responsive feeding methods when their children have avid or poor appetites and are already either gaining weight too rapidly or too slowly. The only way to really find this out is through a randomized trial. A recent review of all randomized trials to prevent overweight and obesity in infancy and childhood concluded that the most promising trials were those that focused on responsive feeding as well as diet.[2]

The most important trial to date on responsive feeding during complementary feeding and appetite regulation is NOURISH, which randomized 352 Australian women to receive twelve group sessions on how to feed responsively and what foods their babies should be given when they were between four and seven months old (six sessions) and again when they were thirteen to sixteen months old (six sessions).[3] Another 346 moms were randomized to be in the control group—they had access to all the usual health services but no extra information on feeding. At two years of age the toddlers whose moms were in the intervention group had better appetite control—they were less food responsive, had better satiety sensitivity and were less likely to emotionally overeat (wanting to eat when feeling upset, anxious or annoyed).[4] They were also less fussy with regard to food. Many of these effects were still there when the children were three to four years old—they were still less food responsive and more satiety sensitive.[5] The intervention did not have a big effect on children's weights, however.[6] At five years of age there were slightly fewer children with overweight in the intervention group, but this difference was not considered statistically significant (meaning it could have been due to chance). Nevertheless, it showed that responsive feeding can have long-lasting effects on appetite.

How to Feed Your Toddler Responsively

As mentioned in Chapter 6, responsive feeding involves feeding your child only when he is hungry and stopping as soon as he indicates to you that he is full. The good news is that, now that your child is older, it is much easier to read his hunger and satiety signals—these gestures tend to be far easier to read in a toddler than a baby, probably because he will sometimes just tell you, so you don't have to rely solely on his body language.

Hunger Cues from Around Twelve Months of Age

- leaning toward food
- visually tracking food
- excited arm and leg movements
- opening his mouth as the spoon approaches
- asking for or pointing toward food

Satiety Cues from Around Twelve Months of Age

- shaking head to say "no more"
- using words like "all done" and "get down"
- playing with food or throwing food
- pushing food or plate away

However, for toddlers and young children, responsive feeding gets a little bit more complicated than simply looking out for his hunger and fullness signals—it involves much more than that. Broadly speaking, it means you taking care not to be too controlling or dominating in feeding interactions with your child and of his "food world." This certainly doesn't mean giving him free rein and letting him rule mealtimes —overindulgence and lack of control can lead to nothing short of chaos with a two-year-old! At the same time, a laissez-faire approach to feeding, or being uninvolved or disinterested, means he won't get the support that he needs to nurture good eating habits. In order for your child to develop effective appetite regulation, healthy food preferences and a good relationship with food, he needs to learn which foods are nutritious and safe to eat, what hunger and fullness feel like, and that he should only eat when he is hungry and stop when he feels full. You are an important part of this learning process.

The trick is to find the right balance—not being too controlling, but not leaving everything up to him. In practice, this will mean making sure that you respond appropriately to your child's needs when he signals them to you—not ignoring them and then overruling him—and giving him a sense that he has *some* control over how he eats (how much and how often) and what food he chooses to eat, while also setting some boundaries (like anything with young children). Children differ in their natural dispositions toward food—some have hearty appetites and want to eat all the time, while others are harder to feed—and different types of eaters pose very different challenges for you as a parent. We will discuss specific tips for different types of eaters in detail on pages 271–86 and offer tailored strategies that you can use to manage eager eaters and very picky ones.

However, there are a few principles of responsive feeding that are important to follow, whatever your child's appetite and eating style:

1. **Let your child decide how much to eat—don't pressure him.**
   Although it can be tempting to pressure your child to finish the meal that you have spent ages preparing, don't make him finish everything on the plate or encourage him to eat more if he has indicated that he is full. This will help him to learn what fullness feels like and to stop eating in response to his satiety. Encourage him to have autonomy over his intake by self-feeding—this may mean accepting there will be some mess!

2. **Avoid excessive restriction of food and use covert rather than overt ways to restrict your child's intake.**
   As he gets older your child will begin to have more autonomy around his eating. This, of course, means that it can be difficult to monitor your child's eating when he goes to parties and there are cakes, chips and other foods high in sugar and fat freely available. At times you may have to simply accept that your child will indulge, but the key is not to make these foods out of bounds. Birthday parties don't happen every day (although they can be every weekend when they are little!), and it is fine for your child to enjoy these foods from time to time. As we mentioned in Chapter 8, being overly restrictive with certain foods

can backfire, and your child may be more likely to want the foods he is never allowed. If you allow foods high in sugar and/or fat but limit them, hopefully when he attends parties he won't go over the top. Try to restrict foods in a covert way—for example, by not keeping too much chocolate in the house—rather than in an overt way—for example, by eating chocolate in front of him but not allowing him any. This will make your life easier insofar as it will minimize pestering, but it will also guard against the "forbidden-fruit effect"—your child wanting more than ever the food that he isn't allowed.

3. **Offer him a range of nutritious foods to choose from.**
   Offering your child a choice of nutritious options will help him to feel like he has some control over *what* he eats and will teach him to make decisions about food for himself. If you offer your child two or three alternatives, it will also soften the blow of saying no to something that he wants. You can read more on this on page 270.

4. **Offer him age-appropriate portion sizes.**
   Make sure you pay attention to the portions of food that you serve your child at meals and for snacks (see page 260). Some toddlers will eat more if served larger portions, simply because the food is there and they can. In addition, it is good to teach your child what an appropriate portion of food looks like; this will lay the groundwork for when he gets older and makes decisions about portion sizes for himself.

5. **Offer food only in response to hunger, or because it is a snack or mealtime, not for any other reason.**
   This means making sure you only feed your child because he needs the nourishment, not because you want to soothe him if he is upset, control his behavior or distract him. If your child learns to eat only in response to hunger, it will support him not only in developing good appetite regulation, but it will also help to ensure that he develops a healthy relationship with food and doesn't come to rely on it as a source of comfort or entertainment. A good strategy is to provide food in the context of regular mealtimes and snack times (see number 10).

6. **Give him lots of praise when he eats nutritious foods that he is reluctant to eat or even try.**
   To your toddler, your praise is a reward worth working for. If he sees that you are pleased with him when he tries certain foods, he will be more likely to do it again next time. This is a fundamental part of

becoming familiar with a food and learning to like it—repeated tastes of a food result in increased exposure and ultimately liking. Expect that he will refuse some foods; this is normal in toddlerhood. If he refuses to eat something, don't make a fuss or try to coax him. Just offer it again tomorrow.

7. **Use nonfood rewards to incentivize him to try a nutritious new food that he is reluctant to eat or to eat a food he doesn't like.**

   Nonfood rewards are a great way to motivate your child to try a food he is suspicious of or refuses to eat. Stickers, badges and star charts work well for some children. You could also give your child a token each time he tries the food, and once he has earned a certain number he can win a nonfood prize (e.g., a game, toy, outing or coloring book). But children differ a lot in how they respond to rewards; you know your child best and will have a good idea about what motivates him. Be sure never to use his favorite food as a bribe to get him to eat nutritious foods he doesn't like—it may result in him disliking the nutritious food even more and increasing his desire for his favorite food, which has now become a reward as well as something that tastes good.

8. **Make sure there are no distractions.**

   Distractions, such as the television or other screens, should be avoided during mealtimes so that your child is able to focus on eating, the taste and texture of the food and the feeling of fullness as he eats.

9. **Be a good model for him yourself.**

   It is important when it comes to healthy eating that you act as a role model by eating healthy foods yourself in front of and with your child. This is the most important way that he will learn about which foods are safe and good to eat. As your child gets older, an important part of this is allowing him to participate in family mealtimes (see pages 267–68). You can also include him in food shopping and preparing meals and snacks. All of these activities are opportunities to teach him about eating healthily. But being a good role model is not just about your behavior; it also involves you having a healthy attitude toward food and eating and using positive language to describe foods. Talking about the nutritional value of foods is a great way to get kids interested in healthy eating.

10. **Establish structured mealtime and snack routines.**

    Try to get into a routine whereby your toddler has three meals each day that are always served at the same time, and two snacks (one midmorning and one midafternoon). This will mean that your child learns what to expect in terms of food and is less likely to pester you for food when it's not a set time to eat. It's really important not to skip meals—a child with an avid appetite will be extremely hungry and may then overcompensate at the next meal, while a child who has a poor appetite may not sufficiently compensate at the next meal. In particular, eating a healthy breakfast is an important habit for your toddler to develop (see pages 268–69). We would also advise limiting mealtimes to thirty minutes. This is plenty of time for children to get all the nutrition they need; dragging out a mealtime for a picky eater will only lead to a battle of wills. There are many more effective strategies for encouraging healthy eating for picky eaters on pages 279–83.

Feeding your child responsively may seem quite a difficult task, and sometimes you will just want an easy life and give in to what your child will or will not eat, but following these tips will help your child to be more in tune with his feelings of hunger and fullness and less fussy, and you will feel more confident about how often and how much he should be eating.

FAMILY MEALTIMES

Eating together as a family appears to benefit children's health and well-being in numerous ways. This is probably not that surprising given that communal eating plays a socially valuable function in virtually every human society. Children who participate in shared family mealtimes have better language development and academic achievement, greater well-being, and better-quality diets.[7] This is probably because "table talk" by parents and older siblings exposes young children to a large and sophisticated vocabulary, problem-solving conversations, parental support, family cohesion and varied nutrition—among other benefits. A recent analysis of seventeen different studies explored the nutritional health of 182,836 children aged two to seventeen years who participated in family mealtimes with varying frequency.[8] The analysis found that children who ate with their family three or more times per week were more likely to have healthier eating patterns and be in the healthy weight range than children who ate fewer than three family meals together. Importantly, too, they were less likely to engage in disordered eating , such as bingeing or using extreme weight control strategies (e.g., diet pills and skipping meals). Another study of two- to five-year-old children found that children's vegetable consumption and liking reflected the extent to which they ate the same food as their parents at mealtimes.[9] This highlights the importance of eating together, giving your child the same food that you eat and modeling healthy eating behaviors in front of your child by eating the same food as he does. Because of the observational design of these studies we cannot know for certain if it is the family meal itself that is responsible for these benefits, or if the types of families who choose to eat their meals together provide all sorts of other advantages to their children that mean they do well in life. But it would seem a wise idea to do this as often as you can, if it works for your family.

However, we do appreciate that it is not always possible to sit down together and eat as a family when work schedules, childcare and other commitments don't allow it. But, if possible, try to get into a routine where you have a meal together once or a few times a week—for example, dinner together at home every Wednesday or breakfast together every Saturday morning. A family meal doesn't have to include anyone other than you and your toddler, but if there are other family members, encourage them to join in as often as they can. The most important thing is that you or someone else sits down with your toddler and eats with him, as often as possible, so that he can watch you eat and learn about foods and behaviors during mealtimes. Family meals also provide time to engage in conversation and spend quality time together. Even if you are not eating with your child, it is still an opportunity to talk, and you can engage with him about what he is eating. The same applies with grandparents and babysitters; it doesn't necessarily have to be immediate family. When you have your meal, aim to sit down together without the television on so that there are no distractions.

BREAKFAST—AN IMPORTANT MEAL

Try to always make time for your child to eat breakfast. Concentration and performance at nursery or school can suffer if a child is hungry and lacking in energy. One review of forty-five studies evaluated the effects of breakfast on children's cognitive performance, and the evidence indicated that breakfast consumption is more beneficial than skipping breakfast, particularly among children who are less well-nourished (such as picky eaters).[10] There is also research to suggest that children who skip breakfast tend to be at slightly increased risk of developing overweight. A review of sixteen observational studies involving almost 60,000 children and adolescents from Europe looked at the evidence on the effects of breakfast consumption on weight.[11] Thirteen of the studies consistently showed that children who regularly ate breakfast were less likely to develop overweight or obesity. Because these were observational studies and not randomized controlled trials, it could, of course, be the case that children and adolescents who were already gaining weight quickly were more likely to skip breakfast in an attempt to control their weight, or it could indicate that skipping breakfast leads to children feeling hungry and overcompensating by eating too much later in the day. Either way, it seems important to ensure that children do not skip breakfast.

Breakfast cereals can be a good source of energy and are usually fortified with vitamins and minerals including iron. However, there are many that contain a lot of sugar and salt, so be aware of these. Good options are plain cereals such as bran flakes, puffed rice or shredded wheat, as these are lower in sugar and contain fiber. Oatmeal with fruit is an excellent option for breakfast.

TAKE YOUR CHILD FOOD SHOPPING

A great way of helping your child learn which foods are nutritious and which are less so is to involve him when you buy and prepare food. It will also help him to become familiar with the appearance and texture of different foods, which is an important part of encouraging children to try new foods.

Some parents avoid taking their children with them to do the family food shopping because of "pester power"—children pressure parents to buy certain foods, often those that they have seen advertised on television. However, if you can fend off this pressure, then taking your child with you to do the family food shop can be very beneficial. It gives you an opportunity to show him that you read food labels and to teach him about the different food groups and making healthy choices. He can contribute toward choosing foods for the family meals and will feel like his input is valued.

Involving your child in the preparation of meals—for example, by washing fresh vegetables and measuring and counting ingredients— also gives him an understanding of how meals are prepared, and he may be more inclined to try the food if he has seen how it has been made. It will also provide a "norm" of eating food that has been prepared from scratch.

OFFER HEALTHY CHOICES

From about the age of two your child will be able to verbalize which foods he likes and dislikes, and which foods he does and doesn't want to eat. But remember that the choices you offer him will influence what he likes and what he will eat, as well. If you give your child total control over what to choose for his meal, there is a strong chance that he will opt for something that doesn't include vegetables. Fish fingers and fries are much more appealing for many young children than, for example, fresh fish with vegetables and boiled new potatoes. Similarly, if you offer a choice between a bag of chips and an apple, most children would choose the chips (adults struggle with these choices, too, even though we know and understand that there are health benefits to choosing the apple over the chips). Therefore, it is important to think about the choices you offer. At a mealtime, for example, offering a choice of broccoli or carrots, rather than broccoli or fries, means that your child will probably end up eating some fresh vegetables. But remember as well to make sure that you always include some food that he likes at every meal.

How to Feed Different Types of Eaters

Responsive feeding and good mealtime habits are important for all children, regardless of what type of eater they are—those with an eager appetite who like big portions and want to eat constantly; those who have a poorer appetite, low interest in food and are fussy; and those who are in between. However, different types of eaters also present unique challenges to parents. There is currently no science to guide us—studies linking responsive feeding with appetite and weight never look at whether different strategies work better for different types of eaters. But ensuring that you feed responsively can be challenging if you have a child with a voracious appetite or one who seems to not want anything at all. The strategies you use will need to be tailored for your child. It's important to learn what type of eater you have, so that you can then feed your child using responsive strategies that will be effective for him.

What Gemini has shown us is that some toddlers are much better at regulating their food intake than others. This is based on their appetite or the type of eater they are: "eager eaters" (those with an avid appetite who have a tendency to eat too much) or "picky eaters" (those with a poor appetite who have a tendency to eat too little). There are distinct eating behaviors that each type of child engages in that can be difficult to manage, and we provide suggestions for how to deal with the key challenges of each.

EAGER EATERS

Children with a hearty appetite tend to be less sensitive to their internal feelings of fullness, are very food responsive, eat quickly and are more likely to develop a tendency to use food for comfort. We know from our research and others that babies and children with these characteristics are at increased risk of gaining excessive weight over time, because these behaviors can lead to overeating, so management early in life is important.[12] In particular, in Gemini we found that toddlers with lower satiety sensitivity consumed larger portions every time they ate, but they didn't compensate for the larger portions by eating less often throughout the day.[13] Another experimental study of one hundred US five- to six-year-olds found that while all children ate more when they were offered larger portions, the children who were not very satiety sensitive and very food responsive ate the most.[14] These studies indicate that children with a more avid appetite are particularly vulnerable to overeating if given larger portions. Many health professionals suggest using your child's appetite to gauge how much food he needs, but this is not straightforward, because a child who is food responsive and less sensitive to his satiety will eat beyond fullness, if given the opportunity. As a parent in this situation, with a seemingly ravenous child, how do you know if you have given him enough or too much? Your child might be indicating that he is still hungry, when in fact he may have had enough food but carries on eating because the food tastes good and because it is there. And what do you do if your child eats everything that you provide for him, and then always says he is still hungry for more? We call this "plate-clearing."

How to Manage Plate-Clearing

If your child will eat everything he is served, this can be very fulfilling for you as a parent and often allays any concerns that he is not eating enough. However, it is important to be mindful of serving large portions. We recommend using the MyPlate portion size guidance and advise you against getting into the habit of providing large portions of food for your child. Start with a reasonable portion (based on the guidelines for his age); if he finishes it and then asks for seconds, ask him if he is still hungry and suggest he wait a few minutes to let his food go down. This will give his satiety time to kick in (we know from research that the hormones that control satiety take ten to fifteen minutes to be released in response to food intake and take effect[15]). If he is still hungry after waiting ten minutes, you could offer him a small portion more or a low-energy-density snack, such as vegetables or fruit. These foods take a while to eat because they require a lot of chewing and will give him more time to feel satiated. They tend also to be high in fiber so are filling. Children with an avid appetite tend to eat very quickly, and this affects their ability to feel full. Eating quickly also reflects a person's enthusiasm to eat that particular food—we all eat super-delicious food faster than we eat blander food—so food-responsive children tend to eat faster, especially when the food tastes really good. But the problem with eating too quickly is that we outpace the biological mechanisms that control our satiety, and it is easy to eat too much before we realize we have had enough because our feelings of fullness come into effect too late. A recent review of twenty-two studies concluded that we eat more food when we eat it quickly rather than slowly, and that slowing down eating rate is a helpful and effective strategy for reducing the amount of food we eat.[16] Many of these studies used elegant experimental designs, providing convincing evidence that slowing down eating really does help prevent overeating. So, if your child has a tendency to eat quickly, it is a good idea to encourage him to slow down the pace. This is no easy task, but some of the following strategies might work (you'll soon figure out what works best for your particular child):

- Teach him to put his spoon or fork down between bites, as this will allow more time for him to feel full after each mouthful.

- Encourage him to have a sip of water throughout the meal to introduce pauses.

- Cut his food up into smaller pieces that he can eat one at a time so it takes him longer to eat the whole meal.

- Remind him to chew his food properly before he swallows it.

- Give him low-energy-density foods that require a lot of chewing and that he can eat larger portions of, such as lean meat or fish and vegetables. Try to limit processed energy-dense foods, such as macaroni and cheese. It is easy to eat large quantities of these quickly before feeling full.

In general, different types of foods vary in how filling they are and how long they will keep us full for. The glycemic index of food (GI; discussed on page 43) determines how much insulin we produce in response to eating it, and there is a considerable body of research showing that low-GI meals and snacks also keep us fuller for longer in the short term.[17] Offering your child low-GI foods might therefore be a good strategy to help him to feel fuller for longer, so it's worth giving them a try. However, bear in mind that not all foods with a low-GI are nutritious; for example, chocolate is low-GI because the high fat content slows down the absorption of the carbohydrates. So, make sure that any low-GI foods you offer are also healthy. The following are examples of nutritious low-GI foods.

- Most fruit and vegetables
- Whole grain cereals, such as oatmeal
- Whole grain and rye bread
- Pulses, such as beans, lentils and peas
- Milk
- Basmati or quick-cooking rice
- Pasta and noodles
- Sweet potatoes

We would caution against routinely serving your child second portions—always wait for him to indicate he is hungry before offering him more. If he is participating in family meals with you, remember that he will be watching you and the rest of the family as part of the process through which he learns about how to eat. If you tend to serve yourselves large portions and routinely have seconds or thirds, your child will also want them and will come to regard this as normal and may develop this habit, too. A good tip to guard against this is putting leftovers away as soon as you have served everyone, to avoid temptation (out of sight, out of mind), and use them for another meal. It is also probably a good idea not to get into the habit of always offering dessert, and only offer it if your child is hungry. If you offer it at every meal, he may start to expect sweet foods after each meal and take this habit with him throughout life. However, if you think he is still hungry, some fruit and yogurt is a great option.

It is especially important for a child with an avid appetite that you never encourage him to clear his plate or to eat past the point at which he indicates to you that he is full. He needs to be supported in learning what fullness feels like and to stop eating when he has those sensations. In the modern environment where we are served large portions, if a young child learns always to clear his plate, he may learn to overeat as he grows into adulthood. He should be guided by his internal feelings of satiety, not the amount of food left on the plate or on the table.

We recommend limiting the amount of time your child eats in front of the television or while playing on an iPad or mobile phone. There has been research to suggest that this may be linked to overeating.[18]

One possible reason is because children focus on the external stimulus rather than on their internal feelings of fullness and are then unaware how much they are eating. How often have you been to the movies and gotten through an entire tub of popcorn without even realizing? Or demolished half a package of cookies in front of the television and have no memory of eating them? Another possible reason why media use has been linked to overeating is exposure to food advertisements, which can make food-responsive children hungry. Imaginative experimental studies have shown that children eat more after they have watched food ads and that the effect is much greater for more food-responsive children and those with overweight.[19] Having the television on while your child is eating could prime him to want to eat more. He may also start to associate watching television with eating. Food ads aren't only on television—they also dominate the internet—so be aware that your child will be exposed to these regardless of the type of media he interacts with, as he gets older.

We would also encourage you to start talking openly with your child about hunger and fullness as early as possible. Explain to him what a full tummy feels like and that it is something to pay attention to while he is eating, and to stop when his tummy feels full. A fantastic experimental study by a US researcher showed that it is possible to train preschool children (three- to four-year-olds) to improve their ability to self-regulate their food intake by teaching them how to recognize their feelings of hunger and satiety and pay close attention to them when starting and stopping eating.[20] The children were taught what the signs of hunger are (a rumbling and empty-feeling stomach), what eating to fullness feels like (stomach extension and satisfaction) and what the consequences of overeating feel like once satiety has been passed (stomach discomfort). They were taught basic things about eating—biting, chewing, swallowing and where the food then goes. Researchers used a doll with a transparent stomach to teach them about how the doll might be feeling with different amounts of food in her stomach. The six-week program led to improved appetite regulation for all of the children—both those who were initially prone to overeating as well as those who were initially prone to undereating.

Top Tips for Plate-Clearing

- Serve age-appropriate portions to your toddler—these will be a lot smaller than an adult portion.

- Use the portion sizes recommended by MyPlate to guide you.

- Do not encourage plate-clearing.

- Do not routinely offer second helpings; only offer them if your child indicates he is still hungry.

- Encourage your child to wait ten to fifteen minutes after eating to check he is still hungry before offering him more food.

- Put leftovers away (out of sight, out of mind).

- Only offer a dessert if your child is still hungry.

- Try to avoid technology during meal times to focus attention on hunger and fullness.

- Offer foods with a low-GI that are also high in fiber, such as oatmeal, beans or whole grain bread (see page 43 for more on GI); these may help your child feel fuller for longer.

- Encourage slower eating to allow time for your child to feel full.

- Encourage your child to take sips of water throughout the meal.

- Talk to your child about hunger and fullness—explain what it feels like and that it's important to stop eating when his tummy feels full.

How to Manage Snacking

From Gemini we know that more food-responsive toddlers eat more frequently,[21] and one of the challenges that parents face with a food-responsive child is that they are constantly asking for snacks. They may also ask for more-palatable foods (those high in fat and sugar that taste really good), often in response to seeing or smelling something appetizing and wanting it. As a parent of a toddler who loves his food, you might be struggling with what sort of snacks to offer and how much and how often to give them. Most parents tend to offer their toddler three meals (breakfast, lunch and dinner) and two snacks per day, and this is what we would recommend. So, how do you deal with your child if he wants snacks constantly throughout the day?

If your child is very food responsive, seeing, smelling or tasting delicious food will make him want to eat it. We all do this to some extent (have you ever ordered your favorite dessert in a restaurant, even if you're full after the main course?), but some of us find temptation much harder to resist than others. Some toddlers will therefore want to eat something nice when they see it and can get very upset or annoyed if they can't have it. The problem is that in the current food environment we are bombarded with food cues—it is virtually impossible to walk down a main street without a waft of something nice finding its way up your nose . . . and your toddler's. While you can't necessarily protect your child from food cues in the wider environment, you can certainly control your food environment at home and what he sees you eating.

If your toddler has a tendency to want to eat all the time, some level of restriction over what and how much he eats is necessary. Unfortunately, the world we live in today has meant that you will come up against this challenge more and more as he gets older and gains increasing independence to interact with the outside world. So, it's wise to get some strategies in place early, but restriction should never be too extreme. The most effective strategy is probably not to have foods in the house that you don't want your child to eat (see covert restriction, pages 203–04).[22] But this is not realistic for everyone and may feel a bit draconian. If this is the case for you, do try to control the sheer volume of these foods that you have in your home and keep them out of sight (for example, in a cupboard) so your child doesn't have to sit and ogle them! We would suggest having a bowl of fruit and ready-to-eat vegetables available, as your child will then learn that those are the foods he is able to have, and it will help to encourage healthy eating. If a bag of chips is on the side next to a fruit bowl, which one are most children likely to choose? Do also bear in mind that you are your child's model. If there are foods you don't want him to eat, then don't eat them yourself in front of him. Wait until you are on your own (after he has gone to bed or is having a nap). If not, you will end up having to say no to him and dealing with the consequences! But in general, some access to these foods is fine; it's about setting limits and boundaries—some foods should only be eaten in moderation.

Controlling your home food environment is one thing, but what do you do if you are out and about and your child is asking for food? We would still suggest that you limit the number of snacks your child regularly eats, regardless of whether they are healthy snacks or not. We know from Gemini that children who snack more often do not compensate enough for these additional snacks by reducing the amount they eat at mealtimes, and this can lead to them eating too much on a daily basis. And small amounts add up over time if this happens regularly. But we appreciate that it isn't always possible or easy to say no, and if your child is genuinely hungry then you need to provide something for him to snack on. In this situation we would suggest that you offer a nutritious snack that is low in energy density and has a low GI (such as fruit)—we have provided healthy-snack ideas on page 256. If your child has a tendency to ask for foods when you are out (such as at the supermarket), then you could preempt this by taking a healthy snack with you.

When you are on the go and haven't brought your own snack for your child, try to purchase food items that are in small snack packs, as this puts a limit on the portion size. It can be difficult to determine what an appropriate portion looks like if you have a large bag of rice cakes, for example, and as we mentioned earlier, children are likely to eat more when there is more available. Consider how much your child has already eaten when you offer him snacks; for example, offer smaller snacks if he has had a large lunch. It can be difficult not to give in to requests for food because you worry that your child is hungry, but try not to offer food if the request is being made in response to a food cue, such as walking past a bakery or the candy aisle in the supermarket. Only offer snacks if your child is genuinely hungry—for example, if it has been a few hours since he last ate. A good way to test this is to offer him a drink of water (it might simply be that he is thirsty, not hungry) and if he is still hungry, then offer him a healthy snack. But also remember that snacks can be a great way of getting more fruit and veggies into your child!

Top Tips for Snacking

- Put more-palatable snacks away (out of sight, out of mind).
- Have fruit and vegetables available and on display: Keep the fruit bowl stocked.
- Try to limit the number of snacks to two per day: one in the morning and one in the afternoon.
- Offer low-GI snacks that are also lower in energy density.
- Buy snack packs rather than large packs—the more there is available, the more children will eat.
- Decide on snack sizes according to how much your child has eaten already that day: Use an age-appropriate portion size.
- Try to avoid offering snacks when your child is responding to food cues; make sure he is genuinely hungry.

PICKY EATERS

While some children show a great interest in food and are prone to overeating, there are others who are far less interested in food, and some who are also very picky about what they will eat. These children are known as fussy eaters (the term *food neophobia* is also sometimes used, but this is more of a reluctance to try new or unfamiliar foods). Fussy eating can be a great worry for some parents and often leads to concerns that their child is not getting the right nutrition. Fussy eating becomes a lot more common as children approach two years of age and is seen in as many as 50 percent of toddlers.[23] If you have a child who seems incredibly fussy about what he eats at this age, even though he seemed to eat perfectly well when he was younger, you are not alone! A large US study of children found that fussy eating increased as children reached two years of age.[24] Children this age were less likely to eat vegetables and more likely to eat energy-dense foods, such as sugary cereals and fries. This resulted in a lack of variety in their diet. As omnivores, humans are capable of consuming a wide variety of different foods. This makes us extremely adaptable but also means we must quickly learn to distinguish between safe and poisonous foods. In this context, fussiness makes sense—fear or refusal of unknown foods (neophobia) protects against harm. Because it emerges shortly after babies start to walk (usually in the second year of life), it is thought to prevent newly mobile toddlers from eating harmful substances. As such, you should expect some fussiness to emerge around toddlerhood—this is totally normal. The types of foods children tend to become wary of are vegetables and fruit; protein foods that require a lot of biting and chewing (such as unprocessed pieces of meat or fish); mixed foods (such as pasta sauces); foods with "bits" in it (such as yogurt with pieces of fruit); and slimy foods (such as gravy). They tend to be fine with yellow or beige foods, including carbohydrate-based foods such as bread, cereal, cookies, chips and processed meat. And frustratingly, it is not uncommon for children to refuse to eat foods that they seemed to like before, simply because there is a small deviation in appearance or texture. So, what do you do if your child is suspicious of most new foods and won't even eat the foods that he seemed to like before? Fussiness can be one of the most challenging aspects of parenting a toddler, but scientists have tested a few strategies that seem to work pretty well with most children.

How to Manage Fussiness

Research from our group has shown that fussy toddlers are pressured to eat more by their parents.[25] We also found that fussy toddlers in Gemini were having more formula and, more often than not, "follow-on" formulas (instead of or as well as cow's milk) at two years than nonfussy toddlers.[26] These children also ate less solid food. Their mothers perceived this to be because their child was not interested in food and reported using the formula to provide their child with nutrients and to make sure they were getting enough calories. However, there is the real possibility that the toddlers were full up on milk so they were not hungry for solid food and were not being given the opportunity to develop healthy eating behaviors and become less fussy through exposure to different foods. We would therefore not recommend using milk to compensate for low food intake and instead focus on the following strategies to help your child develop healthy eating habits. If you introduce your child to a wide variety of foods, there is no need for nor any evidence of benefits to using fortified milks, such as "toddler" milks (see Chapter 5). In fact, it's really important to ensure your child is hungry at mealtimes. A child with a poor appetite will feel too full to eat a proper meal if he has had a snack too close to the meal being offered. The snack can even be a glass of milk or juice. So, make sure meals and snacks are spaced out during the day and that snacks are not too filling. It is certainly not a good idea to let your child graze on snacks throughout the day—limit him to two snacks and three meals served at the same time each day.

Parents of fussy eaters often report struggling at mealtimes and, as a result, they limit their child's exposure to new or disliked foods. However, as we explained in Chapter 9, food preferences develop through exposure, which increases familiarity and reduces the fear factor, making children more likely to try the food. With repeated tasting, children eventually accept and like those particular foods. It comes as a surprise to many parents to discover that toddlers may need to be exposed to a disliked food fifteen times before they are even willing to try it. This is because neophobia during toddlerhood makes it harder to accept new food (much harder than when they were babies). Don't be tempted to replace the disliked food with something your child does like; for example, don't remove the broccoli and give fries instead—this is what we call negative reinforcement. Your child's dislike of broccoli will be reinforced because it is taken away and replaced with something he sees as better. Of course, it can be very demoralizing when you have cooked or prepared food for your child and he won't eat it, but if each time he rejects a food it's replaced with something that he does like, then it stands to reason that he will keep rejecting foods he's not that keen on. It's best not to get into the habit of giving in to what your child does and doesn't like. You are the parent, and sometimes being tough is in your child's best interests. But while it is good to keep introducing your child to new foods and flavors and including foods you know he doesn't like, always provide some foods that you know he likes, as well. This will ensure he eats something, and it will make him feel as though he has some control over his eating and less anxious at the meal; it will help to keep your anxieties at bay, too.

It's important not to reward the consumption of disliked food with your child's favorite food. For example, don't tell him that if he eats all of his broccoli he can have some ice cream. This reinforces the fact that the broccoli is not something to be enjoyed—it only gets eaten because he wants the ice cream. This will not improve your child's liking of the broccoli; in fact, it will probably just enhance his liking of the ice cream because it has now acquired the lofty status of a reward, as well as tasting good. Instead, try rewarding with something other than food if your child eats, or at least tries, the broccoli, such as a sticker, badge or a new toy (see page 266).

One of the first studies to explore the combination of rewards with exposure was conducted by our department at UCL in 2010.[27] Four- to six-year-olds were given a taste of a vegetable they disliked every day for twelve days, and they either received a physical reward (sticker), social reward (praise) or no reward. There was also a control group in which children were not given a disliked vegetable over the twelve days. The children who were given a reward ate more of the disliked vegetable than those who were simply given the vegetable with no reward or not given the vegetable at all. Within Gemini we ran something similar called "Tiny Tastes."[28] When they were three years old, a sample of children was randomized either to be given daily tastes of a disliked vegetable over fourteen days in their home with a sticker reward if they tasted it or not to be given daily tastings at all (the control group). The children who were given daily tastings of the vegetable and a reward ate far more of it and liked it far more, compared to those in the control group. Asking your toddler to try a disliked vegetable, or a vegetable they have not had before, and offering a nonfood reward is an excellent way of improving his acceptance of vegetables and other problem foods. A recent high-quality review of studies that have tested which methods are most effective for getting preschool children (aged two to five years) to increase their vegetable consumption concluded that repeated tastings of disliked vegetables combined with a nonfood reward are two of the strategies that work the best.[29]

New or disliked foods can also be introduced outside of a mealtime, and we would recommend that you do this if meals have become a battleground! If you and your child have come to associate mealtimes with stress and anxiety, then it's a good idea to try out new foods in a totally different context. Here is a simple and effective technique for fussy eaters that you can try anywhere—at home or even in a park or playground. Play this game at snack time when your child is hungry.

- Choose a vegetable that you would like your child to eat or that your child does not like.
- Show your child the whole vegetable, name it and say that you are both going to have a small taste of it.
- Cut two small pieces—one for you and one for your child.
- Try your piece and say how delicious it is.
- Ask your child to taste their piece—and if he doesn't want to, tell him he can spit it out if he really doesn't like it.
- Give lots of praise if he tastes it and give him a sticker or an alternative nonfood reward.
- Repeat with the same vegetable every day for up to fifteen days, depending on how long it takes for your child to accept it.
- Choose another vegetable and start again.

We must stress that it is important to use nonfood rewards, such as stickers or praise, rather than offering your child a food you know he likes as a reward. Try not to use food for any reason other than to satisfy his hunger (see page 205). It is important not to use food to soothe, for example, offering your child his favorite food if he is upset, or to use food to control behavior (for example, offering his favorite food if he sits quietly). This is likely to enhance the liking of that food and potentially make it more difficult to get your child to eat the foods he does not like.

How to Keep Mealtimes Stress-Free

Mealtimes can be stressful if your child will not eat a certain food or does not try everything he is served. One way to overcome this is to provide a nutritious balanced meal and allow your child to serve himself, or at least play a part in what he is served and how much. There is then less pressure on him, and you can relax a bit knowing that he may not be eating everything on offer, but what he does have is healthy.

Feel free to put a new or disliked vegetable on your child's plate every day even if he doesn't eat it for several days in a row. This process will help to familiarize him with it—what it looks and feels like—and eventually he is likely to try it. Modeling is also a very useful strategy to improve your child's acceptance of healthy foods. This is particularly important when it comes to new or problem foods. If he sees that you dislike a certain food, he will regard it with suspicion and is likely to reject it, too. Try to show him that nutritious foods are safe to eat, enjoyable and a routine part of everyday life. You can't expect your child to do something you are not prepared to do yourself.

It's important not to pressure your child to eat or to clear his plate. Some children can become very anxious when they are forced to eat certain foods, and those foods then become associated with anxiety. The effect you intend to have (your child eating the food) will in fact be the opposite (your child will not want to eat it now, and possibly not in the future either). Try to have a relaxed attitude toward feeding (as hard as that might be sometimes!). If your child doesn't want to eat something, that is fine—you can try again another day and repeat the exposure. And if he tries a new food but doesn't like it, it is fine for him to spit it out. Some children need to try new foods several times before they're willing to eat them happily. Each tasting occasion will help. He may simply refuse to try a food, and that is fine, too. As difficult as it can be not to lose your temper when you have tried everything to get your child to eat, children start to associate ill feeling and conflict with certain foods. They are then likely to avoid those foods even more, so do try not to get upset with your child or punish him by removing his favorite foods (for example, saying, "If you don't eat your vegetables you won't get dessert") or privileges (for example, saying, "If you don't eat your broccoli you won't be going to the playground"). This may actually reinforce your child's desire *not* to eat the disliked foods. In fact, pressuring him to eat is not a good idea with any food—even one that he likes. If he has had enough, let him finish eating.

Eating past satiety for a child with a small appetite can feel very unpleasant, and it will make him feel stressed.

There is a growing trend for parents with fussy eaters to disguise the flavor of vegetables among other foods. Though it's very tempting to "hide" vegetables among other flavors—for example, in a sauce or by adding a flavor that's more appealing, such as the sweetness of fruit—this means that your child will not actually taste the flavor of the vegetables. Your child needs to identify the flavors and textures to get used to them and like them. It is also not uncommon for parents to try to make food look more appealing to children—for example, by making smiley faces on the plate with the vegetables. This is fine—we as adults tend to enjoy food more if it is well presented, hence why many chefs add fancy garnishes to their dishes. If your child is more likely to eat a carrot if it is a "nose" on the plate, then go ahead and do this.

Whatever food you end up offering your child for a meal, bear in mind that children with a poor appetite can easily feel overwhelmed by food. Make sure that you provide small portions that look manageable to him and cut the food up into little pieces so he can eat a small amount at a time. You can always offer him some more if he indicates to you that he is still hungry. It may seem counterintuitive to limit the length of a meal when your child eats slowly and doesn't eat much at all. But limiting the total mealtime to thirty minutes will help to reduce your child's anxiety levels because he knows that the ordeal is time-limited. Dragging out the meal past this length of time is unlikely to result in him eating any more.

Lastly, if things have become really difficult at mealtimes and there are two parents, then try getting the least stressed parent to sit and eat with your child. You can also try getting another adult to eat with your child instead; this can be a grandparent, a babysitter or friend. This can sometimes help to alleviate the anxiety for both you and your child and break the association between stress and meals.

And, finally, don't give up! Most children go through a period of being a bit difficult with food and with meals, and it's normal for some days to be harder than others. But rest assured that fussy eating is very common in toddlerhood, and the vast majority of toddlers do grow out of it. And in the meantime, there are lots of strategies that you can try to make things a bit easier.

Top Tips for Picky Eaters

- Praise your child when he tries a nutritious new food or eats something he says he dislikes. Reward him with praise—let him know you are happy that he has eaten something he doesn't like (for some children this can be quite an achievement).

- Reward your child with stickers, a badge, a reward chart or a token (or another nonfood reward that you know your child likes) if he tries a new food or eats a disliked food. Children learn to associate eating the disliked foods with something positive and rewarding, and that positive reinforcement can lead to liking. But never reward food with food.

- Try offering your child a little piece of the new/disliked food every day alongside other foods that he will eat.

- Offer small portions so that your child does not get overwhelmed by a large amount of food.

- Eat the new/disliked foods with your child and model healthy eating behavior. Remember, you are your child's best teacher.

- Ensure the family eats the same foods, but try to allow your child to serve himself.

- Limit the meal to thirty minutes. A long, drawn-out meal will stress everyone out and is unlikely to result in your child eating more.

Having read about these different eating styles, can you identify these behaviors in your child—plate-clearing, constant snacking or fussiness? Parents tend to be able to identify with one or other of these, but there are children who simply do not fit into a category. You may have no concerns at all about your child's eating habits and simply want some general advice on how to help your toddler develop healthy eating habits and a good relationship with food. If that's the case, you can still make use of the tips we have provided here as they apply to all children.

For example, generally it is a good idea not to routinely offer second helpings, not to have energy-dense foods on display at home and to praise your child for trying nutritious new foods.

If you can identify with one of these eating styles and you implement some of the tips we have provided, remember it's not always going to be easy. You may start out with the best of intentions, but children can be rather willful; if your child is pestering you for food, you may find yourself becoming impatient and just giving in to his requests, or if your child will not eat what you have served, you may become worried that he is not eating enough and give him his favorite food. This is normal, but tomorrow is another day and you can try again. All is not lost if you give up sometimes.

THE BOTTOM LINE

- Establish a mealtime and snack routine, feeding at the same time each day.
- Don't let your toddler skip meals; always offer him breakfast.
- Include your child in food shopping, preparation and family meals.
- Feed your child responsively.
- Understanding your child's appetite is key; use feeding strategies that are tailored to his eating styles. There will be an element of trial and error, but the more you experiment the more you will grow in confidence.
- If you have a "plate-clearer," be mindful of portion sizes and second helpings and do not encourage plate-clearing.
- If you have a "snacker," put more-palatable snacks out of sight.
- If you have a "fussy eater," do not pressure him to eat and do not use food to control his behavior, such as offering him his favorite food if he eats a disliked food.

Final Thoughts

Our mission with this book was to provide you with everything you need to know about food and feeding for the first 1,000 days from a *scientific perspective*, to help you support your child in developing lifelong healthy eating habits. As such, we have tried to give you the facts, not the fads, about feeding, dispel some of the commonly believed myths and correct misinformation that we know is out there.

We now know quite a lot from science about where appetite and food preferences come from, how they develop and why they're important. One thing is for sure—healthy eating is about both *what* and *how* your child eats. And we hope we have armed you with lots of useful strategies and tips that you can use to help your baby develop a good relationship with food as you navigate your way through the first 1,000 days. Here are our final tips on *what* and *how* to feed.

The Bottom Line on *What* to Feed

The first 1,000 days offer a window of opportunity for "setting" your baby's food preferences—you can help him learn to like nutritious foods, such as vegetables and fruit, so that he is more likely to eat them willingly without making a fuss. The keys to liking are familiarity and feeling sure that foods are safe. This process may start as early as pregnancy, possibly continues during breastfeeding, and is more firmly established when your baby is introduced to solid foods.

Do...

1. **Eat the foods you want your baby to eat when you are pregnant.**
   Your baby may start to get a taste for vegetables and fruit (and other

foods) through your own diet when you are pregnant, and then from your breast milk if he receives this.

2. **If you would like to breastfeed him, it's a great option.**
   Breastfeeding will help protect your baby from infections and may provide other health benefits, too. But if you need to use formula (either exclusively or alongside breastfeeding) you can feel assured that formula is a safe way to feed your baby.

   Seek help and support early on if you are struggling to breastfeed in the first few days or weeks and want to continue. This can make the difference between giving up and carrying on. Every breastfeeding counts, so celebrate each one. It doesn't have to be all or nothing—there are benefits to partial breastfeeding, too.

3. **Don't wait until later than six months to introduce solid foods.**
   If your baby is healthy, then start solid foods around six months of age in order to make sure that you make the most of his openness to new flavors and textures and that he gets the nutrients he needs and has timely oral development for speech.

4. **Use a bitter vegetable as his first food.**
   During complementary feeding, start with lots of different vegetables and try to choose bitter-tasting ones (such as spinach) over sweet ones (such as carrot) initially. Once your baby has had a taste for sweet foods, it might be harder to convince him that the bitter-tasting foods will be just as nice. Don't disguise vegetables in sauces and don't mix them with fruit. Babies and toddlers need to get to know what each separate vegetable tastes like and become familiar with its texture.

5. **Persevere with new foods.**
   You may have to offer a new food up to fifteen times to get your toddler to like it, but repeated tasting is the most effective way for you to increase his liking for foods, especially those he doesn't seem keen on.

6. **Praise him for eating new nutritious foods.**
   Give him lots of praise and encouragement. This will act as a reward for the behavior and will make him more likely to want to do it again.

7. **Reward him with a nonfood for trying a new nutritious food or a food he doesn't like.**
   Stickers and other age-appropriate nonfood rewards work well for most young children when it comes to motivating them to try new

foods. You could even try a star chart so your child can see his progress.

8. **Lead by example and eat what you want him to eat.**
Once your baby starts solid foods, he will be looking to you as his main source of information about what foods are safe to eat. You need to show him by happily eating and enjoying nutritious foods in front of him. If you give your baby the impression that you don't like what you are eating, you can be sure he will trust you on this! He will copy your behavior. That's how he learns.

9. **Have fruit and vegetables available as snacks and always on show.**
Your baby is more likely to eat them if they are readily available, such as in a fruit bowl, and if he can see them. It will also help him to become more familiar with them, which will help him to accept them and like them.

10. **Provide lots of variety.**
Make sure you give your baby the opportunity to try as many different flavors and textures as you can—this is the best way to ensure he will eat a varied diet now and later.

Don't . . .

1. **Reward nonliked food with his favorite food in order to get him to try something.**
This is not a good way to get him to eat nutritious foods—it only serves to make him think the nutritious food is so dreadful that it requires a reward to be given and increases his desire for his favorite food, which becomes both a reward as well as a nice-tasting food.

2. **Replace food with milk.**
If you have a picky eater who has a poor appetite, the temptation is to keep giving him milk to ensure he's getting enough calories. But this usually means he fills up on milk and has even less of an appetite for proper food. Persevere with the solid foods using the techniques we have provided in this book and try to limit the milk to sensible amounts.

3. **Replace food with any food substitute.**
Never use a food substitute (such as a food-replacement shake or similar) unless instructed to do so by your pediatrician. These are packed with sugar and will only hinder your baby's ability to develop

healthy eating habits. He needs to learn how to eat proper food, not avoid it by having a substitute. This will only make it harder to get him to eat a varied and healthy diet.

4. **Make a separate meal for your toddler.**
   The best way to model healthy eating behavior is to eat the same food with your child at the table. There is no need to buy special snacks for toddlers or make them separate meals—they can eat whatever you eat, just in smaller portions and with no sugar or salt added.

5. **Order something off the children's menu.**
   Your child doesn't need special kids' meals in any context. He can have a smaller portion of most adult meals, as long as they don't have added salt or sugar. He can have a small portion of the meal you order yourself, and this will mean he gets used to eating the types of foods and meals that adults eat.

The Bottom Line on *How* to Feed

Babies and toddlers are all different when it comes to milk and food—some have hearty appetites, while others are picky eaters, and this is partly down to their genes. These eating styles bring with them unique feeding challenges for you as a parent. *How* to feed your baby or toddler means making sure you know what type of feeder your baby is and responding to him appropriately through *responsive feeding*. Babies and toddlers who have a hearty appetite will have a tendency to overeat, especially in response to larger portions and food cues, such as sight, smell or taste. They need to be supported in learning to pay attention to their feelings of hunger and fullness, stopping eating as soon as they are full, being offered age-appropriate portions and making sure they are offered healthy snacks that are low in energy density if regularly hungry. Children with a poor appetite will struggle to eat a proper meal if they have filled up on other snacks beforehand (this includes milk) and tend to be more reluctant to eat vegetables, fruit and protein foods (meat and fish). They need to be supported by not being pressured to eat certain foods, by being praised if they try a nutritious new food and being offered smaller portions so that they are not overwhelmed by a large amount of food. It goes without saying that parents need to use different strategies with the two types of children, but there are some general tips that will apply to all children.

Do...

1. **Learn to read your baby's or toddler's hunger and fullness signals.**
   Crying on its own doesn't signal hunger—hunger cues cluster together, and crying is only one indication. Hunger and fullness cues are easier to read in toddlers than young babies, but try to get to know your baby's cues from Day 1.

2. **Offer food only in response to hunger or at a meal or snack.**
   Don't feed your baby or toddler for any reason other than hunger or because it is a meal or snack time—for example, for comfort or to keep them quiet. This may be very difficult to do when you know feeding will soothe him, but there are other ways to comfort your baby or toddler without offering food. Always try these first.

3. **Stop feeding your baby or toddler as soon as he signals he is full.**
   Trust your baby on this—he will let you know. A baby or toddler with a hearty appetite doesn't need much encouragement to feed beyond fullness and will do so given the chance. This will lead to overeating. Pressuring a baby with a poor appetite to keep on feeding or eating after he is full will make him feel stressed and can even lead to food aversions.

4. **Provide baby- or toddler-sized portions.**
   Make sure that you provide appropriate portion sizes for your child—this includes the amount of milk offered in a bottle (if you bottle-feed him), as well as meals and snacks. If he has a hearty appetite, he will have a tendency to eat whatever is there. This means you need to provide the right amount so you don't encourage him to overeat. Picky eaters can feel overwhelmed by too much food on their plates, so offer meals and snacks that look manageable.

Don't...

1. **Use food to control your child's emotions or behavior.**
   Don't use your child's favorite foods as a bribe to make him behave, keep him quiet or soothe him if he is upset or cranky. This may teach him to use food in order to regulate his emotions rather than learning positive strategies for coping.

2. **Have too many sugary and fatty foods in the house.**

   If you have them on show, he will want them. If you lock them in a cupboard, he will want them even more because they are then seen as "forbidden." The best way to get around this problem is not to have them in the house in the first place, at least not all the time, and in limited quantities.

3. **Make a fuss about all the fuss.**

   Try not to lose control. This is easier said than done—babies and toddlers' eating can be maddening at times, especially when they won't eat what you have prepared for them. But if you get stressed, your baby will, too, and this can intensify the stress around mealtimes, leading to food refusal.

4. **Eat with the television or computer on.**

   Fussy feeders are easily distracted and may have far more interest in watching television or playing on the iPad than eating their meat and veggies. And children who are less sensitive to satiety are more likely to eat too much if they are distracted by the television. This is because they are preoccupied with the screen, and it prevents them from paying attention to their food and the feeling of fullness while eating. Food advertising can also act as a food cue for food-responsive children and can make them want to eat more.

Some Final Reflections

In writing this book, we have had a chance to reflect at length on what science has shown us about how your baby's eating behavior develops in his first 1,000 days. In writing every chapter, we have been struck by how extraordinary the human body is. Your amniotic fluid is already a bath of flavors that may prepare your baby for the outside world, helping him to learn what foods are safe to eat when the time comes. Breast milk may do this, too, but so much more than that, as well—it provides sustenance and immunity, and fuels your baby's brain development.

The "terrible twos" are so-called for a reason—toddlers are renowned for being fusspots and, for some parents, mealtimes can become a bit of a misery. But even this frustrating developmental phase serves an important function—being naturally suspicious of potentially harmful substances is probably nature's way of protecting an extremely vulnerable newly mobile person from eating things he shouldn't. We hope we have given you some tips that will help you work with your baby, at each stage of his development, to support him on his journey into the grown-up world of eating.

We've also felt incredibly privileged that so many parents have shared their experiences of feeding their little ones with us. A couple of the stories we listened to moved us to tears. There is little in life that brings more intensity of emotion than a tiny baby or toddler who won't feed. This was one of our motivations behind writing this book—to give you some tips that will help things go as smoothly as possible. But things don't always go to plan and there is help available—don't struggle alone; do seek advice and support if you need it. If you have tried everything and you are at a loss, take your baby or toddler to your pediatrician.

A final message we want to leave you with is that it's never too late to intervene. Clare is a prime example—a random social intervention as an adult meant she finally started eating properly after nineteen years! So, never lose hope. Even if things have gone well so far, you may face new challenges as your baby or toddler grows into an older child. With increasing age comes independence, and sometimes defiance! And you will be less able to control what and how your child eats at school. But laying the groundwork now will help him to establish healthy eating habits that set him up for life.

The Eating Behaviour Questionnaires

The Baby Eating Behaviour Questionnaire (BEBQ) (birth to six months)

This questionnaire will give you an idea about the type of milk-feeder your baby is—whether he has a big or a small appetite. Answering these questions will help you to understand him and the feeding strategies that might suit him best. The questions are about all the different aspects of his appetite during his first few months of life, when he is still being fed milk only. How would you describe his feeding style at a *typical daytime feed*? Answer each statement using any of the following response options: *never, rarely, sometimes, often* or *always*. Instructions about how to interpret your answers are on pages 296–97.

MILK RESPONSIVENESS

- *My baby frequently wants more milk than I provide.*
- *If allowed to, my baby would take too much milk.*
- *Even when my baby has just eaten well he is happy to feed again if offered.*
- *My baby is always demanding a feed.*
- *If given the chance, my baby would always be feeding.*
- *My baby can easily take a feed within thirty minutes of the last one.*

ENJOYMENT OF FEEDING

- *My baby seems contented while feeding.*
- *My baby loves milk.*
- *My baby becomes distressed while feeding.* *
- *My baby enjoys feeding time.*

SATIETY RESPONSIVENESS

- *My baby gets full easily.*
- *My baby gets full before taking all the milk I think he should have.*
- *My baby finds it difficult to manage a complete feeding.*
- *My baby has a big appetite.* *

SLOWNESS IN FEEDING

- *My baby finishes feeding quickly.* *
- *My baby takes more than thirty minutes to finish feeding.*
- *My baby feeds slowly.*
- *My baby sucks more and more slowly during the course of a feed.*

SCORING INSTRUCTIONS FOR THE BEBQ

Look at your general responses for each aspect of appetite—for example, did you tend to answer *always* for most of the statements for milk responsiveness?

Your baby has a *big appetite* if:

- You answered mainly *often* or *always* for statements relating to milk responsiveness and enjoyment of feeding, except for the statement with an asterisk, to which you answered either *rarely* or *never*. This pattern of responses means your baby is very milk responsive and derives a lot of pleasure from feeding.

- You answered mainly *rarely* or *never* for satiety responsiveness and slowness in feeding, except for the statements with an asterisk, to which you answered either *often* or *always*. This pattern of responses means your baby is not very sensitive to his internal satiety and feeds quickly.

Your baby has a *small appetite* if:

- You answered mainly *rarely* or *never* for milk responsiveness and enjoyment of feeding, except for the statement with an asterisk, to which you answered either *often* or *always*. This means your baby is not very milk responsive and has low interest in feeding.

- You answered mainly *often* or *always* for satiety responsiveness and slowness in feeding, except for the statements with an asterisk, to which you answered either *rarely* or *never*. This means your baby is very sensitive to his internal satiety and feeds slowly.

The Child Eating Behaviour Questionnaire (CEBQ) (twelve months and up)

This questionnaire will give you an idea about the type of eater your toddler is—whether he has a big or a small appetite. Answering these questions will help you to understand him and the feeding strategies that might suit him best. The questions are about all the different aspects of his appetite for solid food. How would you describe his eating styles on a *typical day*? Answer each statement using any of the following response options: *never, rarely, sometimes, often* or *always*. Instructions about how to interpret your answers are on page 299.

FOOD RESPONSIVENESS

- *My child is always asking for food.*
- *Given the choice, my child would eat most of the time.*
- *Even when my child has just eaten well, he is happy to eat again if offered.*
- *If allowed to, my child would eat too much.*

ENJOYMENT OF FOOD

- *My child looks forward to mealtimes.*
- *My child loves food.*
- *My child is interested in food.*
- *My child enjoys eating.*

SATIETY RESPONSIVENESS

- *My child leaves food on his plate or in the jar at the end of a meal.*
- *My child gets full before his meal is finished.*
- *My child cannot eat a meal if he has had a snack just before.*
- *My child gets full easily.*
- *My child has a big appetite.* *

SLOWNESS IN EATING

- *My child finishes his meal quickly.* *
- *My child eats slowly.*
- *My child takes more than thirty minutes to finish a meal.*
- *My child eats more and more slowly during the course of a meal.*

EMOTIONAL OVEREATING

- *My child eats more when irritable.*
- *My child eats more when grumpy.*
- *My child eats more when upset.*

EMOTIONAL UNDEREATING

- *My child eats less when angry.*
- *My child eats more when he is happy.* *
- *My child eats less when upset.*

FOOD FUSSINESS

- *My child refuses new foods at first.*
- *My child enjoys a wide variety of foods.* *
- *My child enjoys tasting new foods.* *
- *My child is difficult to please with meals.*
- *My child decides that he does not like a food even without tasting it.*
- *My child is interested in tasting food he has not tasted before.* *

SCORING INSTRUCTIONS FOR THE CEBQ

Look at your general responses for each aspect of appetite—for example, did you tend to answer *always* for most of the statements for food responsiveness?

Your child has a *big appetite* if:

- You answered mainly *often* or *always* for statements relating to food responsiveness, enjoyment of feeding and emotional overeating. This pattern of responses means your toddler is very food responsive, derives a lot of pleasure from eating and has a tendency to want to eat more when he is upset or annoyed.

- You answered mainly *rarely* or *never* for satiety responsiveness, slowness in feeding, emotional undereating and food fussiness, except for the statements with an asterisk, to which you answered either *often* or *always*. This pattern of responses means your toddler is not very sensitive to his internal satiety, eats quickly, doesn't lose his appetite even when he's upset or annoyed and will eat most foods without a fuss.

Your child has a *small appetite* if:

- You answered mainly *rarely* or *never* for food responsiveness, enjoyment of feeding and emotional overeating. This means your toddler is not very food responsive, has low interest in food and doesn't take much comfort from food when he is upset or annoyed.

- You answered mainly *often* or *always* for satiety responsiveness, slowness in feeding, emotional undereating and food fussiness, except for the statements with an asterisk, to which you answered either *rarely* or *never*. This means your toddler is very sensitive to his internal satiety, feeds slowly, tends to lose his appetite when he has been very upset or annoyed and is picky about what foods he is willing to eat or even try.

REFERENCES

INTRODUCTION

1. 1,000 Days, "Why 1,000 Days," thousanddays.org.

2. A. S. Dekaban, "Changes in Brain Weights During the Span of Human Life: Relation of Brain Weights to Body Heights and Body Weights," *Annals of Neurology* 4, no. 4 (1978): 345–56.

3. UNICEF, "The First 1,000 Days of Life: The Brain's Window of Opportunity," unicef-irc.org.

CHAPTER 1

1. J. Wardle et al., "Development of the Children's Eating Behaviour Questionnaire," *Journal of Child Psychology and Psychiatry* 42, no. 7 (2001): 963–70.

2. C. H. Llewellyn et al., "Development and Factor Structure of the Baby Eating Behaviour Questionnaire in the Gemini Birth Cohort," *Appetite* 57, no. 2 (2011): 388–96.

3. J. Ashcroft et al., "Continuity and Stability of Eating Behaviour Traits in Children," *European Journal of Clinical Nutrition* 62, no. 8 (2008): 985–90.

4. C. M. Taylor, "Picky/Fussy Eating in Children: Review of Definitions, Assessment, Prevalence and Dietary Intakes," *Appetite* 95 (2015): 349–59.

5. C. H. van Jaarsveld et al., "Appetite and Growth: A Longitudinal Sibling Analysis," *JAMA Pediatrics* 168, no. 4 (2014): 345–50.

6. P. L. Quah et al., "Prospective Associations of Appetitive Traits at 3 and 12 Months of Age with Body Mass Index and Weight Gain in the First 2 Years of Life," *BMC Pediatrics* 15 (2015): 153.

7. S. Carnell and J. Wardell, "Appetite and Adiposity in Children: Evidence for a Behavioral Susceptibility Theory of Obesity," *American Journal of Clinical Nutrition* 88, no. 1 (2008): 22–29.

   H. Croker, L. Cooke and J. Wardell, "Appetitive Behaviours of Children Attending Obesity Treatment," *Appetite* 57, no. 2 (2011): 525–29.

   K. N. Parkinson et al., "Do Maternal Ratings of Appetite in Infants Predict Later Child Eating Behaviour Questionnaire Scores and Body Mass Index?" *Appetite* 54, no. 1 (2010): 186–90.

   E. F. Sleddens, S. P. Kremers and C. Thijs, "The Children's Eating Behaviour Questionnaire: Factorial Validity and Association with Body Mass Index in Dutch Children Aged 6–7." *International Journal of Behavioral Nutrition and Physical Activity* 5 (2008): 49.

   J. C. Spence et al., "Examining Behavioural Susceptibility to Obesity Among Canadian Pre-School Children: The Role of Eating Behaviours," *International Journal of Pediatric Obesity* 6, no. 2-2 (2010): e501–7.

   V. Viana, S. Sinde and J. C. Saxton, "Children's Eating Behaviour Questionnaire: Associations with BMI in Portuguese Children," *British Journal of Nutrition* 100, no. 2 (2008): 445–50.

L. Webber et al., "Eating Behaviour and Weight in Children," *International Journal of Obesity* 33, no. 1 (2009): 21–28.

8. J. L. Harris et al., *FACTS 2017: Food Industry Self-Regulation After 10 Years: Progress and Opportunities to Improve Food Advertising to Children,* UCONN Rudd Center for Food Policy and Obesity, 2017, uconnruddcenter.org/facts2017.

9. E. J. Boyland et al., "Advertising as a Cue to Consume: A Systematic Review and Meta-Analysis of the Effects of Acute Exposure to Unhealthy Food and Nonalcoholic Beverage Advertising on Intake in Children and Adults," *American Journal of Clinical Nutrition* 103, no. 2 (2016): 519–33.

10. Harris et al., *FACTS 2017.*

11. American Academy of Pediatrics, "Where We Stand: Screen Time" (2016), healthychildren.org/English/family-life/Media/Pages/Where-We-Stand-TV -Viewing-Time.aspx.

12. H. Syrad, "Appetitive Traits and Food Intake Patterns in Early Life," *American Journal of Clinical Nutrition* 103, no. 1 (2016): 231–35.

13. Ibid.

14. R. E. Kron, J. Ipsen and K. E. Goddard, "Consistent Individual Differences in the Nutritive Sucking Behavior of the Human Newborn," *Psychosomatic Medicine* 30, no. 2 (1968): 151–61.

15. K. G. Dewey and B. Lönnerdal, "Infant Self-Regulation of Breast Milk Intake," *Acta Paediatrica Scandinavica* 75, no. 6 (1986): 893–98.

     K. G. Dewey et al., "Maternal Versus Infant Factors Related to Breast Milk Intake and Residual Milk Volume: The DARLING Study," *Pediatrics* 87, no. 6 (1991): 829–37.

     R. F. Drewett and M. Wooridge, "Milk Taken by Human Babies from the First and Second Breast," *Physiology and Behavior* 26, no. 2 (1981): 327–29.

16. R. M. Milstein, "Responsiveness in Newborn Infants of Overweight and Normal Weight Parents," *Appetite* 1, no. 1 (1980): 65–74.

17. W. S. Agras et al. "Does a Vigorous Feeding Style Influence Early Development of Adiposity?" *Journal of Pediatrics* 110, no. 5 (1987): 799–804.

     A. J. Stunkard et al., "Predictors of Body Size in the First 2 Y of Life: A High-Risk Study of Human Obesity," *International Journal of Obesity and Related Metabolic Disorders* 28, no. 4 (2004): 503–13.

18. C. H. Llewellyn et al., "Nature and Nurture in Infant Appetite: Analysis of the Gemini Twin Birth Cohort," *American Journal of Clinical Nutrition* 91, no. 5 (2010): 1172–79.

19. M. W. Schwartz et al., "Central Nervous System Control of Food Intake," *Nature* 404, no. 6778 (2000): 661–71.

20. I. S. Farooqi, "Defining the Neural Basis of Appetite and Obesity: From Genes to Behaviour," *Clinical Medicine (London)* 14, no. 3 (2014): 286–89.

     G. S. Yeo and L. K. Heisler, "Unravelling the Brain Regulation of Appetite: Lessons from Genetics," *Nature Neuroscience* 15, no. 10 (2012): 1343–49.

21. M. Herle et al., "The Home Environment Shapes Emotional Eating in Childhood," *Child Development* 89, no. 4 (2018): 1423–34.

     M. Herle et al., "Emotional Over- and Under-Eating in Early Childhood Are Learned Not Inherited," *Scientific Reports* 7 (2017): 9092.

22. M. Herle, A. Fildes and C. H. Llewellyn, "Emotional Eating Is Learned Not Inherited in Children, Regardless of Obesity Risk," *Pediatric Obesity* 13, no. 10 (2018): 628–31.

23. S. Steinsbekk et al., "Emotional Feeding and Emotional Eating: Reciprocal Processes and the Influence of Negative Affectivity," *Child Development* 89, no. 4 (2018): 1234–46.

24. R. Lozano et al., "Global and Regional Mortality from 235 Causes of Death for 20 Age Groups in 1990 and 2010: A Systematic Analysis for the Global Burden of Disease Study 2010," *Lancet* 380, no. 9859 (2012): 2095–128.

25. S. E. Cusick and M. K. Georgieff, "The Role of Nutrition in Brain Development: The Golden Opportunity of the 'First 1,000 Days,'" *Journal of Pediatrics* 175 (2016): 16–21.

    J. Lanigan and A. Singhal, "Early Nutrition and Long-Term Health: A Practical Approach," *Proceedings of the Nutrition Society* 68, no. 4 (2009): 422–29.

26. Cusick and Georgieff, "The Role of Nutrition in Brain Development."

27. Lanigan and Singhal, "Early Nutrition and Long-Term Health."

28. J. A. Mennella and N. K. Bobowski, "The Sweetness and Bitterness of Childhood: Insights from Basic Research on Taste Preferences," *Physiology and Behavior* 152 (2015): 502–7.

29. G. Harris and S. Mason, "Are There Sensitive Periods for Food Acceptance in Infancy?" *Current Nutrition Reports* 6, no. 2 (2017): 190–96.

30. A. M. Craigie et al., "Tracking of Obesity-Related Behaviours from Childhood to Adulthood: A Systematic Review," *Maturitas* 70, no. 3 (2011): 266–84.

31. A. Fildes et al., "Nature and Nurture in Children's Food Preferences," *American Journal of Clinical Nutrition* 99, no. 4 (2014): 911–17.

32. A. Fildes, C. H. M. van Jaarsveld, L. Cooke, J. Wardle and C. H. Llewellyn, "Common Genetic Architecture Underlying Young Children's Food Fussiness and Liking for Vegetables and Fruit." *American Journal of Clinical Nutrition* 103, no. 4 (2016): 1099–1104.

33. L. Cooke, "The Importance of Exposure for Healthy Eating in Childhood: A Review," *Journal of Human Nutrition and Dietetics* 20, no. 4 (2007): 294–301.

34. J. A. Mennella and A. K. Ventura, "Understanding the Basic Biology Underlying the Flavor World of Children," *Current Zoology* 56, no. 6 (2010): 834–41.

35. J. A. Mennella, A. Johnson and G. K. Beauchamp, "Garlic Ingestion by Pregnant Women Alters the Odor of Amniotic Fluid," *Chemical Senses* 20, no. 2 (1995): 207–9.

36. S. R. Crystal and I. L. Bernstein, "Infant Salt Preference and Mother's Morning Sickness," *Appetite* 30, no. 3 (1998): 297–307.

37. Mennella and Ventura, "Understanding the Basic Biology Underlying the Flavor World of Children."

PART 1

1. U. Ramakrishnan et al., "Effect of Women's Nutrition Before and During Early Pregnancy on Maternal and Infant Outcomes: A Systematic Review," *Paediatric and Perinatal Epidemiology* 26, no. S1 (2012): 285–301.

CHAPTER 2

1. Ramakrishnan et al., "Effect of Women's Nutrition Before and During Early Pregnancy on Maternal and Infant Outcomes: A Systematic Review."

2. M. G. Ross and M. Desai, "Developmental Programming of Appetite/Satiety," *Annals of Nutrition and Metabolism* 64, no. S1 (2014): 36–44.

3. P. D. Gluckman and M. A. Hanson, "Developmental and Epigenetic Pathways to Obesity: An Evolutionary-Developmental Perspective," *International Journal of Obesity* 32, no. S7 (2008): S62–71.

 D. R. Grattan, "Fetal Programming from Maternal Obesity: Eating Too Much for Two?" *Endocrinology* 149, no. 11 (2008): 5345–47.

4. Mennella, Johnson and Beauchamp, "Garlic Ingestion by Pregnant Women."

5. J. A. Mennella, C. P. Jagnow and G. K. Beauchamp, "Prenatal and Postnatal Flavor Learning by Human Infants," *Pediatrics* 107, no. 6 (2001): e88–93.

6. Institute of Medicine (IOM), *Weight Gain During Pregnancy: Reexamining the Guidelines* (Washington, DC: National Academies Press, 2009).

7. Ibid.

8. R. F. Goldstein et al., "Association of Gestational Weight Gain with Maternal and Infant Outcomes: A Systematic Review and Meta-Analysis," *JAMA* 317, no. 21 (2017): 2207–25.

9. IOM, *Weight Gain During Pregnancy.*

10. Ibid.

11. Ibid.

12. Ibid.

13. M. A. Kominiarek and P. Rajan, "Nutrition Recommendations in Pregnancy and Lactation," *Medical Clinics of North America* 100, no. 6 (201): 1199–215.

14. Institute of Medicine (IOM), *Dietary Reference Intakes for Energy, Carbohydrate, Fiber, Fat, Fatty Acids, Cholesterol, Protein, and Amino Acids* (Washington, DC: National Academies Press, 2005).

15. R. P. Mensink, *Effects of Saturated Fatty Acids on Serum Lipids and Lipoproteins: A Systematic Review and Regression Analysis* (Geneva, Switzerland: World Health Organization, 2016).

16. R. Zhang et al., "Effects of Low-Glycemic-Index Diets in Pregnancy on Maternal and Newborn Outcomes in Pregnant Women: A Meta-Analysis of Randomized Controlled Trials," *European Journal of Nutrition* 57, no. 1 (2018): 167–77.

17. IOM, *Dietary Reference Intakes for Energy, Carbohydrate, Fiber, Fat, Fatty Acids, Cholesterol, Protein, and Amino Acids.*

18. C. Zhang et al., "Dietary Fiber Intake, Dietary Glycemic Load, and the Risk for Gestational Diabetes Mellitus," *Diabetes Care* 29, no. 10 (2006): 2223–30.

 C. Qiu et al., "Dietary Fiber Intake in Early Pregnancy and Risk of Subsequent Preeclampsia," *American Journal of Hypertension* 21, no. 8 (2008): 903–9.

19. IOM, *Dietary Reference Intakes for Energy, Carbohydrate, Fiber, Fat, Fatty Acids, Cholesterol, Protein, and Amino Acids.*

20. L. M. De-Regil et al., "Effects and Safety of Periconceptional Oral Folate Supplementation for Preventing Birth Defects," *Cochrane Database of Systematic Reviews* no. 12 (2015): CD007950.

21. American College of Obstetricians and Gynecologists (ACOG), "Nutrition During Pregnancy," acog.org/Patients/FAQs/Nutrition-During-Pregnancy.

22. Institute of Medicine (IOM), *Dietary Reference Intakes for Thiamin, Riboflavin, Niacin, Vitamin B6, Folate, Vitamin B12, Pantothenic Acid, Biotin, and Choline* (Washington, DC: National Academy Press, 1998).

23. L. Kaiser L and L. H. Allen, "Position of the American Dietetic Association: Nutrition and Lifestyle for a Healthy Pregnancy Outcome," *Journal of the American Dietetic Association* 108, no. 3 (2008): 553–61.

24. Office of Dietary Supplements, National Institutes of Health, "Vitamin D: Fact Sheet for Health Professionals," ods.od.nih.gov/factsheets /VitaminD-HealthProfessional.

25. R. L. Bailey et al., "Estimation of Total Usual Calcium and Vitamin D Intakes in the United States," *Journal of Nutrition* 140, no. 4 (2010): 817–22.

26. L. De-Regil et al., "Vitamin D Supplementation for Women During Pregnancy," *Cochrane Database of Systematic Reviews* 1 (2016): CD008873.

W. G. Bi et al., "Association Between Vitamin D Supplementation During Pregnancy and Offspring Growth, Morbidity, and Mortality: A Systematic Review and Meta-Analysis," *JAMA Pediatrics* 172, no. 7 (2018): 635-645.

27. IOM, *Dietary Reference Intakes for Calcium and Vitamin D* (Washington, DC: National Academies Press, 2011).

28. IOM, *Dietary Reference Intakes for Vitamin C, Vitamin E, Selenium, and Carotenoids* (Washington, DC: National Academies Press, 2000).

29. IOM, *Dietary Reference Intakes for Vitamin A, Vitamin K, Arsenic, Boron, Chromium, Copper, Iodine, Iron, Manganese, Molybdenum, Nickel, Silicon, Vanadium, and Zinc* (Washington, DC: National Academy Press, 2001).

30. Ibid.

31. T. O. Scholl, "Maternal Iron Status: Relation to Fetal Growth, Length of Gestation and the Neonate's Iron Endowment," *Nutrition Reviews* 69, no. S1 (2011): S23–29.

32. Z. Mei et al., "Assessment of Iron Status in US Pregnant Women from the National Health and Nutrition Examination Survey (NHANES), 1999–2006," *American Journal of Clinical Nutrition* 93, no. 6 (2011): 1312–20.

33. IOM, *Dietary Reference Intakes for Vitamin A, Vitamin K, Arsenic, Boron, Chromium, Copper, Iodine, Iron, Manganese, Molybdenum, Nickel, Silicon, Vanadium, and Zinc.*

34. American College of Obstetricians and Gynecologists, "ACOG Practice Bulletin No. 95: Anemia in Pregnancy," *Obstetrics and Gynecology* 112, no. 1 (2008): 201–7.

35. Centers for Disease Control and Prevention (CDC), "Recommendations to Prevent and Control Iron Deficiency in the United States," *MMWR Recommendations and Reports* 47 (1998): 1–29.

36. IOM, *Dietary Reference Intakes for Vitamin A, Vitamin K, Arsenic, Boron, Chromium, Copper, Iodine, Iron, Manganese, Molybdenum, Nickel, Silicon, Vanadium, and Zinc.*

Burke, Leon and Suchdev, "Identification, Prevention and Treatment of Iron Deficiency."

37. J. P. Peña-Rosas et al., "Daily Oral Iron Supplementation During Pregnancy," *Cochrane Database of Systematic Reviews* no. 7 (2015): CD004736.

38. G. J. Hofmeyr, "Calcium Supplementation During Pregnancy for Preventing Hypertensive Disorders and Related Problems," *Cochrane Database of Systematic Reviews* no. 6 (2014): CD001059.

39. American College of Obstetrics and Gynecologists, *Hypertension in Pregnancy* (Washington, DC: ACOG, 2013).

40. K. L. Caldwell et al., "Iodine Status of the U.S. Population, National Health and Nutrition Examination Survey, 2005–2006 and 2007–2008," *Thyroid* 21, no. 4 (2011): 419–27.

E. N. Pearce et al., "Dietary Iodine in Pregnant Women from the Boston, Massachusetts Area," *Thyroid* 14, no. 4 (2004): 327–28.

41. S. C. Bath et al., "Effect of Inadequate Iodine Status in UK Pregnant Women on Cognitive Outcomes in Their Children: Results from the Avon Longitudinal Study of Parents and Children (ALSPAC)," *Lancet* 283, no. 9889 (2013): 331–37.

42. IOM, *Dietary Reference Intakes for Vitamin A, Vitamin K, Arsenic, Boron, Chromium, Copper, Iodine, Iron, Manganese, Molybdenum, Nickel, Silicon, Vanadium, and Zinc.*

43. D. V. Becker et al., "Iodine Supplementation for Pregnancy and Lactation-United States and Canada: Recommendations of the American Thyroid Association." *Thyroid* 16, no. 10 (2006): 949–51.

44. A. M. Leung, E. N. Pearce and L. E. Braverman, "Iodine Content of Prenatal Multivitamins in the United States," *New England Journal of Medicine* 360, no. 9 (2009): 939–40.

45. US Department of Health and Human Services (HHS) and US Department of Agriculture (USDA), *2015–2020 Dietary Guidelines for Americans*, 8th ed. (Washington, DC: US Government Printing Office, 2015).

46. Ibid.

47. Food and Drug Administration (FDA), "Meat, Poultry and Seafood from Food Safety for Moms to Be."

48. CDC, "*Listeria* (Listeriosis): People at Risk—Pregnant Women and Newborns," cdc.gov/listeria/risk-groups /pregnant-women.html.

49. R. F. Lamont et al., "Listeriosis in Human Pregnancy: A Systematic Review," *Journal of Perinatal Medicine* 39, no. 3 (2011): 227–36.

50. CDC, "Listeria (Listeriosis)."

51. Lamont et al., "Listeriosis in Human Pregnancy."

52. CDC, "Listeria (Listeriosis)."

53. FDA, "Preventing Listeriosis in Pregnant Hispanic Women in the U.S.," fda.gov.

54. J. L. Jones et al., "Rate of Congenital Toxoplasmosis in Large Integrated Health Care Setting, California, USA, 1998–2012," *Emerging Infectious Diseases* 20, no. 9 (2014): 1573–74.

55. FDA, "Preventing Listeriosis in Pregnant Hispanic Women in the US."

56. Food and Drug Administration (FDA), "Enjoying Homemade Ice Cream Without the Risk of Salmonella Infection," fda.gov.

57. FDA, "Meat, Poultry and Seafood from Food Safety for Moms to Be," fda.gov.

58. K. P. Stillerman et al., "Environmental Exposures and Adverse Pregnancy Outcomes: A Review of the Science," *Reproductive Sciences* 15, no. 7 (2008): 631–50.

59. FDA, "Eating Fish: What Pregnant Women and Parents Should Know," fda.gov.

60. D. C. Greenwood et al., "Caffeine Intake During Pregnancy and Adverse Birth Outcomes: A Systematic Review and Dose-Response Meta-Analysis," *European Journal of Epidemiology* 29, no. 10 (2014): 725–34.

61. L. Fenster, "Caffeinated Beverages, Decaffeinated Coffee, and Spontaneous Abortion," *Epidemiology* 8, no. 5 (1997): 515–23.

62. B. H. Bech et al., "Effect of Reducing Caffeine Intake on Birth Weight and Length of Gestation: Randomised Controlled Trial." *BMJ* 334, (2007): 409.

63. ACOG, "Nutrition During Pregnancy."

64. J. Patra et al., "Dose-Response Relationship Between Alcohol Consumption Before and During Pregnancy and the Risks of Low Birthweight, Preterm Birth and Small for Gestational Age (SGA): A Systematic Review and Meta-Analyses," *BJOG* 118, no. 12 (2011): 1411–21.

65. A. L. Flak et al., "The Association of Mild, Moderate, and Binge Prenatal Alcohol Exposure and Child Neuropsychological Outcomes: A Meta-Analysis," *Alcoholism, Clinical and Experimental Research* 38, no. 1 (2014): 214–26.

66. L. Mamluk et al., "Low Alcohol Consumption and Pregnancy and Childhood Outcomes: Time to Change Guidelines Indicating Apparently 'Safe' Levels of Alcohol During Pregnancy? A Systematic Review and Meta-Analyses," *BMJ Open* 7, no. 7 (2017): e015410.

67. HHS and USDA, *2015–2020 Dietary Guidelines for Americans.*

American College of Obstetricians and Gynecologists, "Alcohol and Women," acog.org/Patients/FAQs/Alcohol-and-Women.

68. Rethinking Drinking: Alcohol and Your Health, "What's a 'Standard' Drink?" rethinkingdrinking.niaaa.nih.gov.

69. S. Michie et al., "Effective Techniques in Healthy Eating and Physical Activity Interventions: A Meta-Regression," *Health Psychology* 28, no. 6 (2009): 690–701.

J. M. Spahn et al., "State of the Evidence Regarding Behavior Change Theories and Strategies in Nutrition Counseling to Facilitate Health and Food Behavior Change," *Journal of the American Dietetic Association* 100, no. 6 (2010): 879–91.

M. J. Brown et al., "A Systematic Review Investigating Healthy Lifestyle Interventions Incorporating Goal Setting Strategies for Preventing Excess Gestational Weight Gain," *PLOS ONE* 7, no. 7 (2012): e39503.

70. L. E. Burke et al., "The Effect of Electronic Self-Monitoring on Weight Loss and Dietary Intake: A Randomized Behavioral Weight Loss Trial," *Obesity* 19, no. 2 (2011): 338–44.

71. T. R. Einarson, C. Pikwo and G. Koren, "Quantifying the Global Rates of Nausea and Vomiting of Pregnancy: A Meta Analysis," *Journal of Population Therapeutics and Clinical Pharmacology* 20, no. 2 (2012): e171–83.

72. S. M. Flaxman and P. W. Sherman, "Morning Sickness: A Mechanism for Protecting Mother and Embryo," *Quarterly Review of Biology* 75, no. 2 (2000): 113–48.

   M. Davis, "Nausea and Vomiting of Pregnancy: An Evidence-Based Review," *Journal of Perinatal and Neonatal Nursing* 18, no. 4 (2004): 312–28.

73. A. Matthews et al., "Interventions for Nausea and Vomiting in Early Pregnancy," *Cochrane Database of Systematic Reviews* no. 9 (2015): CD007575.

74. K. C. Allison et al., "Psychosocial Characteristics and Gestational Weight Change Among Overweight, African American Pregnant Women," *Obstetrics and Gynecology International* (2012): 878607.

CHAPTER 3

1. J. Villar et al., "Monitoring the Postnatal Growth of Preterm Infants: A Paradigm Change," *Pediatrics* 141, no. 2 (2018): e20172467.

2. Ibid.

3. American Academy of Pediatrics (AAP), "Sample Hospital Breastfeeding Policy for Newborns," aap.org/en-us/advocacy-and-policy/aap-health-initiatives /Breastfeeding/Documents/Hospital_Breastfeeding_Policy.pdf.

4. V. J. Flaherman et al., "Early Weight Loss Nomograms for Exclusively Breastfed Newborns," *Pediatrics* 135, no. 1 (2015): e16–23.

5. J. R. Miller et al., "Early Weight Loss Nomograms for Formula Fed Newborns," *Hospital Pediatrics* 5, no. 5 (2015): 263–68.

6. I. M. Paul et al., "Weight Change Nomograms for the First Month After Birth," *Pediatrics* 138, no. 6 (2016): e20162625.

7. Ibid.

8. Ibid.

9. C. Wright and K. Parkinson, "Postnatal Weight Loss in Term Infants: What Is 'Normal' and Do Growth Charts Allow for It?" *ADC Fetal and Neonatal Edition* 89, no. 3 (2004): F254–57.

10. "AAP Schedule of Well-Child Care Visits," healthychildren.org.

11. G. Wang et al., "Weight Gain in Infancy and Overweight or Obesity in Childhood Across the Gestational Spectrum: A Prospective Birth Cohort Study," *Scientific Reports* 6 (2016): 29867.

12. C. Druet et al., "Prediction of Childhood Obesity by Infancy Weight Gain: An Individual-Level Meta-Analysis," *Paediatric and Perinatal Epidemiology* 26, no. 1 (2012): 19–26.

13. R. W. Leunissen et al., "Timing and Tempo of First-Year Rapid Growth in Relation to Cardiovascular and Metabolic Risk Profile in Early Adulthood," *JAMA* 301, no. 21 (2009): 2234–42.

14. D. Charalampopoulos et al., "Age at Menarche and Risks of All-Cause and Cardiovascular Death: A Systematic Review and Meta-Analysis," *American Journal of Epidemiology* 180, no. 1 (2014): 29–40.

   F. R. Day, "Puberty Timing Associated with Diabetes, Cardiovascular Disease and Also Diverse Health Outcomes in Men and Women: The UK Biobank Study," *Scientific Reports* 5 (2015): 11208.

K. K. Ong et al., "Infancy Weight Gain Predicts Childhood Body Fat and Age at Menarche in Girls," *Journal of Clinical Endocrinology and Metabolism* 94, no. 5 (2009): 1527–32.

15. L. Johnson et al., "Genetic and Environmental Influences on Infant Growth: Prospective Analysis of the Gemini Twin Birth Cohort," *PLOS ONE* 6, no. 5 (2011): e19918.

C. H. Llewellyn et al., "Inherited Behavioral Susceptibility to Adiposity in Infancy: A Multivariate Genetic Analysis of Appetite and Weight in the Gemini Birth Cohort," *American Journal of Clinical Nutrition* 95, no. 3 (2012): 633–39.

16. Ong, "Catch-Up Growth in Small for Gestational Age Babies."

17. E. Ross et al., "Failure to Thrive: Case Definition and Guidelines for Data Collection, Analysis and Presentation of Maternal Immunisation Safety Data," *Vaccine* 35, no. 48 (2017): 6483–91.

18. C. Larson-Nath and V. F. Biank, "Clinical Review of Failure to Thrive in Pediatric Patients," *Pediatric Annals* 45, no. 2 (2016): e46–49.

19. M. C. Rudolf and S. Logan, "What Is the Long Term Outcome for Children Who Fail to Thrive? A Systematic Review," *Archives of Disease in Childhood* 90, no. 9 (2005): 925–31.

S. S. Corbett and R. F. Drewett, "To What Extent Is Failure to Thrive in Infancy Associated with Poorer Cognitive Development? A Review and Meta-Analysis," *Journal of Child Psychology and Psychiatry* 45, no. 3 (2004): 641–54.

E. C. Perrin et al., "Criteria for Determining Disability in Infants and Children: Failure to Thrive," Evidence Report Summary 72 (Rockville, MD: Agency for Healthcare Research and Quality, 2003).

A. M. Emond et al., "Weight Faltering in Infancy and IQ Levels at 8 Years in the Avon Longitudinal Study of Parents and Children," *Pediatrics* 120, no. 4 (2007): e1051–58.

20. Shields, Wacogne and Wright, "Weight Faltering and Failure to Thrive in Infancy and Early Childhood."

21. Ibid.

22. Ibid.

Larson-Nath and Biank, "Clinical Review of Failure to Thrive in Pediatric Patients."

23. Larson-Nath and Biank, "Clinical Review of Failure to Thrive in Pediatric Patients."

24. C. Wright, J. Loughridge and G. Moore, "Failure to Thrive in a Population Context: Two Contrasting Studies of Feeding and Nutritional Status," *Proceedings of the Nutrition Society* 59, no. 1 (2000): 37–45.

K. N. Parkinson, C. M. Wright and R. F. Drewett, "Mealtime Energy Intake and Feeding Behaviour in Children Who Fail to Thrive: A Population-Based Case-Control Study," *Journal of Child Psychology and Psychiatry* 45, no. 5 (2004): 1030–35.

R. F. Drewett, M. Kasese-Hara and C. Wright, "Feeding Behaviour in Young Children Who Fail to Thrive," *Appetite* 40, no. 1 (2003): 55–60.

A. Emond et al., "Postnatal Factors Associated with Failure to Thrive in Term Infants in the Avon Longitudinal Study of Parents and Children," *Archives of Disease in Childhood* 92, no. 2 (2007): 115–19.

C. M. Wright, K. N. Parkinson and R. F. Drewett, "How Does Maternal and Child Feeding Behavior Relate to Weight Gain and Failure to Thrive? Data from a Prospective Birth Cohort," *Pediatrics* 117, no. 4 (2006): 1262–69.

P. McDougall et al., "The Detection of Early Weight Faltering at the 6–8-Week Check and Its Association with Family Factors, Feeding and Behavioural Development," *Archives of Disease in Childhood* 94, no. 7 (2009): 549–52.

25. Rhys Blakely, "Birth of the Big One," *The Times*, July 13, 2011, thetimes.co.uk.

    Rachel Porter, "Why Are Today's Babies Being Born So BIG?" *Daily Mail*, August 4, 2011.

26. S. M. Donahue et al., "Trends in Birth Weight and Gestational Length Among Singleton Term Births in the United States: 1990–2005," *Obstetrics and Gynecology* 115, no. 2 (2010): 357–64.

    J. M. Catove et al., "Race Disparities and Decreasing Birth Weight: Are All Babies Getting Smaller?" *American Journal of Epidemiology* 183, no. 1 (2016): 15–23.

27. E. Oken, "Secular Trends in Birthweight," in *Recent Advances in Growth Research: Nutritional, Molecular and Endocrine Perspectives,* ed. M. W. Gillman, P. D. Gluckman and R. G. Rosenfeld (Basel: Karger, 2013), 103–114.

    Office for National Statistics, "Mean, Median and Quantiles for Live Births Born to Mothers Aged Between 20 and 41 and Birthweight Between 300g and 5,000g, 1990 to 2014," ons.gov.uk.

28. Donahue et al., "Trends in Birth Weight and Gestational Length Among Singleton Term Births."

    Catove et al., "Race Disparities and Decreasing Birth Weight."

29. Ibid.

30. L. Belbasis et al., "Birth Weight in Relation to Health and Disease in Later Life: An Umbrella Review of Systematic Reviews and Meta-Analyses," *BMC Medicine* 14, no. 1 (2016): 147.

31. M. S. Kramer, "Determinants of Low Birth Weight: Methodological Assessment and Meta-Analysis," *Bulletin of the World Health Organization* 65, no. 5 (1987): 663–737.

CHAPTER 4

1. American Academy of Pediatrics, "Breastfeeding and the Use of Human Milk," *Pediatrics* 129, no. 3 (2012): e827–84.

   World Health Organization, *Infant and Young Child Nutrition: Global Strategy on Infant and Young Child Feeding: Report by the Secretariat* (World Health Organization, 2002).

2. B. Young, "Formula Feeding Exposure Not Homogenous," *Pediatrics* 140, no. 3 (2017).

3. M. S. Kramer et al., "Promotion of Breastfeeding Intervention Trial (PROBIT): A Randomized Trial in the Republic of Belarus," *JAMA* 285, no. 4 (2001): 413–20.

4. C. G. Victora et al., "Breastfeeding in the 21st Century: Epidemiology, Mechanisms, and Lifelong Effect," *Lancet* 387, no. 10017 (2016): 475–90.

5. B. L. Horta and C. G. Victora, *Short-Term Effects of Breastfeeding: A Systematic Review on the Benefits of Breastfeeding on Diarrhoea and Pneumonia Mortality* (World Health Organization, 2013).

6. G. Bowatte et al., "Breastfeeding and Childhood Acute Otitis Media: A Systematic Review and Meta-Analysis," *Acta Paediatrica* 104, no. 467 (2015): 85–95.

7. S. Ip et al., "Breastfeeding and Maternal and Infant Health Outcomes in Developed Countries," *Evidence Report/Technology Assessment* 153 (Rockville, MD: Agency for Healthcare Research and Quality, 2007).

8. K. Stordal et al., "Breastfeeding and Infant Hospitalisation for Infections: Large Cohort and Sibling Analysis," *Journal of Pediatric Gastroenterology and Nutrition* 65, no. 2 (2017): 225–31.

9. B. J. Stoll et al., "Trends in Care Practices, Morbidity, and Mortality of Extremely Preterm Neonates, 1993–2012," *JAMA* 314, no. 10 (2016): 1039–51.

10. M. Quigley and W. McGuire, "Formula Versus Donor Breast Milk for Feeding Preterm or Low Birth Weight Infants," *Cochrane Database of Systematic Reviews* 6 (2018): CD002971.

11. F. R. Hauck et al., "Breastfeeding and Reduced Risk of Sudden Infant Death Syndrome: A Meta-Analysis," *Pediatrics* 128, no. 1 (2011): 103–10.

12. J. M. D. Thompson et al., "Duration of Breastfeeding and Risk of SIDS: An Individual Participant Data Meta-Analysis," *Pediatrics* 140, no. 5 (2017): e20171324.

13. Kramer et al., "Promotion of Breastfeeding Intervention Trial (PROBIT)."

14. R. S. Horne et al., "Comparison of Evoked Arousability in Breast and Formula Fed Infants," *Archives of Disease in Childhood* 89, no. 1 (2004): 22–25.

15. M. M. Vennemann et al., "Does Breastfeeding Reduce the Risk of Sudden Infant Death Syndrome?" *Pediatrics* 123, no. 3 (2009): e406–10.

     C. C. Blackwell and D. M. Weir, "The Role of Infection in Sudden Infant Death Syndrome," *FEMS Immunology and Medical Microbiology* 25, nos. 1–2 (1999): 1–6.

16. Centers for Disease Control and Prevention, "Sudden Unexpected Infant Death and Sudden Infant Death Syndrome: Data and Statistics," cdc.gov/sids/data.htm.

17. C. G. Victora et al., "Breastfeeding in the 21st Century."

     Kramer et al., "Promotion of Breastfeeding Intervention Trial (PROBIT)."

     C. G. Colen and D. M. Ramey, "Is Breast Truly Best? Estimating the Effects of Breastfeeding on Long-Term Child Health and Wellbeing in the United States Using Sibling Comparisons," *Social Science and Medicine* 109 (2014): 55–65.

18. Kramer et al., "Promotion of Breastfeeding Intervention Trial (PROBIT)."

     M. S. Kramer et al., "Effect of Prolonged and Exclusive Breast Feeding on Risk of Allergy and Asthma: Cluster Randomised Trial," *BMJ* 335, no. 7624 (2007): 815.

     C. Flohr et al., "Effect of an Intervention to Promote Breastfeeding on Asthma, Lung Function, and Atopic Eczema at Age 16 Years: Follow-Up of the PROBIT Randomized Trial," *JAMA Pediatrics* 172, no. 1 (2018): e174064.

19. E. L. Amitay and L. Keinan-Boker, "Breastfeeding and Childhood Leukemia Incidence: A Meta-Analysis and Systematic Review," *JAMA Pediatrics* 169, no. 6 (2015): e151025.

20. M. Greaves, "A Causal Mechanism for Childhood Acute Lymphoblastic Leukaemia," *Nature Reviews, Cancer* 18, no. 8 (2018): 526.

21. D. A. Siegel et al., "Rates and Trends of Pediatric Acute Lymphoblastic Leukemia—United States, 2001–2014," *Morbidity and Mortality Weekly Report* 66, no. 36 (2017): 950–54.

22. B. L. Horta, C. Loret de Mola and C. G. Victora, "Long-Term Consequences of Breastfeeding on Cholesterol, Obesity, Systolic Blood Pressure and Type 2 Diabetes: A Systematic Review and Meta-Analysis," *Acta Paediatrica* 104, no. 467 (2015): 30–37.

23. Centers for Disease Control and Protection, "Childhood Obesity Facts," cdc.gov /obesity/data/childhood.html.

24. M. J. Brion et al., "What Are the Causal Effects of Breastfeeding on IQ, Obesity and Blood Pressure? Evidence from Comparing High-Income with Middle-Income Cohorts," *International Journal of Epidemiology* 40, no. 3 (2011): 670–80.

25. Colen and Ramey, "Is Breast Truly Best?"

26. M. S. Kramer et al., "Effects of Prolonged and Exclusive Breastfeeding on Child Height, Weight, Adiposity, and Blood Pressure at Age 6.5 Y: Evidence from a Large Randomized Trial," *American Journal of Clinical Nutrition* 86, no. 6 (2007): 1717–21.

    R. M. Martin et al., "Effects of Promoting Longer-Term and Exclusive Breastfeeding on Adiposity and Insulin-Like Growth Factor-I at Age 11.5 Years: A Randomized Trial," *JAMA* 309, no. 10 (2013): 1005–13.

    R. M. Martin et al., "Effects of Promoting Long-Term, Exclusive Breastfeeding on Adolescent Adiposity, Blood Pressure, and Growth Trajectories: A Secondary Analysis of a Randomized Clinical Trial," *JAMA Pediatrics* 171, no. 7 (2017): e170698.

27. Quigley and McGuire, "Formula Versus Donor Breast Milk for Feeding Preterm or Low Birth Weight Infants."

28. Horta, Loret de Mola and Victora, "Long-Term Consequences of Breastfeeding on Cholesterol, Obesity, Systolic Blood Pressure and Type 2 Diabetes."

29. R. M. Martin et al., "Effects of Promoting Longer-Term and Exclusive Breastfeeding on Cardiometabolic Risk Factors at Age 11.5 Years: A Cluster-Randomized, Controlled Trial," *Circulation* 129, no. 3 (2013): 321–29.

30. Horta, Loret de Mola and Victora, "Long-Term Consequences of Breastfeeding on Cholesterol, Obesity, Systolic Blood Pressure and Type 2 Diabetes."

31. Kramer et al., "Effects of Prolonged and Exclusive Breastfeeding on Child Height, Weight, Adiposity, and Blood Pressure at Age 6.5 Y."

    Martin et al., "Effects of Promoting Long-Term, Exclusive Breastfeeding on Adolescent Adiposity, Blood Pressure, and Growth Trajectories."

32. A. Singhal et al., "Breastmilk Feeding and Lipoprotein Profile in Adolescents Born Preterm: Follow-Up of a Prospective Randomised Study," *Lancet* 363, no. 9421 (2004): 1571–78.

    A. Singhal, T. J. Cole and A. Lucas, "Early Nutrition in Preterm Infants and Later Blood Pressure: Two Cohorts After Randomised Trials," *Lancet* 357, no. 9254 (2001): 413–19.

33. C. Hoefer and M. C. Hardy, "Later Development of Breast Fed and Artificially Fed Infants: Comparison of Physical and Mental Growth," *JAMA* 92, no. 8 (1929): 615–19.

34. K. G. Dewey et al., "Effects of Exclusive Breastfeeding for Four Versus Six Months on Maternal Nutritional Status and Infant Motor Development: Results of Two Randomized Trials in Honduras," *Journal of Nutrition* 131, no. 2 (2001): 262–67.

 M. Verstergaard et al., "Duration of Breastfeeding and Developmental Milestones During the Latter Half of Infancy," *Acta Paediatrica* 88, no. 12 (1999): 1327–32.

35. B. L. Horta, C. Loret de Mola and C. G. Victora, "Breastfeeding and Intelligence: A Systematic Review and Meta-Analysis," *Acta Paediatrica* 104, no. 467 (2015): 14–19.

36. M. Richards, R. Hardy and M. E. Wadsworth, "Long-Term Effects of Breast-Feeding in a National Birth Cohort: Educational Attainment and Midlife Cognitive Function," *Public Health Nutrition* 5, no. 5 (2002): 631–35.

 R. M. Martin et al., "Breast Feeding in Infancy and Social Mobility: 60-Year Follow-Up of the Boyd Orr Cohort," *Archives of Disease in Children* 92, no. 4 (2007): 317–21.

37. C. G. Victora et al., "Breastfeeding and School Achievement in Brazilian Adolescents," *Acta Paediatrica* 94, no. 11 (2005): 1656–60.

 C. G. Victora et al., "Association Between Breastfeeding and Intelligence, Educational Attainment, and Income at 30 Years of Age: A Prospective Birth Cohort Study from Brazil," *Lancet Global Health* 3, no. 4 (2015): e199–205.

38. E. Evenhous and S. Reilly, "Improved Estimates of the Benefits of Breastfeeding Using Sibling Comparisons to Reduce Selection Bias," *Health Services Research* 40, no. 6 (2005): 1781–802.

39. G. Der, G. D. Batty and I. J. Deary, "Effect of Breast Feeding on Intelligence in Children: Prospective Study, Sibling Pairs Analysis, and Meta-Analysis," *BMJ* 333, no. 7575 (2006): 945.

40. M. S. Kramer et al., "Breastfeeding and Child Cognitive Development: New Evidence from a Large Randomized Trial," *Archives of General Psychiatry* 65, no. 5 (2008): 578–84.

41. G. Der, G. Batty and I. Deary, "Results from the PROBIT Breastfeeding Trial May Have Been Overinterpreted," *Archives of General Psychiatry* 65, no. 12 (2008): 1456–57.

42. S. Yang et al., "Breastfeeding During Infancy and Neurocognitive Function in Adolescence: 16-Year Follow-Up of the PROBIT Cluster-Randomized Trial," *PLOS Medicine* 15, no. 4 (2018): e1002554.

43. Quigley and McGuire, "Formula Versus Donor Breast Milk for Feeding Preterm or Low Birth Weight Infants."

44. R. Chowdhury et al., "Breastfeeding and Maternal Health Outcomes: A Systematic Review and Meta-Analysis," *Acta Paediatrica* 104, no. 467 (2015): 96–113.

 M. S. Kramer and R. Kakuma, "Optimal Duration of Exclusive Breastfeeding," *Cochrane Database of Systematic Reviews* 8 (2012): CD003517.

45. K. Britt and R. Short, "The Plight of Nuns: Hazards of Nulliparity," *Lancet* 379, no. 9834 (2012): 2322–23.

46. Chowdhury et al., "Breastfeeding and Maternal Health Outcomes."

47. American Cancer Society, "Lifetime Risk of Developing or Dying from Cancer," cancer.org.

48. Centers for Disease Control and Prevention (CDC), "United States Cancer Statistics Data Visualizations Tool," based on November 2017 submission data (1999–2015), cdc.gov/cancer/uscs/dataviz/index.htm.

49. M. L. Plasilova et al., "Features of Triple-Negative Breast Cancer: Analysis of 38,813 Cases from the National Cancer Database," *Medicine* 95, no. 35 (2016): e4614.

50. F. Islami et al., "Breastfeeding and Breast Cancer Risk by Receptor Status: A Systematic Review and Meta-Analysis," *Annals of Oncology* 26, no. 12 (2015): 2398–407.

51. Chowdhury et al., "Breastfeeding and Maternal Health Outcomes."

52. American Cancer Society, "Key Statistics for Ovarian Cancer," cancer.org.

53. CDC, "United States Cancer Statistics Data Visualizations Tool."

54. D. Aune et al., "Breastfeeding and the Maternal Risk of Type 2 Diabetes: A Systematic Review and Dose-Response Meta-Analysis of Cohort Studies," *Nutrition, Metabolism, and Cardiovascular Diseases* 24, no. 2 (2014): 107–15.

55. K. L. Bobrow et al., "Persistent Effects of Women's Parity and Breastfeeding Patterns on Their Body Mass Index: Results from the Million Women Study," *International Journal of Obesity* 37, no. 5 (2013): 712–17.

56. E. Oken et al., "Effects of an Intervention to Promote Breastfeeding on Maternal Adiposity and Blood Pressure at 11.5 Y Postpartum: Results from the Promotion of Breastfeeding Intervention Trial, a Cluster-Randomized Controlled Trial," *American Journal of Clinical Nutrition* 98, no. 4 (2013): 1048–56.

57. C. C. Dias and B. Figueiredo, "Breastfeeding and Depression: A Systematic Review of the Literature," *Journal of Affective Disorders* 171 (2015): 142–54.

58. Chowdhury et al., "Breastfeeding and Maternal Health Outcomes."

59. C. E. Neville et al., "The Relationship Between Breastfeeding and Postpartum Weight Change: A Systematic Review and Critical Evaluation," *International Journal of Obesity* 38, no. 4 (2014): 577–90.

60. M. Bartick and C. Reyes, "Las dos cosas: An Analysis of Attitudes of Latina Women on Non-Exclusive Breastfeeding," *Breastfeeding Medicine* 7, no. 1 (2012): 19–24.

61. L. R. Mitoulas et al., "Efficacy of Breast Milk Expression Using an Electric Breast Pump," *Journal of Human Lactation* 18, no. 4 (2002): 344–52.

62. V. J. Flaherman et al., "Effect of Early Limited Formula on Duration and Exclusivity of Breastfeeding in At-Risk Infants: An RCT," *Pediatrics* 131, no. 6 (2013): 1059–65.

   V. J. Flaherman et al., "The Effect of Early Limited Formula on Breastfeeding, Readmission, and Intestinal Microbiota: A Randomised Clinical Trial," *Journal of Pediatrics* 196 (2018): 84–90.

Z. Stranak et al., "Limited Amount of Formula May Facilitate Breastfeeding: Randomized, Controlled Trial to Compare Standard Clinical Practice Versus Limited Supplemental Feeding," *PLOS ONE* 11, no. 2 (2016): e0150053.

63. Centers for Disease Control and Prevention (CDC), "Breastfeeding Among US Children Born 2009–2015, CDC National Immunization Survey," cdc.gov/breastfeeding/data/nis_data/results.html.

64. F. McAndrew et al., *Infant Feeding Survey 2010* (Health and Social Care Information Centre, 2012).

65. E. C. Odom et al., "Reasons for Earlier than Desired Cessation of Breastfeeding," *Pediatrics* 131, no. 3 (2013): e726–32.

66. CDC, "Chapter 3. Infant Feeding," in *Infant Feeding Practices Study II* (Centers for Disease Control and Prevention, 2017).

67. Ibid.

68. D. J. Chapman and R. Pérez-Escamilla, "Identification of Risk Factors for Delayed Onset of Lactation," *Journal of the American Dietetic Association* 99, no. 4 (1999): 450–54.

   K. G. Dewey et al., "Risk Factors for Suboptimal Infant Breastfeeding Behavior, Delayed Onset of Lactation, and Excess Neonatal Weight Loss," *Pediatrics* 112, no. 3 (2003): 607–9.

   S. L. Matias et al., "Risk Factors for Early Lactation Problems Among Peruvian Primiparous Mothers," *Maternal and Child Nutrition* 6, no. 2 (2010): 120–33.

   L. A. Nommsen-Rivers et al., "Delayed Onset of Lactogenesis Among First-Time Mothers Is Related to Maternal Obesity and Factors Associated with Ineffective Breastfeeding," *American Journal of Clinical Nutrition* 92, no. 3 (2010): 574–84.

   E. Brownell et al., "Delayed Onset Lactogenesis II Predicts the Cessation of Any or Exclusive Breastfeeding," *Journal of Pediatrics* 161, no. 4 (2012): 608–14.

69. N. M. Hurst, "Recognizing and Treating Delayed or Failed Lactogenesis II," *Journal of Midwifery and Women's Health* 52, no. 6 (2007): 588–94.

70. E. LaFleur, "What Causes a Low Milk Supply During Breastfeeding?" mayoclinic.org.

71. S. Lee and S. L. Kelleher, "Biological Underpinning of Breastfeeding Challenges: The Role of Genetics, Diet, and Environment on Lactation Physiology," *American Journal of Physiology, Endocrinology and Metabolism* 311, no. 2 (2016): E405–22.

72. M. Neifert et al., "The Influence of Breast Surgery, Breast Appearance, and Pregnancy-Induced Breast Changes on Lactation Sufficiency as Measured by Infant Weight Gain," *Birth* 17, no. 1 (1990): 31–38.

73. Lee and Kelleher, "Biological Underpinning of Breastfeeding Challenges."

74. Hurst, "Recognizing and Treating Delayed or Failed Lactogenesis II."

75. L. R. Mitoulas et al., "Efficacy of Breast Milk Expression Using an Electric Breast Pump."

76. O. E. Savenije and P. L. Brand, "Accuracy and Precision of Test Weighing to Assess Milk Intake in Newborn Infants," *Archives of Disease in Childhood, Fetal and Neonatal Edition* 91, no. 5 (2006): F330–322.

77. American Academy of Pediatrics, "Making Sure Your Baby Is Getting Enough Milk," healthychildren.org.

78. D. Elad et al., "Biomechanics of Milk Extraction During Breast-Feeding," *Proceedings of the National Academy of Sciences of the USA* 111, no. 14 (2014): 5230–35.

79. N. H. Lauersen and E. Stukane, *The Complete Book of Breast Care* (New York: Fawcett Columbine, 1998).

80. B. Rinker, M. Veneracion and C. P. Walsh, "The Effect of Breastfeeding on Breast Aesthetics," *Aesthetic Surgery Journal* 28, no. 5 (2008): 534–37.

81. M. B. Ramamurthy et al., "Effect of Current Breastfeeding on Sleep Patterns in Infants from Asia-Pacific Region," *Journal of Paediatrics and Child Health* 48, no. 8 (2012): 669–74.

82. I. M. Paul et al., "INSIGHT Responsive Parenting Intervention and Infant Sleep," *Pediatrics* 138, no. 1 (2016): e20160762.

83. A. E. Rudzik, L. Robinson-Smith and H. L. Ball, "Discrepancies in Maternal Reports of Infant Sleep vs. Actigraphy by Mode of Feeding," *Sleep Medicine* 49 (2018): 90–98.

84. A. Brown and V. Harries, "Infant Sleep and Night Feeding Patterns During Later Infancy: Association with Breastfeeding Frequency, Daytime Complementary Food Intake, and Infant Weight," *Breastfeeding Medicine* 10, no. 5 (2015): 246–52.

85. National Conference of State Legislatures, "Breastfeeding State Laws," ncsl.org /research/health/breastfeeding-state-laws.aspx.

86. Ibid.

87. S. N. Hester et al., "Is the Macronutrient Intake of Formula-Fed Infants Greater than Breast-Fed Infants in Early Infancy?" *Journal of Nutrition and Metabolism* (2012): 891201.

88. J. C. Kent, "How Breastfeeding Works," *Journal of Midwifery and Women's Health* 52, no. 6 (2007): 564–70.

89. Office of Dietary Supplements (ODS), National Institutes of Health, "Vitamin D: Fact Sheet for Health Professionals," ods.od.nih.gov/factsheets /VitaminD-HealthProfessional.

90. C. R. Wagenr, F. R. Greer and the Section on Breastfeeding and Committee on Nutrition, "Prevention of Rickets and Vitamin D Deficiency in Infants, Children, and Adolescents," *Pediatrics* 122, no. 5 (2008): 1142–52.

91. ODS, "Vitamin D: Fact Sheet for Health Professionals."

92. AAP, "Vitamin D & Iron Supplements for Babies: AAP Recommendations—Where We Stand: Iron Supplements" (2016), healthychildren.org/english/ages-stages /baby/feeding-nutrition/pages/vitamin-iron-supplements.aspx.

93. F. Savino et al., "Ghrelin, Leptin and IGF-I Levels in Breast-Fed and Formula-Fed Infants in the First Years of Life," *Acta Paediatrica* 94, no. 5 (2005): 531–37.

   F. Savino and S. A. Liguori, "Update on Breast Milk Hormones: Leptin, Ghrelin and Adiponectin," *Clinical Nutrition (Edinborough)* 27, no. 1 (2008): 42–47.

   S. Aydin et al., "Presence of Obestatin in Breast Milk: Relationship Among

Obestatin, Ghrelin, and Leptin in Lactating Women," *Nutrition* 24, nos. 7–8 (2008): 689–93.

94. F. Hassiotou and D. T. Geddes, "Programming of Appetite Control During Breastfeeding as a Preventative Strategy Against the Obesity Epidemic," *Journal of Human Lactation* 30, no. 2 (2014): 136–42.

95. Ibid.

96. J. A. Mennella, C. P. Jagnow and G. K. Beauchamp, "Prenatal and Postnatal Flavor Learning by Human Infants," *Pediatrics* 107, no. 6 (2001): e88.

97. J. A. Mennella and A. K. Ventura, "Understanding the Basic Biology Underlying the Flavor World of Children," *Current Zoology* 56, no. 6 (2010): 834–41.

98. L. J. Cooke et al., "Demographic, Familial and Trait Predictors of Fruit and Vegetable Consumption by Pre-School Children," *Public Health Nutrition* 7, no. 2 (2004): 295–302.

L. M. Möller et al., "Infant Nutrition in Relation to Eating Behaviour and Fruit and Vegetable Intake at Age 5 Years," *British Journal of Nutrition* 109, no. 3 (2013): 564–71.

A. T. Galloway, Y. Lee and L. L. Birch, "Predictors and Consequences of Food Neophobia and Pickiness in Young Girls," *Journal of the American Dietetic Association* 103, no. 6 (2003): 692–98.

99. Ibid.

100. L. Kaiser and L. H. Allen, "Position of the American Dietetic Association: Nutrition and Lifestyle for a Healthy Pregnancy Outcome," *Journal of the American Dietetic Association* 108, no. 3 (2008): 553–61.

101. IOM, *Dietary Reference Intakes for Thiamin, Riboflavin, Niacin, Vitamin B6, Folate, Vitamin B12, Pantothenic Acid, Biotin, and Choline.*

102. U. von Schenck, C. Bender-Götze and B. Koletzko, "Persistence of Neurological Damage Induced by Dietary Vitamin B-12 Deficiency in Infancy," *Archives of Disease in Childhood* 77, no. 2 (1997): 137–39.

103. IOM, *Dietary Reference Intakes for Thiamin, Riboflavin, Niacin, Vitamin B6, Folate, Vitamin B12, Pantothenic Acid, Biotin, and Choline.*

104. M. A. Hanson et al., "The International Federation of Gynecology and Obstetrics (FIGO) Recommendations on Adolescent, Preconception, and Maternal Nutrition: 'Think Nutrition First,'" *International Journal of Gynaecology and Obstetrics* 131, no. S4 (2015): S213–53.

105. Ibid.

106. Ibid.

107. British Dietetic Association, "Iodine Facts," bda.uk.com/foodfacts/iodine_facts.

108. Ibid.

CHAPTER 5

1. Centers for Disease Control and Prevention (CDC), "Breastfeeding Among US Children Born 2009–2015, CDC National Immunization Survey."

2. Brown and Harries, "Infant Sleep and Night Feeding Patterns During Later Infancy."

3. US Food and Drug Administration (FDA), "FDA Takes Final Step on Infant Formula Protections," fda.gov.

4. Code of Federal Regulations, Title 21, Chapter I, Subchapter B, Parts 106, 107, ecfr. gov.

5. FDA, "How US FDA's GRAS Notification Program Works," fda.gov.

6. C. K. Green Corkins and T. Shurley, "What's in the Bottle? A Review of Infant Formulas," *Nutrition in Clinical Practice* 31, no. 6 (2016): 723–29.

7. R. W. Walker and M. I. Goran, "Laboratory Determined Sugar Content and Composition of Commercial Infant Formulas, Baby Foods and Common Grocery Items Targeted to Children," *Nutrients* 7, no. 7 (2015): 5850–67.

8. J. Moskin, "For an All-Organic Formula, Baby, That's Sweet," *The New York Times*, May 19, 2008.

9. M. Weber et al., "Lower Protein Content in Infant Formula Reduces BMI and Obesity Risk at School Age: Follow-Up of a Randomized Trial," *American Journal of Clinical Nutrition* 99, no. 5 (2014): 1041–51.

10. K. Simmer, "Long-Chain Polyunsaturated Fatty Acid Supplementation in Infants Born at Term," *Cochrane Database of Systematic Reviews* 3 (2017): CD000376.

11. European Food Safety Authority (EFAS), "Scientific Opinion on the Essential Composition of Infant and Follow-On Formulae," *EFSA Journal* 12, no. 7 (2014): 3760.

12. C. R. Martin, P. Ling and G. L. Blackburn, "Review of Infant Feeding: Key Features of Breast Milk and Infant Formula," *Nutrients* 8, no. 5 (2016): 279.

13. Z. Weizman and A. Alsheikh, "Safety and Tolerance of a Probiotic Formula in Early Infancy Comparing Two Probiotic Agents: A Pilot Study," *Journal of the American College of Nutrition* 25, no. 5 (2006): 415–19.

14. EFSA, "Essential Composition of Infant and Follow-On Formulae."

15. Ibid.

16. P. F. Belamarich, R. E. Bochner and A. D. Racine, "A Critical Review of the Marketing Claims of Infant Formula Products in the United States," *Clinical Pediatrics (Phila)* 55, no. 5 (2016): 437–42.

17. FDA, *A Food Labeling Guide* (College Park, MD: Office of Nutrition and Food Labeling, FDA, 2013).

18. EFSA, "Essential Composition of Infant and Follow-On Formulae."

19. Centers for Disease Control and Prevention (CDC), "Learn About *Cronobacter* Infection," cdc.gov/features/cronobacter/index.html.

20. J. Vicini et al., "Survey of Retail Milk Composition as Affected by Label Claims Regarding Farm-Management Practices," *Journal of the American Dietetic Association* 108, no. 7 (2007): 1198–203.

21. Green Corkins and Shurley, "What's in the Bottle?"

22. Consumer Reports, "Baby Formula Buying Guide," consumerreports.org.

23. P. Lucassen, "Colic in Infants," *BMJ Clinical Evidence* (2010): 309.

24. C. S. Chung, S. Yamini and P. R. Trumbo, "FDA's Health Claim Review: Whey-Protein Partially Hydrolyzed Infant Formula and Atopic Dermatitis," *Pediatrics* 132, no. 2 (2012): e408–14.

25. American Academy of Pediatrics (AAP), "Choosing an Infant Formula," healthychildren.org.

26. R. J. Boyle et al., "Hydrolysed Formula and Risk of Allergic or Autoimmune Disease: Systematic Review and Meta-Analysis," *BMJ* 352 (2016): i974.

27. A. Horvath, P. Dziechciarz and H. Szajewska, "The Effect of Thickened-Feed Interventions on Gastroesophageal Reflux in Infants: Systematic Review and Meta-Analysis of Randomized Controlled Trials," *Pediatrics* 122, no. 6 (2008): e1267–77.

28. J. A. Martinez and M. P. Ballew, "Infant Formulas," *Pediatrics in Review* 32, no. 5 (2011): 179–89.

29. M. B. Heyman, "Lactose Intolerance in Infants, Children, and Adolescents," *Pediatrics* 118, no. 3 (2006): 1279–86.

30. Ibid.

31. Ibid.

32. AAP, "Choosing an Infant Formula."

33. Lucassen, "Colic in Infants."

34. Committee on Toxicity of Chemicals in Food, Consumer Products and the Environment, *Phytoestrogens and Health* (Food Standards Agency, 2003).

35. ESPGHAN Committee on Nutrition et al., "Soy Protein Infant Formulae and Follow-On Formulae: A Commentary by the ESPGHAN Committee on Nutrition," *Journal of Pediatric Gastroenterology and Nutrition* 42, no. 4 (2006): 352–61.

36. J. Bhatia and F. Greer, "Use of Soy Protein-Based Formulas in Infant Feeding," *Pediatrics* 121, no. 5 (2008): 1062–68.

37. Ibid.
    R. S. Zeiger et al., "Soy Allergy in Infants and Children with IgE-Associated Cow's Milk Allergy," *Journal of Pediatrics* 134, no. 5 (1999): 614–22.

38. J. Bhatia et al., "Use of Soy Protein-Based Formulas in Infant Feeding," *Pediatrics* 121, no. 5 (2008): 1062–68.

39. D. J. Hill et al., "Manifestations of Milk Allergy in Infancy: Clinical and Immunologic Findings," *Journal of Pediatrics* 109, no. 2 (1986): 270–76.

40. C. T. Cordle, "Soy Protein Allergy: Incidence and Relative Severity," *Journal of Nutrition* 134, no. 5 (2004): 1213S–19S.

41. AAP, "Hypoallergenic Infant Formulas," *Pediatrics* 106, no. 2 (2000): 346–49.

42. Martinez and Ballew, "Infant Formulas."
    Green Corkins and Shurley, "What's in the Bottle?"

43. I. C. Teller et al., "Post-Discharge Formula Feeding in Preterm Infants: A Systematic Review Mapping Evidence About the Role of Macronutrient Enrichment," *Clinical Nutrition* 35, no. 4 (2016): 791–801.
    L. Young et al., "Nutrient-Enriched Formula Versus Standard Term Formula for Preterm Infants Following Hospital Discharge," *Cochrane Database of Systematic Reviews* 3 (2012): CD004696.

44. J. Lemale et al., "Replacing Breastmilk or Infant Formula with a Nondairy Drink in Infants Exposes Them to Severe Nutritional Complications," *Acta Paediatrica* 107, no. 10 (2018): 1829–29.

45. FDA, "FDA Takes Final Step on Infant Formula Protections."

46. American Academy of Pediatrics, "How to Safely Prepare Formula with Water," healthychildren.org.

47. World Health Organization, *How to Prepare Formula for Bottle-Feeding at Home* (WHO/FAO, 2007).

48. CDC, "Learn About *Cronobacter* Infection."

CHAPTER 6

1. C. H. Llewellyn et al., "Nature and Nurture in Infant Appetite: Analysis of the Gemini Twin Birth Cohort," *American Journal of Clinical Nutrition* 91, no. 5 (2010): 1172–79.

2. S. N. Hester et al., "Is the Macronutrient Intake of Formula-Fed Infants Greater than Breast-Fed Infants in Early Infancy?"

3. M. J. Heinig et al., "Energy and Protein Intakes of Breast-Fed and Formula-Fed Infants During the First Year of Life and Their Association with Growth Velocity: The DARLING Study," *American Journal of Clinical Nutrition* 58, no. 2 (1993): 152–61.

4. K. Paul, J. Dittrichová and H. Papousek, "Infant Feeding Behavior: Development in Patterns and Motivation," *Developmental Psychobiology* 29, no. 7 (1996): 563–76.

5. K. I. DiSantis et al., "Do Infants Fed Directly from the Breast Have Improved Appetite Regulation and Slower Growth During Early Childhood Compared with Infants Fed from a Bottle?" *International Journal of Behavioral Nutrition and Physical Activity* 8 (2011): 89.

6. R. Li et al., "Risk of Bottle-Feeding for Rapid Weight Gain During the First Year of Life," *Archives of Pediatrics and Adolescent Medicine* 166, no. 5 (2012): 431–36.

7. R. Li, S. B. Fein and L. M. Grummer-Strawn, "Do Infants Fed from Bottles Lack Self-Regulation of Milk Intake Compared with Directly Breastfed Infants?" *Pediatrics* 125, no. 6 (2010): e1386–93.

8. K. G. Dewey and B. Lönnerdal, "Infant Self-Regulation of Breast Milk Intake," *Acta Paediatrica* 75, no. 6 (1986): 893–98.

9. C. T. Wood et al., "Association Between Bottle Size and Formula Intake in 2-Month-Old Infants," *Academic Pediatrics* 16, no. 3 (2016): 254–59.

10. C. T. Wood et al., "Bottle Size and Weight Gain in Formula-Fed Infants," *Pediatrics* 138, no. 1 (2016): e20154538.

11. G. J. Hollands et al., "Portion, Package or Tableware Size for Changing Selection and Consumption of Food, Alcohol and Tobacco," *Cochrane Database of Systematic Reviews* 9 (2015): CD011045.

12. A. K. Ventura and R. Pollack Golen, "A Pilot Study Comparing Opaque, Weighted Bottles with Conventional, Clear Bottles for Infant Feeding," *Appetite* 85 (2015): 178–84.

13. K. F. Kavanaugh et al., "Educational Intervention to Modify Bottle-Feeding Behaviors Among Formula-Feeding Mothers in the WIC Program: Impact on Infant Formula Intake and Weight Gain," *Journal of Nutrition Education and Behavior* 40, no. 4 (2008): 244–50.

R. S. Gross et al., "Maternal Perceptions of Infant Hunger, Satiety and Pressuring Feeding Styles in an Urban Latina WIC Population," *Academic Pediatrics* 10, no. 1 (2010): 29–35.

R. Li, S. B. Fein and L. M. Grummer-Strawn, "Association of Breastfeeding Intensity and Bottle-Emptying Behaviors at Early Infancy with Infants' Risk for Excess Weight at Late Infancy," *Pediatrics* 122, no. S2 (2008): S77–84.

14. A. K. Ventura, "Associations Between Breastfeeding and Maternal Responsiveness: A Systematic Review of the Literature," *Advances in Nutrition* 8, no. 3 (2017): 495–510.

15. R. Li et al., "Bottle-Feeding Practices During Early Infancy and Eating Behaviors at 6 Years of Age," *Pediatrics* 131, no. S1 (2014): S70–77.

16. I. M. Paul et al., "The Intervention Nurses Start Infants Growing on Healthy Trajectories (INSIGHT) Study," *BMC Pediatrics* 14 (2014): 184.

17. J. S. Savage et al., "Effect of the INSIGHT Responsive Parenting Intervention on Rapid Infant Weight Gain and Overweight Status at Age 1 Year: A Randomized Clinical Trial," *JAMA Pediatrics* 170, no. 8 (2016): 742749.

18. I. M. Paul et al., "Effect of a Responsive Parenting Educational Intervention on Childhood Weight Outcomes at 3 Years of Age: The INSIGHT Randomized Clinical Trial," *JAMA* 320, no 5 (2018): 461–68.

19. S. Anzman-Frasca et al., "Effects of the INSIGHT Obesity Prevention Intervention on Reported and Observed Infant Temperament," *Journal of Developmental and Behavioral Pediatrics*, June 20, 2018 (epub ahead of print).

20. R. Lakshman et al., "Effectiveness of a Behavioural Intervention to Prevent Excessive Weight Gain During Infancy (The Baby Milk Trial): Study Protocol for a Randomised Controlled Trial," *Trials* 16 (2015): 442.

21. R. Lakshman et al., "A Theory-Based Behavioural Intervention to Reduce Formula-Milk Intake and Prevent Excessive Weight Gain During Infancy (The Baby Milk Trial): A Randomised Controlled Trial," *Lancet* 390 (2017): S56.

22. J. C. Lumeng, "Infant Eating Behaviors and Risk for Overweight," *JAMA* 316, no. 19 (2016): 2036–37.

23. A. Fildes, S. Fildes, C. H. M. van Jaarsveld, C. Llewellyn, J. Wardle and A. Fisher, "Parental Control over Feeding in Infancy: Influence of Infant Weight, Appetite and Feeding Method," *Appetite* 91 (2015): 101–6.

24. H. A. Harris et al., "Maternal Feeding Practices and Fussy Eating in Toddlerhood: A Discordant Twin Analysis," *International Journal of Behavioral Nutrition and Physical Activity* 13 (2016): 81.

25. T. M. Dovey et al., "Food Neophobia and 'Picky/Fussy' Eating in Children: A Review," *Appetite* 50, nos. 2–3 (2008): 181–93.

R. Bryant-Waugh et al., "Feeding and Eating Disorders in Childhood," *International Journal of Eating Disorders* 43, no. 2 (2010): 98–111.

26. Research New Zealand Limited, *Responding to Infants' Hunger and Satiety Cues* (Wellington: Health Promotion Agency, 2014).

27. McNally et al., "Communicating Hunger and Satiation in the First 2 Years of Life."

E. A. Hodges et al., "Development of the Responsiveness to Child Feeding Cues Scale," *Appetite* 65 (2013): 210–19.

28. P. Douglas and P. Hill, "Managing Infants Who Cry Excessively in the First Few Months of Life," *BMJ* 343 (2011): d7772.

29. McNally et al., "Communicating Hunger and Satiation in the First 2 Years of Life." Hodges et al., "Development of the Responsiveness to Child Feeding Cues Scale."

30. I. St. James-Roberts, "Infant Crying and Sleeping: Helping Parents to Prevent and Manage Problems," *Primary Care* 35, no. 3 (2008): 547–67.

31. D. Wolke, A. Bilgin and M. Samara, "Systematic Review and Meta-Analysis: Fussing and Crying Durations and Prevalence of Colic in Infants," *Journal of Pediatrics* 185 (2017): 55–61.

32. Ibid.

33. M. Barr, "What Is the Period of PURPLE Crying?" purplecrying.info/what-is-the -period-of-purple-crying.php.

34. Douglas and Hill, "Managing Infants Who Cry Excessively in the First Few Months of Life."

35. R. Y. Moon, "SIDS and Other Sleep-Related Infant Deaths: Evidence Base for 2016 Updated Recommendations for a Safe Infant Sleeping Environment," *Pediatrics* 138, no. 5 (2016): e20162940.

36. A. S. Anderson et al., "Rattling the Plate—Reasons and Rationales for Early Weaning," *Health Education Research* 16, no. 4 (2001): 471–79.

37. D. W. Leger et al., "Adult Perception of Emotion Intensity in Human Infant Cries: Effects of Infant Age and Cry Acoustics," *Child Development* 67, no. 6 (1996): 3238–49.

   J. Lindová, M. Spinka and L. Nováková, "Decoding of Baby Calls: Can Adult Humans Identify the Eliciting Situation from Emotional Vocalizations of Preverbal Infants?" *PLOS ONE* 10, no. 4 (2015): e0124317.

38. American Academy of Pediatrics, "SIDS and Other Sleep-Related Infant Deaths: Evidence Base for 2016 Updated Recommendations for a Safe Infant Feeding Environment," *Pediatrics* 138, no. 5 (2016): e20162940.

39. F. R. Hauck, O. O. Omojokun and M. S. Siadaty, "Do Pacifiers Reduce the Risk of Sudden Infant Death Syndrome? A Meta-Analysis," *Pediatrics* 116, no. 5 (2005): e716–23.

40. N. R. O'Connor et al., "Pacifiers and Breastfeeding: A Systematic Review," *Archives of Pediatrics and Adolescent Medicine* 163, no. 4 (2009): 378–82.

41. R. G. Barr, "Common Features and Principles of Soothing," purplecrying.info.

42. St. James-Roberts, "Infant Crying and Sleeping."

43. M. W. Woolridge and C. Fisher, "Colic, 'Overfeeding', and Symptoms of Lactose Malabsorption in the Breastfed Baby: A Possible Artifact of Feed Management?" *Lancet* 2, no. 8607 (1988): 382–84.

   Douglas and Hill, "Managing Infants Who Cry Excessively in the First Few Months of Life."

   P. S. Douglas, "Diagnosing Gastro-Oesophageal Reflux Disease or Lactose Intolerance in Babies Who Cry a Lot in the First Few Months Overlooks Feeding Problems," *Journal of Paediatrics and Child Health* 49, no. 4 (2013): e252–56.

44. J. Anderson, "Lactose Overload in Babies," Australian Breastfeeding Association, breastfeeding.asn.au/bfinfo/lactose-overload-babies.

45. Douglas, "Diagnosing Gastro-Oesophageal Reflux Disease or Lactose Intolerance in Babies."

46. Ibid.

47. Ibid.

48. Anderson, "Lactose Overload in Babies."

49. N. J. Bergman, "Neonatal Stomach Volume and Physiology Suggest Feeding at 1-H Intervals," *Acta Paediatrica* 102, no. 8 (2013): 773–77.

50. IOM, *Dietary Reference Intakes for Energy, Carbohydrate, Fiber, Fat, Fatty Acids, Cholesterol, Protein, and Amino Acids.*

51. J. C. Kent et al., "Volume and Frequency of Breastfeedings and Fat Content of Breast Milk Throughout the Day," *Pediatrics* 117, no. 3 (2006): e387–95.

52. S. Jain, "How Often and How Much Should Your Baby Eat?" American Academy of Pediatrics, healthychildren.org.

   American Academy of Pediatrics (AAP), "Amount and Schedule of Formula Feedings," healthychildren.org.

53. H. Crawley and S. Westland, *Infant Milks in the UK: A Practical Guide for Health Professionals* (First Steps Nutrition Trust, 2017).

54. S. Jain, "How Often and How Much Should Your Baby Eat?"

   AAP, "Amount and Schedule of Formula Feedings."

CHAPTER 7

1. M. Fewtrell et al., "Complementary Feeding: A Position Paper by the European Society for Paediatric Gastroenterology, Hepatology, and Nutrition (ESPGHAN) Committee on Nutrition," *Journal of Pediatric Gastroenterology and Nutrition* 64, no. 1 (2017): 119–32.

2. American Academy of Pediatrics, "Infant Food and Feeding," aap.org.

3. Ibid.

4. M. Domellöf et al., "Iron Requirements of Infants and Toddlers," *Journal of Pediatric Gastroenterology and Nutrition* 58, no. 1 (2014): 119–29.

5. Centers for Disease Control and Prevention, "Breastfeeding Report Card: United States, 2018," cdc.gov/breastfeeding/data/reportcard.htm.

6. C. M. Barrera et al., "Timing of Introduction of Complementary Foods to US Infants, National Health and Nutrition Examination Survey 2009–2014," *Journal of the Academy of Nutrition and Dietetics* 188, no. 3 (2018): 464–70.

7. L. May et al., *WIC Infant and Toddler Feeding Practices Study—2: Infant Year Report* (Rockville, MD: Westat, 2017).

8. M. S. Kramer and R. Kakuma, *The Optimal Duration of Exclusive Breastfeeding: A Systematic Review* (World Health Organization, 2002), who.int.

   M. S. Kramer and R. Kakuma, "The Optimal Duration of Exclusive Breastfeeding: A Systematic Review," *Advances in Experimental Medicine and Biology* 554 (2004): 63–77.

9. M. S. Kramer and R. Kakuma, "Optimal Duration of Exclusive Breastfeeding," review, *Cochrane Database of Systematic Reviews* 8 (2012): CD003517.

10. K. Stordal et al., "Breastfeeding and Infant Hospitalisation for Infections: Large Cohort and Sibling Analysis," *Journal of Pediatric Gastroenterology and Nutrition* 65, no. 2 (2017): 225–31.

11. W. Qasem, T. Fenton and J. Friel, "Age of Introduction of First Complementary Feeding for Infants: A Systematic Review," *BMC Pediatrics* 15 (2015): 107.

12. D. Ierodiakonou et al., "Timing of Allergenic Food Introduction to the Infant Diet and Risk of Allergic or Autoimmune Disease: A Systematic Review and Meta-Analysis," *JAMA* 316, no. 11 (2016): 1181–92.

13. AAP, "Vitamin D & Iron Supplements for Babies: AAP Recommendations—Where We Stand: Vitamin D Supplements" (2016), healthychildren.org/English /ages-stages/baby/feeding-nutrition/Pages/Vitamin-Iron-Supplements.aspx.

14. Fewtrell et al., "Complementary Feeding."

15. G. Harris and S. Mason, "Are There Sensitive Periods for Food Acceptance in Infancy?" *Current Nutrition Reports* 6, no. 2 (2017): 190–96.

16. H. Coulthard, G. Harris and A. Fogel, "Exposure to Vegetable Variety in Infants Weaned at Different Ages," *Appetite* 78 (2014): 89–94.

17. H. B. Clayton et al., "Prevalence and Reasons for Introducing Infants Early to Solid Foods: Variations by Milk Feeding Type," *Pediatrics* 131, no. 4 (2013): e1108–14.

18. M. D. Nevarez et al., "Association of Early Life Risk Factors with Infant Sleep Duration," *Academic Pediatrics* 10, no. 3 (2010): 187–93.

    M. L. Macknin, S. V. Medendorp and M. C. Maier, "Infant Sleep and Bedtime Cereal," *American Journal of Diseases of Children* 143, no. 9 (1989): 1066–68.

    L. L. Clark and V. A. Beal, "Age at Introduction of Solid Foods to Infants in Manitoba," *Journal of the Canadian Dietetic Association* 42, no. 1 (1981): 72–78.

19. M. R. Perkin et al., "Association of Early Introduction of Solids with Infant Sleep: A Secondary Analysis of a Randomized Controlled Clinical Trial," *JAMA Pediatrics* 172, no. 8 (2018): e180739.

20. H. Coulthard, G. Harris and P. Emmett, "Delayed Introduction of Lumpy Foods to Children During the Complementary Feeding Period Affects Child's Food Acceptance and Feeding at 7 Years of Age," *Maternal and Child Nutrition* 5, no. 1 (2009): 75–85.

CHAPTER 8

1. L. J. Fangupo et al., "A Baby-Led Approach to Eating Solids and Risk of Choking," *Pediatrics* 138, no. 4 (2016): e20160772.

   E. D'Auria et al., "Baby-Led Weaning: What a Systematic Review of the Literature Adds On," *Italian Journal of Pediatrics* 44, no. 1 (2018): 49.

2. A. Brown and M. Lee, "A Descriptive Study Investigating the Use and Nature of Baby-Led Weaning in a UK Sample of Mothers," *Maternal and Child Nutrition* 7, no. 1 (2011): 34-47.

3. R. W. Taylor et al., "Effect of a Baby-Led Approach to Complementary Feeding on Infant Growth and Overweight: A Randomized Clinical Trial," *JAMA Pediatrics* 171, no. 9 (2017): 838–46.

4. R. Laksman, E. A. Clifton and K. K. Ong, "Baby-Led Weaning—Safe and Effective but Not Preventive of Obesity," *JAMA Pediatrics* 171, no. 9 (2017): 832–33.

5. L. Daniels et al., "Impact of a Modified Version of Baby-Led Weaning on Iron Intake and Status: A Randomised Controlled Trial," *BMJ Open* 8, no. 6 (2018): e019036.

6. E. L. Williams et al., "Impact of a Modified Version of Baby-Led Weaning on Infant Food and Nutrient Intakes: The BLISS Randomised Controlled Trial," *Nutrients* 10, no. 6 (2018): 740.

7. M. Fewtrell et al., "Complementary Feeding: A Position Paper by the European Society for Paediatric Gastroenterology, Hepatology, and Nutrition (ESPGHAN) Committee on Nutrition," *Journal of Pediatric Gastroenterology and Nutrition* 64, no. 1 (2017): 119–32.

D'Auria et al., "Baby-Led Weaning."

8. N. Shloim et al., "Parenting Styles, Feeding Styles, Feeding Practices, and Weight Status in 4–12 Year-Old Children: A Systematic Review of the Literature," *Frontiers in Psychology* 6 (2015): 1849.

K. I. DiSantis et al., "The Role of Responsive Feeding in Overweight During Infancy and Toddlerhood: A Systematic Review," *International Journal of Obesity* 35, no. 4 (2011): 480–92.

9. T. M. Dovey et al., "Food Neophobia and 'Picky/Fussy' Eating in Children: A Review," *Appetite* 50, nos. 2–3 (2008): 181–93.

10. P. W. Jansen et al., "Feeding Practices and Child Weight: Is the Association Bidirectional in Preschool Children?" *American Journal of Clinical Nutrition* 100, no. 5 (2014): 1329–36.

P. W. Jansen et al., "Bi-Directional Associations Between Child Fussy Eating and Parents' Pressure to Eat: Who Influences Whom?" *Physiology and Behavior* 176 (2017): 101–6.

11. Jansen et al., "Feeding Practices and Child Weight."

Jansen et al., "Bi-Directional Associations Between Child Fussy Eating and Parents' Pressure to Eat."

12. K. Campbell et al., "Parental Use of Restrictive Feeding Practices and Child BMI Z-Score: A 3-Year Prospective Cohort Study," *Appetite* 55, no. 1 (2010): 84–88.

13. Webber et al., "Child Adiposity and Maternal Feeding Practices."

Jansen et al., "Feeding Practices and Child Weight."

Alfonso et al., "Bidirectional Association Between Parental Child-Feeding Practices and Body Mass Index."

I. P. Derks et al., "Testing the Direction of Effects Between Child Body Composition and Restrictive Feeding Practices: Results from a Population-Based Cohort," *American Journal of Clinical Nutrition* 106, no. 3 (2017): 783–90.

14. J. O. Fisher and L. L. Birch, "Restricting Access to Palatable Foods Affects Children's Behavioral Response, Food Selection, and Intake," *American Journal of Clinical Nutrition* 69, no. 6 (1999): 1264–72.

15. M. Herle, "The Home Environment Shapes Emotional Eating in Childhood," *Child Development* 89, no. 4 (2018): 1423–34.

16. S. Steinsbekk et al., "Emotional Feeding and Emotional Eating: Reciprocal Processes and the Influence of Negative Affectivity," *Child Development* 89, no. 4 (2018): 1234–46.

17. L. L. Birch, D. W. Marlin and J. Rotter, "Eating as the 'Means' Activity in a Contingency: Effects on Young Children's Food Preference," *Child Development* 55, no. 2 (1984): 431–39.

J. Newman and A. Taylor, "Effect of a Means-End Contingency on Young Children's Food Preferences," *Journal of Experimental Child Psychology* 53, no. 2 (1992): 200–216.

18. Hodges et al., "Development of the Responsiveness to Child Feeding Cues Scale."

19. A. K. C. Leung, "Whole Cow's Milk in Infancy," *Paediatrics and Child Health (Oxford)* 8, no. 7 (2003): 419–21.

Fewtrell et al., "Complementary Feeding."

20. Ibid.

21. *Infant Milks: A Simple Guide to Infant Formula, Follow-On Formula and Other Infant Milks* (First Steps Nutrition Trust, 2018).

22. World Health Organization, "Information Concerning the Use and Marketing of Follow-Up Formula," July 17, 2013, who.int/nutrition/topics/WHO_brief_fufandcode_post_17July.pdf.

23. Abbott Laboratories, *Product Information: Pediasure Grow & Gain with Fiber*, abbottnutrition.com/pediasure-grow-and-gain-with-fiber.

CHAPTER 9

1. L. Cooke, "The Importance of Exposure for Healthy Eating in Childhood: A Review," *Journal of Human Nutrition and Dietetics* 20, no. 4 (2007): 294–301.

A. K. Ventura and J. Worobey, "Early Influences on the Development of Food Preferences," *Current Biology* 23, no. 9 (2013): R401–8.

2. L. J. Cooke and J. Wardle, "Age and Gender Differences in Children's Food Preferences," *British Journal of Nutrition* 93, no. 5 (2005): 741–46.

3. C. Barends et al., "Effects of Starting Weaning Exclusively with Vegetables on Vegetable Intake at the Age of 12 and 23 Months," *Appetite* 81 (2014): 193–99.

C. Barends et al., "Effects of Repeated Exposure to Either Vegetables or Fruits on Infant's Vegetable and Fruit Acceptance at the Beginning of Weaning," *Food Quality and Preference* 29, no. 2 (2013): 157–65.

A. S. Maier et al., "Breastfeeding and Experience with Variety Early in Weaning Increase Infants' Acceptance of New Foods for up to Two Months," *Clinical Nutrition (Edinburgh)* 27, no. 6 (2008): 849–57.

4. A. Fildes et al., "An Exploratory Trial of Parental Advice for Increasing Vegetable Acceptance in Infancy," *British Journal of Nutrition* 114, no. 2 (2015): 328–36.

5. A. M. Siega-Riz et al., "New Findings from the Feeding Infants and Toddlers Study 2008," in *Early Nutrition: Impact on Short-and Long-Term Health*, Nestlé Nutrition Institute Workshop, Vol. 68, ed. H. van Goudoever, S. Guandalini and R. E. Kleinman (Basel: Karger, 2011), 83–105.

6. C. Schwartz et al., "Development of Healthy Eating Habits Early in Life: Review of Recent Evidence and Selected Guidelines," *Appetite* 57, no. 3 (2011): 796–807.

S. Niklaus, "Children's Acceptance of New Foods at Weaning: Role of Practices of Weaning and of Food Sensory Properties," *Appetite* 57, no. 3 (2011): 812–15.

I. Nehring et al., "Impacts of In Utero and Early Infant Taste Experiences on Later Taste Acceptance: A Systematic Review," *Journal of Nutrition* 145, no. 6 (2015): 1271–79.

7. Institute of Food Research and Department of Health, *McCance and Widdowson's The Composition of Foods: Seventh Summary Edition* (Royal Society of Chemistry, 2014).

8. US Department of Health and Human Services (HHS) and US Department of Agriculture (USDA), *2015–2020 Dietary Guidelines for Americans*, 8th ed. (Washington, DC: US Government Printing Office, 2015).

9. American Academy of Pediatrics (AAP), "Starting Solid Foods," healthychildren .org.

10. W. H Dietz and L. Stern, eds., *Nutrition: What Every Parent Needs to Know* (American Academy of Pediatrics, 2011).

11. NHS, "Your Pregnancy and Baby Guide: Drinks and Cups for Babies and Toddlers," www.nhs.uk/conditions/pregnancy-and-baby/drinks-and-cups-children.

12. Stanford Children's Health, "Feeding Guide for the First Year," stanfordchildrens .org.

    T. K. Duryea and D. M. Fleischer, "Patient Education: Starting Solid Foods During Infancy (Beyond the Basics)," uptodate.com.

13. "Market Value of Infant Formula and Baby Food in North America in 2016 and 2025," statista.com.

14. Siega-Riz et al., "New Findings from the Feeding Infants and Toddlers Study 2008."

15. K. J. Moding et al., "Variety and Content of Commercial Infant and Toddler Vegetable Products Manufactured and Sold in the United States," *American Journal of Clinical Nutrition* 107, no. 4 (2018): 576–83.

16. AAP, "Starting Solid Foods."

17. AAP, "Botulism," healthychildren.org.

18. K. D. Jackson, L. D. Howie and L. J. Akinbami, "Trends in Allergic Conditions Among Children: United States, 1997–2011," *NCHS Data Brief* 121 (2013): 1–8.

19. National Center for Health Statistics, Centers for Disease Control and Prevention, "Allergies and Hay Fever," cdc.gov/nchs/fastats/allergies.htm.

20. US Food and Drug Administration, "Food Allergies: What You Need to Know," fda.gov.

21. D. Ierodiakonou et al., "Timing of Allergenic Food Introduction to the Infant Diet and Risk of Allergic or Autoimmune Disease: A Systematic Review and Meta-Analysis," *JAMA* 316, no. 11 (2016): 1181–92.

22. A. Togias et al., "Addendum Guidelines for the Prevention of Peanut Allergy in the United States: Report of the National Institute of Allergy and Infectious Diseases–Sponsored Expert Panel," *Allergy, Asthma and Clinical Immunology* 13, no. 1 (2017): 1.

23. D. M. Fleischer et al. "Primary Prevention of Allergic Disease Through Nutritional Interventions," *Journal of Allergy and Clinical Immunology* 1, no. 1 (2013): 29–36.

24. IOM, *Dietary Reference Intakes for Water, Potassium, Sodium, Chloride, and Sulfate* (Washington, DC: National Academies Press, 2005).

25. US Department of Health and Human Services (HHS) and US Department of Agriculture (USDA), "Table A7-1: Daily Nutritional Goals for Age-Sex Groups Based on Dietary Reference Intakes and *Dietary Guidelines* Recommendations," in *2015–2020 Dietary Guidelines for Americans*, 8th ed. (Washington, DC: US Government Printing Office, 2015).

26. L. J. Stein, B. J. Cowart and G. K. Beauchamp, "The Development of Salty Taste Acceptance Is Related to Dietary Experience in Human Infants: A Prospective Study," *American Journal of Clinical Nutrition* 95, no. 1 (2012): 123–29.

27. H. Syrad et al., "Energy and Nutrient Intakes of Young Children in the UK: Findings from the Gemini Twin Cohort," *British Journal of Nutrition* 115, no. 10 (2016): 1843–50.

28. *National Diet and Nutrition Survey: Results from Years 1–4 (Combined) of the Rolling Programme (2008/2009–2011/2012): Executive Summary* (Public Health England, 2014).

29. R. L. Bailey et al., "Total Usual Nutrient Intakes of US Children (Under 48 Months): Findings from the Feeding Infants and Toddlers Study (FITS) 2016," *Journal of Nutrition*, 148, no. 9S (2018): 1557S–66S.

30. C. L. Wagner and F. R. Greer, "Prevention of Rickets and Vitamin D Deficiency in Infants, Children, and Adolescents," *Pediatrics* 122, no. 5 (2008): 1142–52.

31. Department of Agriculture, Agricultural Research Service, Nutrient Data Laboratory, "USDA National Nutrient Database for Standard Reference, Release 27," ars.usda.gov.

32. Office of Dietary Supplements (ODS), National Institutes of Health (NIH), "Vitamin A: Fact Sheet for Health Professionals," ods.od.nih.gov/factsheets /VitaminA-HealthProfessional.

    Office of Dietary Supplements (ODS), National Institutes of Health (NIH), "Vitamin C: Fact Sheet for Health Professionals," ods.od.nih.gov/factsheets /VitaminC-HealthProfessional.

33. Institute of Medicine (IOM), *Dietary Reference Intakes for Vitamin A, Vitamin K, Arsenic, Boron, Chromium, Copper, Iodine, Manganese, Molybdenum, Nickel, Silicon, Vanadium, and Zinc* (Washington, DC: National Academies Press, 2001).

34. IOM, *Dietary Reference Intakes for Vitamin A, Vitamin K, Arsenic, Boron, Chromium, Copper, Iodine, Manganese, Molybdenum, Nickel, Silicon, Vanadium, and Zinc.*

35. N. F. Butte et al., "Nutrient Intakes of US Infants, Toddlers, and Preschoolers Meet or Exceed Dietary Reference Intakes," *Journal of the American Dietetic Association* 110, no. S12 (2010): S27–37.

36. Department of Agriculture, Agricultural Research Service, Nutrient Data Laboratory, "USDA National Nutrient Database for Standard Reference, Release 27," ars.usda.gov.

37. IOM, *Dietary Reference Intakes for Vitamin A, Vitamin K, Arsenic, Boron, Chromium, Copper, Iodine, Manganese, Molybdenum, Nickel, Silicon, Vanadium, and Zinc.*

CHAPTER 10

1. American Academy of Pediatrics (AAP), "Vitamin D & Iron Supplements for Babies: AAP Recommendations—Where We Stand: Iron Supplements" (2016).

2. A. Maier-Nöth et al., "The Lasting Influences of Early Food-Related Variety Experience: A Longitudinal Study of Vegetable Acceptance from 5 Months to 6 Years in Two Populations," *PLOS ONE* 11, no. 3 (2016): e0151356.

3. L. Cooke, "The Importance of Exposure for Healthy Eating in Childhood: A Review," *Journal of Human Nutrition and Dietetics* 20, no. 4 (2007): 294–301.

4. A. Maier et al., "Effects of Repeated Exposure on Acceptance of Initially Disliked Vegetables in 7-Month Old Infants," *Food Quality and Preference* 18, no. 8 (2007): 1023–32.

5. Maier-Nöth et al., "The Lasting Influences of Early Food-Related Variety Experience."

6. L. Chambers, "Complementary Feeding: Vegetables First, Frequently and in Variety," *Nutrition Bulletin* 41, no. 2 (2016): 142–46.

7. Scientific Advisory Committee on Nutrition, *Feeding in the First Year of Life* (SACN, 2018).

8. AAP, "Healthy Fish Choices for Kids," healthychildren.org.

PART 4

1. C. M. Hales et al., "Prevalence of Obesity Among Adults and Youth: United States, 2015–2016," *NCHS Data Brief* no. 288 (2017): 1–8.

2. M. Simmonds et al., "Predicting Adult Obesity from Childhood Obesity: A Systematic Review and Meta-Analysis," *Obesity Reviews* 17, no. 2 (2016): 95–107.

3. M. Geserick et al., "Acceleration of BMI in Early Childhood and Risk of Sustained Obesity," *New England Journal of Medicine* 379, no. 14 (2018): 1303–12.

4. J. Rankin et al., "Psychological Consequences of Childhood Obesity: Psychiatric Comorbidity and Prevention," *Adolescent Health, Medicine and Therapeutics* 7 (2016): 125–46.

5. A. Llewellyn et al., "Childhood Obesity as a Predictor of Morbidity in Adulthood: A Systematic Review and Meta-Analysis," *Obesity Reviews* 17, no. 1 (2016): 56–67.

CHAPTER 11

1. H. Syrad et al., "Energy and Nutrient Intakes of Young Children in the UK: Findings from the Gemini Twin Cohort," *British Journal of Nutrition* 115, no. 10 (2016): 1843–50.

2. IOM, *Dietary Reference Intakes for Energy, Carbohydrate, Fiber, Fat, Fatty Acids, Cholesterol, Protein, and Amino Acids.*

3. US Department of Health and Human Services (HHS) and US Department of Agriculture (USDA), *2015–2020 Dietary Guidelines for Americans*, 8th ed. (Washington, DC: US Government Printing Office, 2015).

4. D. M. Deming et al., "Cross-Sectional Analysis of Eating Patterns and Snacking in the US Feeding Infants and Toddlers Study 2008," *Public Health Nutrition* 20, no. 9 (2017): 1584–92.

5. R. L. Bailey et al., "Total Usual Nutrient Intakes of US Children (Under 48 Months): Findings from the Feeding Infants and Toddlers Study (FITS) 2016," *Journal of Nutrition* 148, no. 9S (2018): 1557S–66S.

6. HHS, *2015–2020 Dietary Guidelines for Americans.*

7. Bailey et al., "Total Usual Nutrient Intakes of US Children (Under 48 Months)."

8. A. L. Günther, A. E. Buyken and A. Kroke, "Protein Intake During the Period of Complementary Feeding and Early Childhood and the Association with Body Mass Index and Percentage Body Fat at 7 Y of Age," *American Journal of Clinical Nutrition* 85, no. 6 (2007): 1626–33.

9. B. Koletzko et al., "High Protein Intake in Young Children and Increased Weight Gain and Obesity Risk," *American Journal of Clinical Nutrition* 103, no. 2 (2016): 303–4.

10. L. Pimpin et al., "Dietary Protein Intake Is Associated with Body Mass Index and Weight up to 5 Y of Age in a Prospective Cohort of Twins," *American Journal of Clinical Nutrition* 103, no. 2 (2016): 389–97.

11. L. Pimpin et al., "Sources and Pattern of Protein Intake and Risk of Overweight or Obesity in Young UK Twins," *British Journal of Nutrition* 120, no. 7 (2018): 820–29.

    L. Pimpin, S. Jebb and G. Ambrosini, "Dairy Protein in the Post-Weaning Phase Is Positively Associated with BMI and Weight up to Five Years of Age," *Appetite* 87 (2015): 398.

12. L. Pimpin et al., "Dietary Intake of Young Twins: Nature or Nurture?" *American Journal of Clinical Nutrition* 98, no. 5 (2013): 1326–34.

    Syrad et al., "Energy and Nutrient Intakes of Young Children in the UK."

13. HHS, *2015–2020 Dietary Guidelines for Americans.*

14. Bailey et al., "Total Usual Nutrient Intakes of US Children (Under 48 Months)."

15. HHS, *2015–2020 Dietary Guidelines for Americans.*

16. American Academy of Pediatrics, "Cow's Milk Alternatives: Parent FAQs," healthychildren.org.

17. HHS, *2012–2020 Dietary Guidelines for Americans.*

18. A. Reynolds, J. Mann, J. Cummings, N. Winter, E. Mete, L. Te Morenga, "Carbohydrate Quality and Human Health: A Series of Systematic Reviews and Meta-Analyses." *Lancet* 393 (2019): 434–45.

19. HHS, *2015–2020 Dietary Guidelines for Americans.*

20. Reynolds et al., "Carbohydrate Quality and Human Health: A Series of Systematic Reviews and Meta-Analyses."

21. C. L. Wagner and F. R. Greer, "Prevention of Rickets and Vitamin D Deficiency in Infants, Children, and Adolescents," *Pediatrics* 122, no. 5 (2008): 1142–52.

    HHS, *2015–2020 Dietary Guidelines for Americans.*

22. Bailey et al., "Total Usual Nutrient Intakes of US Children (Under 48 Months)."

23. HHS, *2015–2020 Dietary Guidelines for Americans.*

24. Bailey et al., "Total Usual Nutrient Intakes of US Children (Under 48 Months)."

25. IOM, *Dietary Reference Intakes for Water, Potassium, Sodium, Chloride, and Sulfate.*

26. HHS, *2015–2020 Dietary Guidelines for Americans.*

27. S. L. Jackson et al., "Prevalence of Excess Sodium Intake in the United States— NHANES, 2009–2012," *Morbidity and Mortality Weekly Report* 64, no. 52 (2016): 1393–97.

28. L. J. Stein, B. J. Cowart and G. K. Beauchamp, "The Development of Salty Taste Acceptance Is Related to Dietary Experience in Human Infants: A Prospective Study," *American Journal of Clinical Nutrition* 95, no. 1 (2012): 123–29.

29. R. L. Rothman et al., "Patient Understanding of Food Labels: The Role of Literacy and Numeracy," *American Journal of Preventative Medicine* 31, no. 5 (2006): 391–98.

30. US Food and Drug Administration, "Food Labeling: Revision of the Nutrition and Supplement Facts Labels," *Federal Register* 81, no. 103 (2016): 33742.

31. M. Rasmussen et al., "Determinants of Fruit and Vegetable Consumption Among Children and Adolescents: A Review of the Literature. Part I: Quantitative Studies," *International Journal of Behavioral Nutrition and Physical Activity* 3 (2006): 22.

32. G. Mrdjenovic and D. A. Levitsky, "Children Eat What They Are Served: The Imprecise Regulation of Energy Intake," *Appetite* 44, no. 3 (2005): 273–82.

33. F. J. Orlet, B. J. Rolls and L. L. Birch, "Children's Bite Size and Intake of an Entrée Are Greater with Large Portions than with Age-Appropriate or Self-Selected Portions," *American Journal of Clinical Nutrition* 77, no. 5 (2003): 1164–70.

34. Mrdjenovic and Levitsky, "Children Eat What They Are Served."

35. K. G. Dewey and B. Lönnderdal, "Infant Self-Regulation of Breast Milk Intake," *Acta Paediatrica* 75, no. 6 (1986): 893–98.

36. G. J. Hollands et al., "Portion, Package or Tableware Size for Changing Selection and Consumption of Food, Alcohol and Tobacco," *Cochrane Database of Systematic Reviews* 9 (2015): CD011045.

37. N. Zlatevska, C.Dubelaar and S. S. Holden, "Sizing Up the Effect of Portion Size on Consumption: A Meta-Analytic Review," *Journal of Marketing* 78, no. 3 (2014): 140–54.

38. C. Piernas and B. M. Popkin, "Food Portion Patterns and Trends Among U.S. Children and the Relationship to Total Eating Occasion Size, 1977–2006," *Journal of Nutrition* 141, no. 6 (2011): 1159–64.

39. H. Syrad et al., "Overweight Very Young Children Consume Larger Meals" (conference abstract for the 2016 European Obesity Summit, Gothenburg, Sweden, June 1–4, 2016).

39. H. Syrad et al., "Meal Size Is a Critical Driver of Weight Gain in Early Childhood," *Scientific Reports* 6 (2016): 28368.

CHAPTER 12

1. K. M. Hurley, M. B. Cross and S. O. Hughes, "A Systematic Review of Responsive Feeding and Child Obesity in High-Income Countries," *Journal of Nutrition* 141, no. 3 (2011): 495–501.

 K. I. DiSantis et al., "The Role of Responsive Feeding in Overweight During Infancy and Toddlerhood: A Systematic Review," *International Journal of Obesity* 35, no. 4 (2011): 480–92.

2. S. A. Redsell et al., "Systematic Review of Randomised Controlled Trials of Interventions That Aim to Reduce the Risk, Either Directly or Indirectly, of Overweight and Obesity in Infancy and Early Childhood," *Maternal and Child Nutrition* 12, no. 1 (2016): 24–38.

3. L. A. Daniels et al, "The NOURISH Randomised Control Trial: Positive Feeding Practices and Food Preferences in Early Childhood—A Primary Prevention Program for Childhood Obesity," *BMC Public Health* 9 (2009): 387.

4. L. A. Daniels, "Child Eating Behavior Outcomes of an Early Feeding Intervention to Reduce Risk Indicators for Child Obesity: The NOURISH RCT," *Obesity* 22, no. 5 (2014): e104–11.

5. A. Magarey et al., "Child Dietary and Eating Behavior Outcomes up to 3.5 Years After an Early Feeding Intervention: The NOURISH RCT," *Obesity* 24, no. 7 (2016): 1537–45.

6. L. A. Daniels et al., "Outcomes of an Early Feeding Practices Intervention to Prevent Childhood Obesity," *Pediatrics* 132, no. 1 (2013): e109–18.

7. M. Story and D. Neumark-Sztainer, "A Perspective on Family Meals: Do They Matter?" *Nutrition Today* 40, no. 6 (2005): 261–66.

8. A. J. Hammons and B. H. Fiese, "Is Frequency of Shared Family Meals Related to the Nutritional Health of Children and Adolescents?" *Pediatrics* 127, no. 6 (2011): e1565–74.

9. C. Sweetman et al., "Characteristics of Family Mealtimes Affecting Children's Vegetable Consumption and Liking," *Journal of the Academy of Nutrition and Dietetics* 111, no. 2 (2011): 269–73.

10. A. Hoyland, L. Dye and C. L. Lawton, "A Systematic Review of the Effect of Breakfast on the Cognitive Performance of Children and Adolescents," *Nutrition Research Reviews* 22, no. 2 (2009): 220–43.

11. H. Szajewska and M. Ruszczynski, "Systematic Review Demonstrating that Breakfast Consumption Influences Body Weight Outcomes in Children and Adolescents in Europe," *Critical Reviews in Food Science and Nutrition* 50, no. 2 (2010): 113–19.

12. C. H. van Jaarsveld et al., "Appetite and Growth: A Longitudinal Sibling Analysis," *JAMA Pediatrics* 168, no. 4 (2014): 345–50.

    P. L. Quah et al., "Prospective Associations of Appetitive Traits at 3 and 12 Months of Age with Body Mass Index and Weight Gain in the First 2 Years of Life," *BMC Pediatrics* 15 (2015): 153.

    K. N. Parkinson et al., "Do Maternal Ratings of Appetite in Infants Predict Later Child Eating Behaviour Questionnaire Scores and Body Mass Index?" *Appetite* 54, no. 1 (2010): 186–90.

13. H. Syrad et al., "Appetitive Traits and Food Intake Patterns in Early Life," *American Journal of Clinical Nutrition* 103, no. 1 (2016): 231–35.

14. M. Mooreville et al., "Individual Differences in Susceptibility to Large Portion Sizes Among Obese and Normal-Weight Children," *Obesity* 23, no. 4 (2015): 808–14.

15. J. Austin and D. Marks, "Hormonal Regulators of Appetite," *International Journal of Pediatric Endocrinology* (2009): 141753.

16. E. Robinson et al., "A Systematic Review and Meta-Analysis Examining the Effect of Eating Rate on Energy Intake and Hunger," *American Journal of Clinicial Nutrition* 100, no. 1 (2014): 123–51.

17. F. R. Bornet et al., "Glycaemic Response to Foods: Impact on Satiety and Long-Term Weight Regulation," *Appetite* 49, no. 3 (2007): 535–53.

    H. Ford and G. Frost, "Glycaemic Index, Appetite and Body Weight," *Proceedings of the Nutrition Society* 69, no. 2 (2010): 199–203.

18. S. Marsh, C. Ni Mhurchu and R. Maddison, "The Non-Advertising Effects of Screen-Based Sedentary Activities on Acute Eating Behaviours in Children, Adolescents, and Young Adults: A Systematic Review," *Appetite* 71 (2013): 259–73.

19. E. J. Boyland et al., "Advertising as a Cue to Consume: A Systematic Review and Meta-Analysis of the Effects of Acute Exposure to Unhealthy Food and Nonalcoholic Beverage Advertising on Intake in Children and Adults," *American Journal of Clinical Nutrition* 103, no. 2 (2016): 5119–533.

    J. C. Halford et al., "Beyond-Brand Effect of Television Food Advertisements on Food Choice in Children: The Effects of Weight Status," *Public Health Nutrition* 11, no. 9 (2008): 897–904.

20. S. L. Johnson, "Improving Preschoolers' Self-Regulation of Energy Intake," *Pediatrics* 106, no. 6 (2000): 1429–35.

21. Syrad et al., "Appetitive Traits and Food Intake Patterns in Early Life."

22. J. O. Fisher and L. L. Birch, "Restricting Access to Palatable Foods Affects Children's Behavioral Response, Food Selection, and Intake," *American Journal of Clinical Nutrition* 69, no. 6 (1999): 1264–72.

23. C. M. Taylor et al., "Picky/Fussy Eating in Children: Review of Definitions, Assessment, Prevalence and Dietary Intakes," *Appetite* 95 (2015): 349–59.

24. B. R. Carruth et al., "Prevalence of Picky Eaters Among Infants and Toddlers and Their Caregivers' Decisions About Offering a New Food," *Journal of the American Dietetic Association* 104, no. S1 (2004): S57–64.

25. L. Webber et al., "Associations Between Children's Appetitive Traits and Maternal Feeding Practices," *Journal of the American Dietetic Association* 110, no. 11 (2010): 1718–22.

    H. A. Harris et al., "Maternal Feeding Practices and Fussy Eating in Toddlerhood: A Discordant Twin Analysis," *International Journal of Behavioral Nutrition and Physical Activity* 13 (2016): 81.

26. H. Syrad et al., "The Role of Infant Appetite in Extended Formula Feeding," *Archives of Disease in Childhood* 100, no. 8 (2015): 758–62.

27. A. Remington et al., "Increasing Food Acceptance in the Home Setting: A Randomized Controlled Trial of Parent-Administered Taste Exposure with Incentives," *American Journal of Clinical Nutrition* 95, no. 1 (2012): 72–77.

28. A. Fildes et al., "Parent-Administered Exposure to Increase Children's Vegetable Acceptance: A Randomized Controlled Trial," *Journal of the Academy of Nutrition and Dietetics* 114, no. 6 (2014): 881–88.

29. C. Nekitsing et al., "Systematic Review and Meta-Analysis of Strategies to Increase Vegetable Consumption in Preschool Children Aged 2–5 Years," *Appetite* 127 (2018): 138–54.

ACKNOWLEDGMENTS

This book is dedicated to our parents and partners, whose love and support have been unwavering throughout.

We would also like to make a special acknowledgment to the late professor Jane Wardle—a world-leading scientist, and our mentor. Jane introduced us to the fascinating world of children's eating behaviors, inspired us and was the brains behind the UK Gemini twin study. She changed our lives and those of many children and families who have benefited from her decades of research.

We must, of course, thank Batya Rosenblum, Beth Bugler, Jennifer Hergenroeder, Jeanne Tao and Matthew Lore for seeing the potential in our research and bringing this to fruition.

We thank our family, friends and all of the parents we spoke to, for sharing their experiences with us and helping to make sure the book includes the information parents really want.

And thank you to the exceptional scientists who took the time to review parts of this book and provide their feedback to help us ensure that the content is accurate and representative of the broad scientific consensus on early nutrition and feeding (all decisions regarding the final content were ours, and we take full responsibility for any errors and omissions).

Many thanks to:

Dr. Ian Paul, professor of pediatrics and public health sciences and chief of the Division of Academic General Pediatrics, Penn State College of Medicine.

Dr. Valerie Flaherman, associate professor of pediatrics, and of epidemiology and biostatistics, Department of Pediatrics, University of California, San Francisco (UCSF); and pediatrician at UCSF's Benioff Children's Hospital.

Dr. Bridget Young, research assistant professor, Department of Pediatrics, Allergy and Immunology, University of Rochester School of Medicine and Dentistry.

Dr. Michael Kramer, professor of pediatrics, and of epidemiology and biostatistics, Department of Epidemiology, Biostatistics and Occupational Health, the Montreal Children's Hospital.

We would also like to thank several scientists who provided feedback on parts of *Baby Food Matters*, the original book published in the UK, on which this book is based:

Atul Singhal, Great Ormond Street Children's Charity Professor of Paediatric Nutrition at University College London's Institute of Child Health, and Honorary Consultant Pediatrician at Great Ormond Street Hospital.

Dr. Alison Fildes, psychologist and research fellow in the School of Psychology at the University of Leeds.

Dr. Helen Croker, research dietician and senior researcher in Great Ormond Street Institute of Child Health, University College London.

Lynne Daniels, emeritus professor in the School of Exercise and Nutrition Sciences, Queensland University of Technology, Australia.

Dr. Jennifer Fildes, general practitioner at Fieldhead Surgery, Leeds.

Dr. Angela Flynn, researcher in the Department of Women and Children's Health, School of Life Course Sciences, King's College London.

We would especially like to thank Dr. Emma Veitch—a mom of two, and science communication professional who has also volunteered in breastfeeding peer-support and published articles on this topic. She provided detailed comments and editorial suggestions on various parts of the book and engaged in numerous thought-provoking and helpful discussions about how best to frame information for parents. Lastly, we would like to thank Marta Jackowska (mom of Julia, eighteen months) and Susie Meisel (mom of Hannah, twelve months), who read and provided feedback on the original UK edition of the book from a mom's point of view.

INDEX

NOTE: Page numbers followed by *t* indicate tables.

on emotional feeding, 25, 205

on essential nutrients, 224

on food preferences, 29–30

on food responsiveness, 21, 152, 276

on nature-nurture debate, 24–25

on parental feeding strategies, 160–61

on positive reinforcement, 282

on satiety responsiveness, 21–22

on typical toddler diet, 242–44, 245, 259, 271, 278, 280

on weight-appetite relationship, 19–20

genetic predisposition

for appetite, 14, 22–26, 77, 152–53, 160, 161

for birth weight, 81, 82

for food preferences, 28–30, 193, 232–33

for milk production, 111

for short stature, 78

gestational diabetes, 36, 44

gestational weight gain, 38–40, 65, 83

ghrelin, 24, 124

glycemic index (GI), 43, 273–74, 278, 279

grapes, 198, 220, 234

growth, during first two years, 67–84

growth charts, 68–71, 75–76

growth rate variability, 71

overview, 67–68, 83–84

rapid weight gain, 76–77

routine weighing, 74–76

weighing method, 71–72

weight faltering (failure to thrive), 78–80

weight loss following birth, 72–74

H

Health Promotion Agency (New Zealand), 163–64

healthy diet. *See* nutrition

hindmilk, 177

honey, 220, 251

hormones, for appetite regulation, 24, 36–37, 124, 177

hunger signals. *See also* eager eaters

of babies, 157, 158, 165, 167–68, 169, 171–72, 208

of toddlers, 261–63, 275, 292

hyperemesis gravidarum, 31, 63

hypothalamus, 24, 36, 37

I

Infant and Toddler Feeding and Practices Study, 187

Infant Feeding Practices Study II (IFPS II), 108, 109

Infant Formula Act of 1980 (revised 1986), 131

infections

breastfeeding as protection from, 92–95, 96–97, 106, 188–89, 289

essential nutrients for prevention of, 225

food safety and, 53, 54–55, 148–50

mastitis, 115–16

pacifier use and, 172

solid food introduction timing and, 186, 188–89

INSIGHT study, 158

Institute of Medicine. *See* National Academy of Medicine (NAM)

INTERGROWTH-21st Preterm Postnatal Growth Standards, 70

iodine, 50, 51, 126–27

iron

breastfed-baby supplementation of, 123, 186, 189, 228

complementary feeding and, 197, 200–201, 225–26, 229, 234

cow's milk and, 209

in formulas, 133–34

pregnancy supplementation of, 47, 48–49, 51

for toddlers, 248

J

juice, 216–17, 254

risk reduction for, 97–98, 158, 269

statistics on, 240–41

omega-3 and -6 fatty acids, 42–43, 134–35, 247

Organic Foods Production Act, 139

ovarian cancer, 103

overeating. *See* eager eaters; emotional over- and undereating

overfeeding, 22, 173, 174, 175–78

overt restrictions, 203–4, 264–65

P

pacifier use, 172–73

pâté, 55

Paul, Ian, 165, 166

peanuts, 189, 198, 220, 221–22, 256, 258

PediaSure Grow & Gain, 211

period of PURPLE crying, 170–71, 173

picky eaters (poor appetite)

characteristics of, 7–9, 16–19

complementary feeding for, 193, 200, 202–8, 232–33

food preferences of, 14, 29–30, 281

influences on, 10, 23–26, 125, 152–53, 160–61

responsive feeding strategies for milk-feeding of, 161, 162–63

responsive feeding strategies for toddlers, 262, 264–67, 269, 279–86, 292–94

underfeeding and, 22, 173, 174–75

weight faltering and, 80

plate-clearing, 272–73, 274, 276, 284–85

polyunsaturated fats (PUFAs), 42–43, 101, 134–35

poor appetite. *See* picky eaters

portion size

age-appropriate, 199, 204–5, 257–60, 265

calorie intake and, 250, 257–58, 260

for eager eaters, 206–7, 272

formula-feeding and, 155, 179–81, 181*t*, 210, 210*t*, 245

on Nutrition Facts label, 250

overview, 291, 292

for picky eaters, 285, 286

for snacking, 278, 279

positive reinforcement

avoidance of food as reward, 158, 205–6, 207, 208, 282–83

for goal achievement, 61–62

physical reward options, 282–83, 286, 289–90

praise as reward, 233, 265–66, 282–83, 286, 289

praise. *See* positive reinforcement

prebiotics, 44, 135–36

preeclampsia, 36, 44, 46, 49

pregnancy

dietary recommendations, 35–36, 40–47, 51–53, 61–63, 65

essential nutrient recommendations, 45–51

food aversions and cravings during, 64–65

foods to avoid during, 40, 43, 52–61, 65

influences on baby food preferences during, 30–31, 36–38

nausea and vomiting during, 31, 63–64

overview, 35, 66, 288–89

structured meal plans for, 62–63

weight gain during, 38–40, 65, 83

preterm delivery, 36, 39, 48, 54, 57–58, 109–10

preterm infants

breastfeeding benefits for, 100

catch-up growth for, 77

essential nutrient recommendations, 123

formula-feeding of, 145, 146–47, 148

growth monitoring of, 69–70

lactose intolerance and, 143

solid food introduction for, 194

studies with, 90, 94, 98, 99, 100

Promotion of Breastfeeding Intervention Trial (PROBIT), in Belarus, 90–91, 93–102, 104, 188

protein
in breast milk, 121, 132
in cow's milk, 132, 144–46, 209
in formulas, 132, 133, 140–41, 144–46
on Nutrition Facts label, 251
preferences for, 29–30, 280
pregnancy requirements, 44, 47, 52
toddler requirements, 244–45, 253
public breastfeeding, 86–87, 121, 129
pulses. *See* beans and legumes
purées, 195–96, 200–201, 220, 229–30,
237

R

Rapley, Gill, 196
reflux (spitting up), 141–42, 174
responsive feeding, for babies
about, 18–19, 155–59
appetite regulation and, 153–55
challenges of, 159–64
cues for, 157, 158, 165, 167–69, 171–72,
208–9
of eager eaters, 161–62, 166, 169–70
how-to advice, 164–67, 179–82
overfeeding, 22, 173, 174, 175–78
overview, 86–87, 152–53, 181–82
of picky eaters, 161, 162–63
of solid foods, 196, 201–9
soothing a nonhungry, fussing baby,
171–74
underfeeding, 22, 173, 174–75
responsive feeding, for toddlers. *See also*
family mealtimes; toddler diet
cues for, 261–63, 275, 292
of eager eaters, 264–67, 271–79
food shopping with toddlers, 269–70
how-to advice, 262–67
overview, 261, 291–93, 297
of picky eaters, 262, 264–67, 269,
279–86, 292–94
research on, 261–62
structure and routines for, 266–68,
291

Responsiveness to Child Feeding Cues
Scale, 208–9
retinol, 47
rewards. *See* positive reinforcement
rice, 44, 47, 142, 235, 245, 253, 274
rice cereal, 169, 213, 217
rickets, 123, 224
Rinker, Brian, 117

S

salt avoidance, 200, 222–23, 230, 248–49,
250, 254–55
satiety responsiveness
of babies, 157, 158, 165, 168, 169, 208–9
baby-led weaning and, 199
of eager eaters, 21–22, 271–73
hormone control of, 24–25, 36–37, 124,
177
measurement of, 13, 15, 296–99
overeating and, 21–22
of picky eaters, 16–17
responsive feeding and, 155–57, 262,
292
of toddlers, 261–63, 271–73, 275, 292
saturated fats, 42, 52, 53, 246–47, 250
screen time, 21–22, 170, 238, 266,
274–75, 293
scurvy, 225
seaweed, 50, 126
seeds, 43–44, 47–48, 126, 220, 236–37,
247, 253
self-feeding, 264, 283–84, 286. *See also*
baby-led weaning
serving size. *See* portion size
shellfish, 56, 221
shopping, with toddlers, 269–70
sleep patterns
breastfed *vs.* formula-fed babies,
118–20, 130
complementary feeding readiness
and, 192
responsive feeding and, 158, 166–67,
173

slowness in eating, 13, 17, 272–73, 285, 298, 299

slowness in feeding, 16, 17, 23–24, 152, 154, 175, 296, 297

small for gestational age (SGA), 56, 58, 77, 81, 82

SMART goals, 62

smoking, 83, 101

snacks and snacking

    for optimal nutrition, 22, 223, 254–57, 265, 276–79, 290

    during pregnancy, 63–65

    routines for, 266–67, 276, 281, 291, 292

social context, for eating. *See* family mealtimes

soda, 52, 57–58, 216–17, 245–46, 251

soft cheeses, 54–55. *See also* dairy products

solid food, introduction of. *See* complementary feeding; first foods

soothing techniques, 158, 166, 168, 171–74

soy-based milk and formulas, 137, 144–45, 147, 211, 253–54

soybeans, 145–46, 221, 236. *See also* beans and legumes

Special Supplemental Nutrition Program for Women, Infants, and Children (WIC), 51, 187, 256–57

spoon-feeding, 195–201, 202, 229–31

St. James-Roberts, Ian, 172

starches, 29, 52, 235, 252

sterilization, for food safety, 92, 138, 148–49, 150–51, 173

sudden infant death syndrome (SIDS), 94–95, 104–6, 171, 172

sugar

    avoidance of, 40, 52, 65, 203–4, 206, 207, 223, 254–55, 293

    in breast milk, 132

    food advertising and, 20–21

    on food labels, 251

    food sources of, 43, 52, 132–33, 211, 216–19, 252

in formulas, 132–33, 143, 144–45

    guidelines for, 245–46

    preferences for, 18, 27, 29–30, 36, 203–4, 214–18, 223

Syrad, Hayley, 4, 9–11

T

taste preferences. *See* eager eaters; food preferences; picky eaters

TASTE study, 215

tea, 48, 57–58

television, 21–22, 170, 238, 266, 274–75, 293

textures

    food preferences and, 28, 30, 190, 285

    introduction of, 28, 190, 193, 195–96, 201, 229–31, 289–90

toddler diet, 242–60. *See also* responsive feeding, for toddlers

    defined, 241

    economic support for, 256–57

    food labels and, 249–52

    optimal nutrition for, 249–52

    overview, 242, 260

    portion size for, 257–60, 265

    snack choices for, 22, 254–57, 265, 276–79, 290

    typical diet, 242–49, 271, 278, 280

toddler milks, 211

toxoplasmosis, 54, 56

trans-fatty acids, 41–42, 246–47, 250

2015–2020 Dietary Guidelines for Americans, 45, 60, 216, 243, 244, 248

twin studies. *See* Gemini study

type 2 diabetes, 76–77, 96, 98–99, 104

U

UK Committee on Toxicity (COT), 144

UK Scientific Advisory Committee on Nutrition, 232

undereating. *See* emotional over- and undereating; picky eaters

underfeeding, 22, 173, 174–75

unsaturated fats, 42–43, 101, 134–35, 247, 250

ABOUT THE AUTHORS

Clare Llewellyn, PhD, is a chartered psychologist and associate professor of obesity at University College London, where she leads the Obesity Research Group and the Gemini twin study. In 2011 she completed her PhD at UCL on the nature and nurture of eating behavior and weight in early life and she has a long-standing fascination with the topic, which probably stems from having been a notoriously fussy eater as a child. A decade ago she helped establish Gemini, the largest twin study ever set up to explore the nature and nurture of eating behavior from the beginning of life. She has published nearly 100 scientific papers, articles and book chapters on this topic and has given over sixty invited talks worldwide at international organizations, such as the American Dietetic Association, the UK Royal Society of Medicine and the European Society for Paediatric Gastroenterology Hepatology and Nutrition. She lives in London with her partner, Andy.

Hayley Syrad, PhD, is a chartered psychologist. She gained a first-class psychology bachelor's degree at the University of Southampton in 2007 and a PhD in behavioral nutrition at the Health Behaviour Research Centre, University College London, in 2016. Her research has focused on the factors influencing *what* and *how* young children eat. She has used real-world dietary data from the largest twin study in the UK (Gemini) to explore children's eating behaviors and has specifically examined the role of appetite and parental feeding practices. She uncovered the finding that children who are more food responsive tend to eat more often, and children with lower sensitivity to satiety tend to eat larger portions. Her research also showed that the portion size served to children can influence how much they consume (larger servings = more consumed), and she was the first researcher to provide evidence of this relationship. Hayley has published a number of articles on infant and toddler feeding.

31901064664669